Discovery and Development of Anti-Cancer Agents from Natural Products

Discovery and Development of Anti-Cancer Agents from Natural Products

Editor: Felix Cliburn

AMERICAN
MEDICAL PUBLISHERS
www.americanmedicalpublishers.com

AMERICAN
MEDICAL PUBLISHERS
www.americanmedicalpublishers.com

Cataloging-in-Publication Data

Discovery and development of anti-cancer agents from natural products / edited by Felix Cliburn.
p. cm.
Includes bibliographical references and index.
ISBN 979-8-88740-064-8
1. Antineoplastic agents. 2. Drug development. 3. Natural products. 4. Drugs--Design.
5. Cancer--Chemotherapy. I. Cliburn, Felix.
RS431.A64 D57 2023
615.798--dc23

American Medical Publishers,
41 Flatbush Avenue,
1st Floor, New York,
NY 11217, USA

ISBN 979-8-88740-064-8 (Hardback)

Contents

Preface

This book has been an outcome of determined endeavour from a group of educationists in the field. The primary objective was to involve a broad spectrum of professionals from diverse cultural background involved in the field for developing new researches. The book not only targets students but also scholars pursuing higher research for further enhancement of the theoretical and practical applications of the subject.

Natural products, with remarkable chemical diversity have played a dominant role in the treatment of human ailments. They are considered as a reservoir of bioactive compounds and are extensively investigated for their therapeutic potentials, most notably in the area of cancer therapy. They cannot function as effective drugs in isolation but they can be converted into a drug through chemical modification. There are a variety of widely-used anticancer agents that originate from natural sources, which are structurally unique and function by novel action mechanisms. Some examples of these natural anticancer agents are camptothecin, irinotecan, vincristine, etoposide and paclitaxel derived from plants; actinomycin D and mitomycin C obtained from bacteria; as well as marine-derived bleomycin. Camptothecin is a naturally occurring quinolone alkaloid isolated from wood and bark of Camptotheca acuminate. It is used as a chemotherapeutic agent for treating leukemia. This book is a compilation of chapters that discuss the most vital concepts and emerging trends in the discovery and development of anti-cancer agents from natural products. It includes contributions of experts and scientists which will provide innovative insights into this area of study.

It was an honour to edit such a profound book and also a challenging task to compile and examine all the relevant data for accuracy and originality. I wish to acknowledge the efforts of the contributors for submitting such brilliant and diverse chapters in the field and for endlessly working for the completion of the book. Last, but not the least; I thank my family for being a constant source of support in all my research endeavours.

Editor

1

An In Vitro Evaluation of the Molecular Mechanisms of Action of Medical Plants from the Lamiaceae Family as Effective Sources of Active Compounds against Human Cancer Cell Lines

Przemysław Sitarek [1,*], Anna Merecz-Sadowska [2], Tomasz Śliwiński [3], Radosław Zajdel [2] and Tomasz Kowalczyk [4]

1 Department of Biology and Pharmaceutical Botany, Medical University of Lodz, 90-151 Lodz, Poland
2 Department of Economic Informatics, University of Lodz, 90-214 Lodz, Poland; anna.merecz-sadowska@uni.lodz.pl (A.M.-S.); radoslaw.zajdel@uni.lodz.pl (R.Z.)
3 Laboratory of Medical Genetics, Faculty of Biology and Environmental Protection, University of Lodz, 90-236 Lodz, Poland; tomasz.sliwinski@biol.uni.lodz.pl
4 Department of Molecular Biotechnology and Genetics, University of Lodz, 90-237 Lodz, Poland; tomasz.kowalczyk@biol.uni.lodz.pl
* Correspondence: przemyslaw.sitarek@umed.lodz.pl

Simple Summary: Plants have been used in folk medicine for thousands of years. The Lamiaceae family is one of the largest families of flowering plants and includes a wide variety of species with biological and medical uses. They are mainly herbs and shrubs with an aromatic scent and rich in valuable compounds of great value in medicine. The article focuses on the assessment of the anticancer properties of extracts, essential oils, and pure compounds derived from various species of the Lamiaceae family and their potential molecular mechanisms of action in in vitro studies against the four most common types of cancer in women and men: breast, lung, prostate, and colon.

Abstract: It is predicted that 1.8 million new cancer cases will be diagnosed worldwide in 2020; of these, the incidence of lung, colon, breast, and prostate cancers will be 22%, 9%, 7%, and 5%, respectively according to the National Cancer Institute. As the global medical cost of cancer in 2020 will exceed about $150 billion, new approaches and novel alternative chemoprevention molecules are needed. Research indicates that the plants of the Lamiaceae family may offer such potential. The present study reviews selected species from the Lamiaceae and their active compounds that may have the potential to inhibit the growth of lung, breast, prostate, and colon cancer cells; it examines the effects of whole extracts, individual compounds, and essential oils, and it discusses their underlying molecular mechanisms of action. The studied members of the Lamiaceae are sources of crucial phytochemicals that may be important modulators of cancer-related molecular targets and can be used as effective factors to support anti-tumor treatment.

Keywords: Lamiaceae; cost-effective natural products; secondary metabolites; cancer; molecular mechanisms of action; in vitro studies

---

1. Introduction

Cancer is an important health problem and leading cause of death globally. The development of cancer is a multistage process that begins with genetic alteration and is followed by abnormal cell proliferation. Carcinogenesis is strictly related to the activation of oncogenes (induction of cell growth) and the inactivation of tumor suppressor genes (repression of cell growth), resulting in a loss of control of cell cycle progression. This initiation stage is followed by progression related to additive mutation within cells, some of which are implicated in even more rapid growth, and the suppression of cancer cell death. As a result of these changes, mature epithelial cancer cells may undergo epithelial–mesenchymal transition (EMT), which is characterized by the reduction of adhesion among cells and increased cell motility. Finally, tumor invasion and metastasis occur, and these are strictly related to angiogenesis, i.e., the process of new blood vessel formation. The progression of angiogenesis depends on the secretion of growth factors by cancer cells. The transformation of normal cells into malignant ones is a complex process regulated at every step by numerous factors, each of which may be a crucial target for anticancer agents [1,2].

The most prevalent form of cancer globally is lung cancer (11.6% of total cases), followed by breast cancer, among women (11.6%), prostate cancer, among men (7.1%), and colorectal cancer (6.1%) [3]. In 2018, more than 18 million cases of cancer were reported, and there were more than 9.6 million deaths globally [4]. In addition, the cost of medical care and economic value of nonmedical expense has been still rising [5].

Research into cancer therapy is currently directed toward the development of new therapeutic strategies and more effective chemotherapeutic factors [6]. An important source of novel effective agents with medicinal potential is the plant kingdom [7]. It is estimated that approximately 35 to 70,000 higher plant species produce secondary metabolites with diverse forms of bioactivity that are widely used in the regulation of signaling and metabolic pathways [8]. One family of particular interest is the Lamiaceae, which includes a number of herb and shrub genera with significant anticancer activities, such as *Salvia* sp., *Thymus* sp., *Origanum* sp., *Melissa* sp., *Plectranthus* sp., or *Scutellaria* sp.; all have been found to possess effective antiproliferative potential against lung, breast, prostate, and colon cancer cells in vitro. They commonly exert their cytotoxicity by promoting cancer cell death, especially via the apoptosis pathway, but they have also been found to influence angiogenesis [9]. Therefore, plant extracts, individual compounds, and essential oils from the Lamiaceae may support treatment as alternative or complementary cancer therapy.

The present paper focuses on the anticancer effects of plant extracts, purified single compounds, and essential oils from selected species of the Lamiaceae family. It discusses their in vitro cytotoxicity toward lung, colon, breast, and prostate cancer cell lines and the underlying mechanisms of action.

2. Criteria for Selection of Experimental Papers

This review was conducted to report work done previously to access the anticancer activity of plants from the Lamiaceae family published from 2015 to 2020. The studies were selected in the electronic databases PubMed/MEDLINE, Scopus, Web of Science, and Google Scholar. The search terms included Lamiaceae alone, and with the following: plant extract, derived compounds, essential oils, cancer, lung cancer cells, colon cancer cells, breast cancer cells, prostate cancer cells, mechanism of action. Published experimental studies reporting extracts, derived compounds, and essential oils from plants belonged to the Lamiaceae family with in vitro activity against lung, colon, breast, and prostate cancer cell lines were included. Research reporting review articles, published in languages other than English, abstract only or without full text access, lacking specific plant names with no reports of clear objective and methodologies, published more than five years ago, using plant species other than Lamiaceae, and cell lines other than lung, colon, breast, and prostate were excluded. The duplicates of articles obtained from the electronic databases were removed. After removal, inclusion/exclusion criteria were checked. Each selected document was examined and the following data were extracted and presented in the table: the scientific names of the species, parts of the plants used for extract preparation, types of extract, class of compounds, or compounds identified in extracts, cancer cell line, and reference. Articles with included mechanisms of action of interested plant extracts, single compounds, and essential oils were discussed in the main text.

3. Cancer

The term cancer is used to refer to a large group of diseases that can affect any part of the body. They are caused by uncontrolled cell proliferation that can take place in different tissues and spread into surrounding and distant organs [10,11]. Cancer occurs by a series of successive mutations in the relevant genes, leading to changes in cell function. Various physical and chemical factors play an obvious role in the formation of gene mutations and the appearance of cancer cells [12].

The first records of cancer date back to the ancient Egyptian and Greek civilizations, where the disease was treated mainly with radical surgery and often ineffective cauterization procedures, leading to the death of patients [13]. Currently, cancer is one of the most commonly occurring conditions and a major public health problem worldwide [14–16]. In 2018, cancer was responsible for approximately 9.6 million deaths [4]. Statistics show that high cancer morbidity and mortality are associated with an increasing incidence of risk factors such as overweight, alcohol abuse, smoking, unhealthy diets, urban air pollution, hepatitis and human papilloma virus, lack of physical activity, or sedentary lifestyle [17,18]. The World Health Organization (WHO) reports that in 2018, the highest percentages of cancer types in men occur in the lung, prostate, and colon, while the greatest prevalence in women is observed in the lung, breast, and colon. The most common types in both men and women were lung (2.09 million cases) and colon cancer (1.80 million cases). The second most common types of cancer were breast cancer in women (2.09 million cases) and prostate cancer in men (1.28 million cases) [14,19,20].

There are two main forms of lung cancer: non-small cell lung cancer (NSCLC; 85% of patients) and small cell lung cancer (SCLS, 15%). In 2018, this cancer caused 1.76 million deaths [14]. It is currently the most lethal malignant tumor in the world, often because it is not detected until the disease progresses significantly, leading to a significant reduction in the patient's quality of life [21,22]. So far, genetic factors leading to increased susceptibility to lung cancer have been poorly studied. First-degree relatives of patients with lung cancer are at increased risk, even after adjusting for smoking habits. The most commonly accepted causes of lung cancer include active cigarette smoking, exposure to passive smoking, pipe and cigar smoking, indoor and outdoor air pollution, radiation, and occupational exposure to factors such as asbestos, nickel, or chromium [23–25]. Among others, important common driver gene mutations in patients with NSCLC are as follows: tumor suppressor genes *TP53* and *PTEN*; *EGFR*, which encodes protein, is involved in cell growth and survival [26]. These genes constitute molecular targets for compounds from the Lamiaceae family.

Another common cancer among women, and one of the leading causes of death, is breast cancer [27]. In 2018, this cancer caused 627,000 deaths [14]. Breast cancer risk is related to many factors including a diet too high in calories leading to obesity, tobacco smoking, hormonal history, exposure to estrogen and progesterone, early first menstruation, and late menopause. All of these factors lead to shorter menstrual cycles and hormone exposure [28]. Genetic predisposition also plays an important role, as approximately 7% of breast cancer cases are hereditary [29]. In turn, mutations in the *BRCA1* and *BRCA2* genes cause as much as 80% of genetic breast cancer [30,31]. BRCAs proteins regulate genes linked to DNA repair, the cell cycle, and apoptosis [32]. Another crucial mutations is that in *TP53*, which is linked with histological grade in breast cancer patients [33].

Prostate cancer is the second most common malignant neoplasm after lung cancer in men around the world [34]. In 2018, this cancer caused 358,989 deaths, this being 3.8% of all deaths caused by cancer in men. About 60% of cases are diagnosed in men over 65. The mean age of diagnosis is 66 years. The disease rarely occurs in people under 40 years of age [35]. The main risk factors for the development of prostate cancer in men can be divided into non-modified and modified factors. Non-modified factors include age, family history, ethnicity, and genetic factors, while the modified ones are obesity, infectious diseases, smoking, hormones, or occupational and external exposure [36–38]. Inherited mutations in specific genes, such as *BRCA1*, *BRCA2*, and *HOXB13*, are the cause of some hereditary prostate cancer cases. HOXB13 protein regulates androgen receptor function [39]. Men with mutations in these genes are at high risk of developing prostate cancer and, in some cases, other cancers during their lifetime [40]. Additionally, other different genes have been implicated in prostate cancer by genetic alteration, depending on types (familial, sporadic, hereditary): *TP53, PTEN,* and protooncogenes *MYC,* which also constitute molecular targets for compounds from the Lamiaceae family [41].

Colorectal cancer is already the second most common cause of cancer death in the world (862,000 deaths) and 65% of all new incidences occur in high-income countries in Europe [14]. This incidence constitutes a 1.51% cumulative risk (assuming the absence of other competing causes of death) of colon cancer among men age 0–74 years, and a 1.12% risk among women. Their cumulative lifetime risks are 1.2% and 0.65%, respectively [3]. Colorectal cancer has been attributed to a number of mutations: mutational inactivation of tumor suppressor genes such as *TP53,* and activation of the oncogene pathway *PI3K.* These genes constitute molecular targets for compounds from the Lamiaceae family [42]. Genetically, colorectal cancer is divided into three categories: sporadic (about 60%) for patients with no family history, family (about 30%) for patients with at least one relative with colorectal cancer or adenoma, and hereditary forms (about 10%) due to the germline inheritance of mutations [43,44]. The development of colorectal cancer is believed to be supported by family history, lack of physical activity, old age, excessive alcohol consumption, high-fat diet, diabetes, and inflammatory bowel diseases, including ulcerative colitis and Crohn's disease [45–47].

4. Cancer and Plants

Plants have been used in folk medicine for thousands of years [48]. The oldest written evidence of the use of medicinal plants in the preparation of medicines was found on a Sumerian Nagpur clay plate, approximately 5000 years old. It contained 12 prescriptions for the preparation of drugs, relating to over 250 different plants, including genera such as *Papaver* sp., *Hyoscyamus* sp., or *Mandragora* sp. containing alkaloids [49]. Medicinal plants are still used in developing countries as the source of healing due to their natural multidirectional action and low cost. The secondary metabolites contained in plants mainly do not play a direct role in their growth but serve as defence compounds against herbivores and microorganisms; therefore, they are required for survival in a specific environment. Most are polyphenols, alkaloids, terpenoids, or polyketides, among which there are a number of subclasses. Some have been found to demonstrate anticancer [50], anti-inflammatory [51], antioxidant [52], antimicrobial [53], antiviral [54] or anti-obesity effects [55]. In addition, while they can act as pure compounds, they also can show synergistic or antagonist effect with enhanced, or weaker, biological properties when administered as plant extracts [56–58].

According to the WHO, some nations still consider plant-based treatments to be the primary source of medicine and developing countries are exploiting the benefits of natural origin compounds for therapeutic purposes [59]. Numerous studies confirm the positive use of such natural compounds in the treatment of many diseases [60]. In turn, medicinal plants are also a valuable source of bioactive anticancer agents [61–66]. If plant-derived compounds can demonstrate selectivity in research, are non-toxic to normal cells, and show cytotoxicity in cancer cell lines, these compounds can be used in clinical trials for further therapeutic development. However, it is worth remembering that chemicals of plant origin may also exert toxic effects on both animals and human organisms in in vivo study [61,67].

The modern search for anticancer drugs from plants began in the 1950s, with the discovery of vinca alkaloids from the genus *Vinca* [68]. This highlights that medicinal plants remain a source of new drugs [69], e.g., vinblastine or vincristine obtained from the *Vinca* sp., paclitaxel from the *Taxus* sp., camptothecin from the *Camptotheca* sp., or podophyllotoxin from *Podophyllum* sp. [48,61,70,71]. These compounds often exert their anticancer activity by inhibiting the proliferation of cancer cells and inducing cell death [67]. Many in vivo and in vitro studies show the activation of apoptosis in various cancer cells, both under the influence of pure compounds and plant extracts [71]. Numerous plant species from different families (Lamiaceae, Fabaceae, Asteraceae, Papaveraceae, Apocynacea etc.) are traditionally used to treat or prevent the development of cancer.

5. The Lamiaceae Family Plants

The Lamiaceae family is one of the largest families of flowering plants and includes a wide variety of species with biological and medical uses. They are mainly herbs and shrubs with an aromatic scent and rich in valuable compounds of great value in natural medicine. Plants of this family are characterized by square stems and opposite leaves [72,73]. The most famous representatives are thyme, mint, oregano, basil, sage, savory, rosemary, hyssop, and lemon balm, which are used as aromatic spices, and some others with more limited uses [74]. Historically, species in the Lamiaceae family have enjoyed a long history of use in flavoring, preserving food, and for medicinal purposes. This family includes about 250 genera and about 7000 species, with the largest genera being *Salvia*, *Scutellaria*, *Stachys*, *Plectranthus*, *Hyptis*, *Teucrium*, *Vitex*, *Thymus*, or *Nepeta* (Figure 1). It is one of the most economically important families with great diversity and cosmopolitan distribution due to the aromatic properties of most of its members [75]. It is well known that each species produces a wide variety of secondary metabolites with strong antibacterial, antioxidant, anti-inflammatory, antiviral or anticancer properties; the oils comprise a complex mixture of bioactive compounds, in which each ingredient contributes to its overall bioactivity [56].

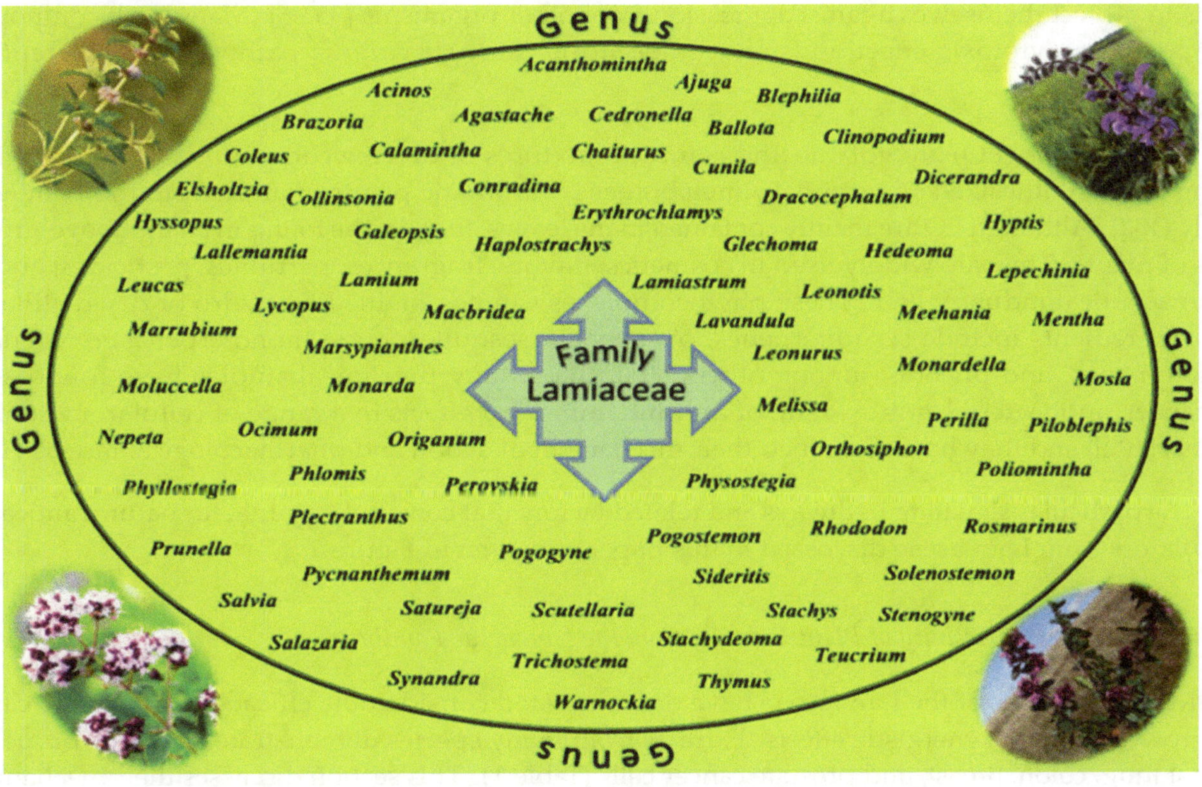

Figure 1. Selected genera belonging to the Lamiaceae family.

5.1. *The Lamiaceae Family as a Source of Valuable Secondary Metabolites with Anti-Cancer Potential*

The first and largest group of secondary metabolites occurring in the Lamiaceae is polyphenols, which are characterized by at least one aromatic ring having hydroxyl groups. Based on their numbers of phenolic groups and structural elements, polyphenols can be divided into phenolic acids, flavonoids, stilbenes, lignans, lignins, coumarins, anthraquinones, and xanthones [76–78]. In the human body, polyphenols exhibit antioxidant properties, which protect against chronic diseases caused by free radicals damaging of tissues and organs [72], as well as various anticancer [79] anti-diabetic [80], neuroprotective [81], anti-inflammatory [82], antiviral [83], antifungal [84] or antibacterial properties [85]. Polyphenols are believed to cause cancer cell death by apoptosis through several mechanisms, such as DNA fragmentation, alteration of the level of apoptotic proteins, and mitochondrial membrane potential and cell cycle arrest [86,87].

Another potent group of secondary compounds is the terpenes, in particular oxygenated terpenoids [88]. In turn, terpenoids are categorized into monoterpenes, sesquiterpenes, diterpenes, sesterpenes, and triterpenes depending on the number of their isoprene units. Diterpenes constitute a diverse class of plant metabolites with more than 10,000 different structures, isolated in the Lamiaceae present about 50 different skeletons [89,90]. Most diterpenes play a critical role in ecological interactions of plants and show interesting biological activities both in vitro and in vivo [91,92], such as antibacterial, antifungal, antiprotozoal, enzyme-inducing, anti-inflammatory, and the modulation of immune cell function and anticancer properties [92,93]. Studies have shown that some diterpenes have significant cytotoxic and cytostatic effects on various cell lines of human origin, interfere with the biochemical pathways of apoptosis and the cell cycle phase, and can influence the expression of proto-oncogenes such as avian myelocytomatosis viral oncogene homolog (c-Myc) and B-cell lymphoma 2 (Bcl-2) [93,94].

Many members of the Lamiaceae also produce alkaloids, which is an extremely diverse chemical group based on a ring structure including a nitrogen atom. Many alkaloids are toxic and are used by plants to protect themselves against aggression from other organisms [95,96]. Many such compounds have a strong cytotoxic effect and induce apoptosis through various pathways in different cell lines [97,98].

Essential oils (EO) are volatile and complex mixtures of diverse compounds, typically with a strong odor, synthesized as secondary metabolites by aromatic plants, mainly from the Lamiaceae family (132). Although EO are mainly contained in the leaves, they can be found in all the above-ground parts of plants. They are widely used in cosmetics, flavors, fragrances, perfumes, pesticides, and the pharmaceutical industry [99]. These phytocomplexes can be obtained by hydro or dry distillation. Their ingredients include sesquiterpenes, oxygenated sesquiterpenes, monoterpenes, oxygenated monoterpenes, and phenols, among others [100,101]. Many preclinical studies have found some anticancer, antibacterial, antioxidant, or anti-inflammatory effects in a range of cellular and animal models [102], and they have examined their mechanism of action and pharmacological targets [101].

The particular signaling pathways and related factors that constitute a target for natural anticancer modulators from Lamiaceae discussed in this paper are given in Figure 2.

5.2. The Anti-Cancer Activity of Plant Extracts from the Lamiaceae Family

Many members of the Lamiaceae have demonstrated considerable efficacy in inhibiting cancer cell growth through synergistic effects. Extracts from many species demonstrate cytotoxic properties against lung, colon, breast, and prostate cancer cells (Table 1). This section discusses their mechanisms of action, which are mainly based on inducing the apoptosis in cancer cells including lung, breast, prostate, and colon cancer.

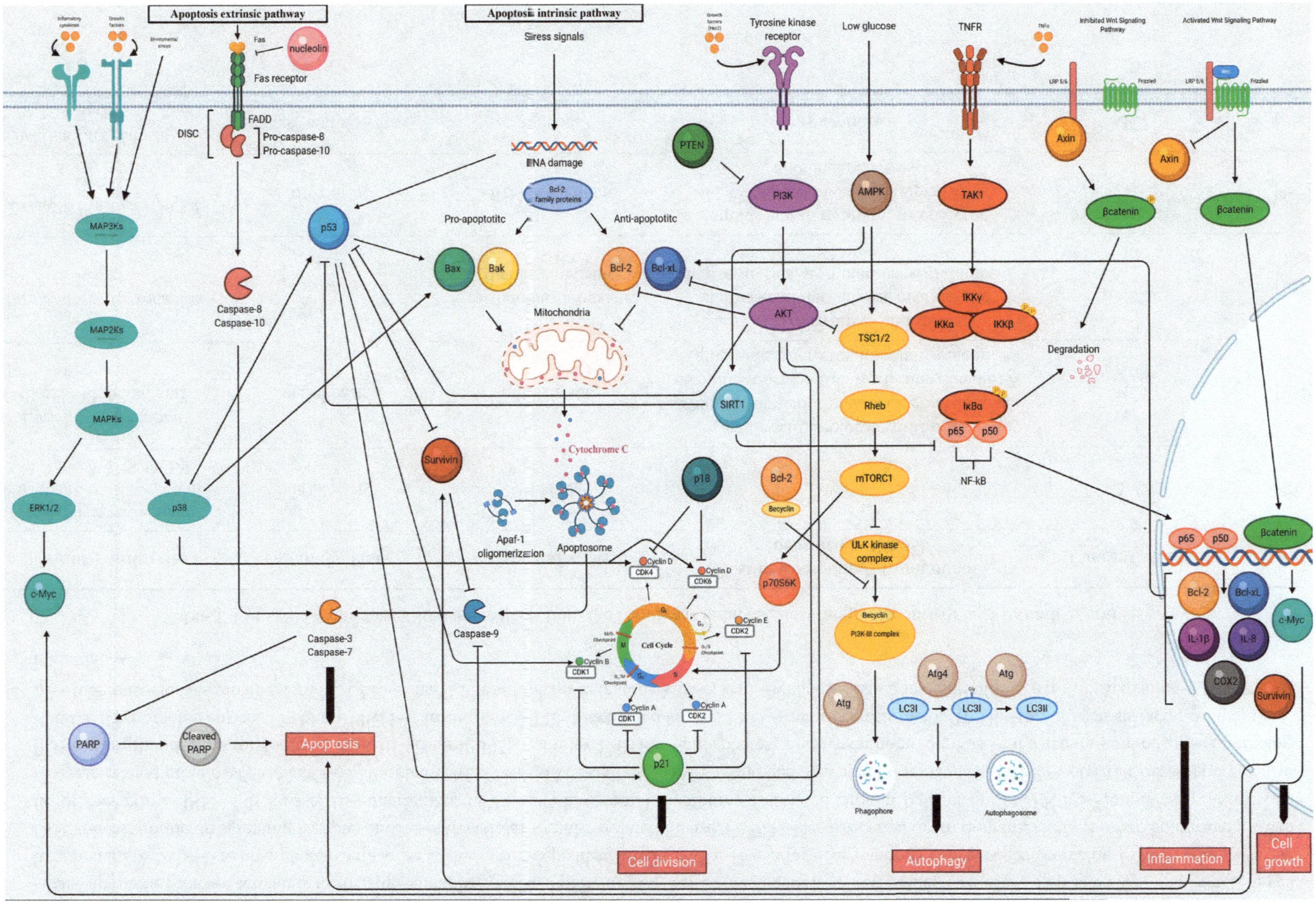

Figure 2. Selected molecular mechanisms of action of extracts, single derived compounds and essential oils from the Lamiaceae family against lung, breast, prostate, and colon cancer cell lines (created by BioRender). Abbreviations Akt—protein kinase B, AMP—adenosine monophosphate, AMPK—AMP-activated protein kinase,

Apaf—apoptotic protease activating factor, Atg—autophagy-related protein, Bak—Bcl-2 homologous antagonist/killer, Bax—Bcl-2 associated X protein, Bcl-2—B-cell lymphoma 2, Bcl-xL—B-cell lymphoma-extra large, CDK—cyclin-dependent kinase, c-Myc—avian myelocytomatosis viral oncogene homolog, COX—cyclooxygenase, DISC—death-inducing signaling complex, ERK—extracellular signal-regulated kinase, FADD—Fas-associated death domain, Her2—human epidermal growth factor receptor 2, IKK—IkB kinase, IL—interleukin, LC3—autophagosomal membrane-associated protein light chain 3, LPR 5/6—low-density lipoprotein receptor–related protein 5/6, MAP2K—MAPK kinase, MAP3K—MAP2K kinase, MAPK—mitogen-activated protein kinase, PARP—poly(ADP-ribose) polymerase, PI3K—phosphatidylinositol 3-kinase, PI3K-III—class III PI3K complex 1, PTEN—phosphatase and tensin homolog, Ras—rat sarcoma viral oncogene homolog, RHEB—Ras homolog enriched in brain, SIRT1—Sirtuin, TAK—TGF-β-activated kinase, TNF—tumor necrosis factor, TNFR—tumor necrosis factor receptor, TSC 1/2—tuberous sclerosis proteins 1 and 2, ULK—Unc-51 like autophagy activating kinase, Wnt—wingless-related integration site. Arrows: Activation—→; Inhibition—⊢.

Table 1. Cytotoxic properties of selected extracts from the Lamiaceae family against lung, colon, breast, and prostate cancer cells.

Name of The Species	Part of the Plant	Type of Extract	Class of Compounds/Compounds Identified in Extract	Cancer Cell Lines	Ref.
Ajuga chamaepitys subsp. chia (Schreb.) = synonym of *Ajuga chia* (Schreb)	aerial parts	ethanolic	-	T-47D	[103]
Cyclotrichium niveum (Boiss.) Manden. and Scheng	aerial parts	ethyl acetate	gallic acid, protocatechuic acid, chlorogenic acid, caffeic acid, gentisic acid, p-coumaric acid, ferulic acid, rutin, luteolin-7 glucoside, quercetin, luteolin, apigenin	MCF-7	[104]
Eremostachys azerbaijanica Rech.f.	rhizomes	methanolic, n-hexane, dichloromethane	fatty acid derivatives and steroids steroids and derivatives, heterocyclic hydrocarbons, sesquiterpenes, and linear alkanes	A549	[105]
Eremostachys azerbaijanica Rech.f.	rhizomes	dichloromethane	steroids and derivatives, heterocyclic hydrocarbons, sesquiterpenes, and linear alkanes	HT-29	[105]
Hymenocrater platystegius Rech.f.	leaves and flowers	aqueous	phenolics	MCF-7	[106]

Table 1. *Cont.*

Name of The Species	Part of the Plant	Type of Extract	Class of Compounds/Compounds Identified in Extract	Cancer Cell Lines	Ref.
Hyptis pectinata L.	leaves	ethanolic	-	MCF-7	[107]
Hyptis pectinate L.	leaves, branches, root	ethanolic	pectinolide J, hyptolide, and pectinolide E	MDA-MB-231	[108]
Lavandula coronopifolia Poir.	aerial parts	petroleum ether, ethyl acetate, chloroform, and ethanol	-	MDA-MB-231	[109]
Lavender angustifolia Mill	leaves	methanolic	phenolics, flavonoids, glycosides	MCF-7	[110]
Melissa officinalis L.	leaves	ethanolic	phenolics and flavonoids	MCF-7, PC-3 and A549	[111]
Melissa officinalis L.	leaves	ethanolic	phenolics: 3-(3,4-dihydroxyphenyl)-lactic acid, caftaric acid, caffeic acid hexoside, fertaric acid, caffeic acid, sulphated rosmarinic acid, yunnaneic acid E, lithospermic acid A isomer, chicoric acid, yunnaneic acid F, salvianolic acid C derivative I, salvianolic acid C derivative II, rosmarinic acid hexoside, sagerinic acid, rosmarinic acid, salvianolic acid A, salvianolic acid C derivative III, lithospermic acid A, salvianolic acid A isomer, salvianolic acid C derivative IV	NCI-H460	[112]
Nepeta bracteata Benth.	flowering shoot	aqueous	phenolics	MCF-7	[106]
Ocimum americanum L.	leaves	ethyl acetate	phenolics, flavonoids, flavanols, tannins, saponins	HCT-116	[113]
Ocimum basilicum var. thyrsiflorum (L.) Benth.	leaves	ethanolic	phenolics and flavonoids: cinnamic acid, gallic acid, methylgallate, ellagic acid, methyl ellagic acid, apigenin, luteolin, vitexin, isovitexin	HCT-116	[114]
Origanum dayi Post.	aerial parts	ethanolic	-	MCF-7 and T47D	[103]

Table 1. *Cont.*

Name of The Species	Part of the Plant	Type of Extract	Class of Compounds/Compounds Identified in Extract	Cancer Cell Lines	Ref.
Origanum majorana L.	aerial parts	ethyl acetate	2-(4-hydroxy phenyl) ethanol, vanillic acid, 4-hydroxybenzoic acid, syringic acid, caffeic acid, vanillin, trans-ferulic acid, luteolin, cinnamic acid	MDA-MB-231 and HT-29	[115]
Origanum syriacum L.	leaves	ethanolic	-	LoVo and SW620	[116]
Orthosiphon aristatus (Blume) Miq.	leaves	methanolic	phenolics	MCF-7	[117]
Orthosiphon pallidus Royle ex Benth.	whole plants	aqueous	-	MCF-7 and MDA-MB-231	[118]
Phlomis viscosa Poiret.	leaves, flowers and stems	ethanolic	diosmin, isovaleraldehyde, 2,4-hexadienal, 2-hexenal, alpha terpinene, 1-octen-3-ol, himachala-2,4-diene, n-octanal, buorbonene, 1-propanal, 2-methyl, cubebene	MCF-7	[119]
Plectranthus amboinicus (Lour.) Spreng	leaves	chloroform	diterpene/7-acetoxy-6-hydroxyroyleanone	MCF-7	[120]
Plectranthus amboinicus (Lour.) Spreng.	leaves	ethanolic	-	MCF-7	[121]
Pogostemon heyneanus Benth.	leaves	chloroform	-	MCF-7 and MDA-MB-231	[121]
Rosmarinus officinalis L.	leaves	ethanolic	flavonoids, diterpenes, triterpenes: apigenin, hispidulin, cirsiliol, diosmetin, cirsimaritin, rosmanol, epiisorosmanol, epirosmanol, genkwanin, miltipolone, carnosol, rosmadial, anemosapogenin, rosmaridiphenol, augustic acid, benthamic acid, carnosic acid, 12-methoxycarnosic acid, shogaol, micromeric acid, hinokione, betulinic acid, ursolic acid	HT-29 and SW480	[122]
Rosmarinus officinalis L.	leaves and flowers	aqueous	phenolics	MCF-7	[106]
Rosmarinus officinalis L.	aerial parts	aqueous	-	Caco-2	[123]
Rosmarinus officinalis L.	leaves	methanolic	terpenes	LoVo	[124]

Table 1. *Cont.*

Name of The Species	Part of the Plant	Type of Extract	Class of Compounds/Compounds Identified in Extract	Cancer Cell Lines	Ref.
Rosmarinus officinalis L.	leaves	methanolic	phenolics and flavonoids, alkaloids, tannins, glycosides	MCF-7	[110]
Rosmarinus officinalis L.	leaves	ethanolic	phenolics: protocatechuic acid, caffeic acid, ellagic acid, ferulic acid, rosemarinic acid, carnosol, carnosic acid	MCF-7	[125]
Salvia fruticosa Mill subsp. *thomasii*	aerial parts	methanolic	luteolin, luteolin 7-O-glucoside, rutin, salvigenin	MCF-7, MDA-MB-231, RKO and Caco-2	[126]
Salvia ballotiflora Benth.	aerial parts	chloroform	-	A549	[127]
Salvia fruticosa Mill	bark	methanolic	-	MCF-7, T-47D and MDA-468	[128]
Salvia fruticosa Mill. (SF.)	aerial parts	aqueous	phenolics and flavonoids: rosmarinic and caffeic acid	Caco-2 and HT-29	[129]
Salvia hispanica L.	seeds	ethanolic	-	A549	[130]
Salvia hispanica L.	seeds	ethanolic	tannins, saponins, flavonoids, alkaloids, proteins, phenols	PC-3	[131]
Salvia officinalis L.	leaves	ethanolic	eucalyptol (1,8-cineole), α-thujone, β-thujone, camphor, β-caryophyllene, α-caryophyllene (α-humulene), viridiflorol, manool	A-549, HT-29	[132]
Salvia officinalis L.	leaves	aqueous	phenolics: caffeic acid, syringic acid, rutin, coumaric acid, vanillin, quercetin, cinnamic acid	MDA-MB-231	[133]

Table 1. *Cont.*

Name of The Species	Part of the Plant	Type of Extract	Class of Compounds/Compounds Identified in Extract	Cancer Cell Lines	Ref.
Salvia pilifera Montbret and Aucher ex Benth.	whole plant	methanolic	fumaric acid, gallic acid, gallocatechin, catechin, oleorufein, 4-hydroxybenzoic acid, caffeic acid, syringic acid, ellagic acid, 3-hydroxy cinnamic acid and protocatechuic acid	DU-145	[134]
Salvia pilifera Montbret et Aucher ex Benth.	mericarps	ethanolic	-	A549	[135]
Salvia verbenaca L.	leaves	ethyl acetate	flavonoids and terpenes	MDA MB-231	[136]
Satureja horvatii subsp. *macrophylla* (Halácsy) Baden.	aerial parts	methanolic	monoterpene hydrocarbons, oxygenated monoterpens, sesquiterpene hydrocarbons, oxygenated sesquiterpenes, monoterpenes, sesquiterpenes: α-thujene, α-pinene, camphene, 1-octen-3-ol, α-myrcene, 3-octanol, α-phellandrene + δ 3-carene, α-terpinene, p-cymene, limonene, 1,8-cineole, cis-ocimene, γ-terpinene, trans sabinene hydrate, terpinolene, linalool, trans-pinocarveol, cis-verbenol, camphor, borneol, terpinene-4-ol, p-cymen-8-ol, α-terpineol, dihydrocarvone, thymol methyl ether, thymoquinone, thymol, carvacrol, caryophyllene, aromadendrene, α-humulene, alloaromadendrene, γ-muurolene, viridiflorene, γ-elemene, b-bisabolene, γ-cadinene, δ-cadinene, (-)-spathulenol, caryophyllene oxide, viridiflorol	A549	[137]
Sideritis ozturkii Aytaç and Aksoy	flower and leaf	methanolic	gallic acid, protocatechuic acid, catechin, 4-hydroxybenzoic acid, caffeic acid, syringic acid, rutin trihydrate, trans-p-coumaric acid, trans-ferulic acid, myricetin, trans-resveratrol, quercetin, trans-cinnamic acid, naringenin, kaempferol	DLD-11	[138]

Table 1. *Cont.*

Name of The Species	Part of the Plant	Type of Extract	Class of Compounds/Compounds Identified in Extract	Cancer Cell Lines	Ref.
Sideritis syriaca L.	leaves	methanolic	phenolic acids: gallic acid, p-hydroxybenzoic acid, cafeic acid, chlorogenic acid, p-coumaric acid, ferulic acid, o-coumaric acid, rosmarinic acid and trans- cinnamic acid	MCF-7	[139]
Teucrium fruticans L.	leaves	ethanol/ethyl acetate/water	-	A549	[140]
Thyme vulgaris L.	leaves	methanolic	phenolics and flavonoids, tannins	MCF-7	[110]
Thymus daenensis Celak.	leaves and stems	ethanolic	-	MCF-7	[141]
Thymus mastichina L.	whole plant	ethanol/ethyl acetate/water	-	A549	[140]
Vitex trifolia L.	leaves	methanol	-	MCF-7	[142]

5.2.1. The Activity of Plant Extracts from the Lamiaceae Family as Modulators of Cell Cycle

The cell cycle events controlling cell duplication and arrest are highly dysregulated in cancer cells. Cell cycle arrest is closely related to the G1/S, G2/M and M phases' checkpoints perturbations. Progression is mediated by the activation and deactivation of cyclin-dependent kinases (CDKs), while activation depends on the presence of activated subunits named cyclins. The levels of cyclins and CDKs are changed in human cancers; for example, the levels of CDK1 and cyclin B1 are reduced in human breast adenocarcinoma (MCF-7) and human colorectal cancer (HCT-116) cell lines following treatment with *Micromeria fruticosa* aerial part extract, resulting in G2/M arrest [143,144]. In addition, treatment with *Melissa officinalis* leaf extract blocked the expression of CDKs 2, 4, and 6 and cyclin D3 in the human colon carcinoma (HT-29 and T84) cell lines, and specifically activated an important CDK inhibitor named p18 [145]; in addition, treatment with *Vitex rotundifolia* fruit extract downregulated cyclin D1 and CDK 4 levels in HCT-116 and human colon adenocarcinoma (SW480) [146]. Manipulation of the cell cycle may induce an apoptotic response [147]. *Ocimum basilicum* leaf extract induced cell cycle arrest in MCF-7 cells [148], and *Salvia miltiorrhiza* root extract induced a G2/M phase arrest in human lung adenocarcinoma (Glc-82) cells [149], as did *Melissa officinalis* leaf extract in HT-29 and T84 cells and *Prunella vulgaris* root extract in human breast carcinoma MCF-5 cells [150]. *Satureja khuzistanica* extract enriched with rosmarinic acid [151] was found to increase the size of the apoptotic sub-G0/G1 population in MCF-7 cells.

5.2.2. The Activity of Plant Extracts from the Lamiaceae Family as Modulators of Apoptosis Signaling

Apoptosis or programmed cell death is a crucial mechanism for maintaining cell homeostasis. The process can be triggered by various conditions, including immune reaction or reactive oxygen species (ROS). The study of *Ocimum sanctum* roots extract suggested that it may increase ROS production in the HCI-H460 lung carcinoma cell line and may decrease viability via apoptosis. The same phenomenon is observed for *Melissa officinalis* leaf extracts against HT-29 and T84 cell lines [145]. That strategy is confirmed by the occurrence of excessive numbers of apoptotic cells [152]. It was concluded that also stress originating from the endoplasmic reticulum may play an important role in triggering apoptosis; for example, *Scutellaria barbata* extract induced human lung cancer (CL1-5) cell death [153].

The signaling mechanisms of apoptotic cell death are divided into two pathways: an intrinsic pathway mediated by mitochondria and an extrinsic one mediated by death receptors. Cell size reduction, membrane blebbing, and apoptotic bodies were observed in HT-29 cells after *Stachys pilifera* leaf extract treatment; these were all signs of apoptosis [154]. MCF-7 cells showed a modified nucleus following incubation with *Caryopteris x clandonensis* stem extract [155], and changes in cell rounding, shrinkage, and detachment from other cells after treatment with *Teucrium mascatense* whole plant extract [156]. Another important future of apoptosis is the translocation of phosphatidylserine phospholipid from the inner to the outer plasma membrane, resulting *inter alia* in recognition by phagocytes [157]; this was observed against HT-29 and T84 cell lines after the administration of *Teucrium mascatense* extract [156] and *Melissa officinalis* leaf extract [145]. *Teucrium flavum* whole plant extracts were found to induce DNA fragmentation in breast carcinoma cells (MDA-MB-231) [158], as well as *Vitex rotundifolia* leaf extract in human breast cancer T-47D cells [159] and *Ocimum sanctum* leaf extract in human prostate adenocarcinoma LNCaP cells [160]; such DNA cleavage is a hallmark of apoptosis. *Perovskia abrotanoides* flower extract has also demonstrated proapoptotic effects against MCF-7 cells [161] and *Salvia chorassanica* root extract against MCF-7 and prostate cancer cells (DU-145) [162].

The treatment of human non-small cell lung carcinoma cells (NCI-H460) with *Ocimum sanctum* root extract [152] and MCF-7 cells with *Teucrium sandrasicum* leaf extract [163] resulted in increased mitochondrial membrane permeability, which is characteristic of the intrinsic pathway. The Bcl-2 protein family also induces a loss of mitochondrial membrane potential. This family is separated into two groups: one, including Bak and Bax, which possesses proapoptotic potential, and another, including Bcl-2 and Bcl-xL, which has antiapoptotic activities. The balance between the two groups influences the progression of apoptosis. The Bcl-2 protein family was found to be modulated by the *Origanum compactum* aerial part extract in A549 cells [164]. Changes in the level of Bcl-2 family members may result in the release of numerous pro-apoptotic molecules. The expression of Bcl-2 protein family members in different lines of human lung cancer cells became unregulated following the administration of extracts from *Salvia milithoriza* roots (Glc-82 cells) [149], *Scutellaria baicalensis* root (H358 and H2087 cells) [165], and *Melissa officinalis* leaves (A549) [166]. A similar result was observed for several human colon cancer cell lines treated with *Coleus amboinicus* leaves (WiDr cells) [167] and *Vitex rotundifolia* fruit (HCT-116, SW480, LoVo and HT-29 cells) extracts [146]. In addition, apoptotic signals have been triggered in breast cancer cell lines after incubation with extracts of *Plectranthus amboinicus* leaves (MCF-7 cells) [120], *Orthosiphon stamineus* leaves (MCF-7 cells) [168], *Melissa officinalis* leaves (MCF-7 cells) [166], *Vitex rotundifolia* leaves (T-47D cells) [159], and *Prunella vulgaris* root (MCF-5 cells) [150]. Changes in the expression level of Bcl-2 family protein are also induced in prostate cancer cell lines by extracts of *Ocimum sanctum* leaves (LNCaP cells) [160], *Dracocephalum palmatum* (PC-3 cells) [169], and *Melissa officinalis* leaves (PC-3) [166].

The insertion of Bax/Bak into the mitochondrial membrane results in the formation of a pore complex and release of cytochrome c into the cytosol from the intermembrane space. In contrast, Bcl-2 and Bcl-xl prevent the release of cytochrome c. Excessive levels of cytochrome c were observed in MCF-7 cells after *Orthosiphon stamineus* leaf extract treatment [168]. Cytochrome c binds to apoptotic protease-activating factor 1 (Apaf-1) to create an apoptosome that activates caspase-9. Caspase-9 was found to be upregulated following treatment with *Coleus amboinicus* leaf extract in WiDr cells [167], *Teucrium sandrasicum* leaf extract in MCF-7 cells [163], *Vitex rotundifolia* leaf extract in T-47D cells [159], *Micromeria fruticose* aerial part extract in MCF-7 cells [144], *Stachys pilifera* leaf extract in HT-29 cell line [154], and *Teucrium chamaedrys* aerial and flowering parts in SW480 cells [170].

Caspase-9 activity results in the activation of the effectors caspase-3 and caspase-7. Caspase-3 and/or caspase-7 activity were observed in the Glc-82, LNCaP, MCF-7, T-47D, MCF-7, and WiDr cell lines following treatment with, respectively, extracts of *Salvia miltiorrhiza* roots [149], *Ocimum sanctum* leaves [160], *Plectranthus amboinicus* leaves [120], *Vitex rotundifolia* leaves [159], *Teucrium mascatense* whole plant [156], and *Coleus amboinicus* leaves [167]. The induction of caspase-3 and/or caspase-7 cleavage was also observed for *Melissa officinalis* leaf extracts against HT-29 and T84 cells [145] and for *Origanum majorana* leaf extract against HT-29 cells [171]. *Dracocephalum palmatum* leaf extract also induced apoptosis according to the intrinsic pathway via the upregulation of activated caspase-3 in PC-3 cells [169]; the same was observed for *Nepeta cataria* aerial parts on PC-3 cells [172] and *Scutellaria baicalensis* whole body extract on H358 and H2087 cell lines [165].

In apoptosis, the detection of poly-ADP-ribose-polymerase (PARP) is an important diagnostic method because it produces specific patterns of proteolytic cleavage fragments [173]. Increased expression of PARP1, a hallmark of apoptotic death, was observed in Glc-82 cells treated with *Salvia miltiorrhiza* roots extract [149], LNCaP cells incubated with *Ocimum sanctum* leaf extract [160], and PC-3 cells interacted with *Nepeta cataria* aerial part extract [172]. PARP activation was also demonstrated after the treatment of *Teucrium mascatense* whole plant extract in MCF-7 cells [156], *Rosmarinus officinalis* leaf extract in A549 cells [174], and *Scutellaria baicalensis* root extract in H358 and H2087 cells [165], suggesting the involvement of mitochondria in the apoptotic signals.

The extrinsic pathway is initiated by the TNF (tumor necrosis factor), TRAIL (TNF-related apoptosis-inducing ligand), and Fas ligands binding to the extracellular domain of death receptors, such as type 1 TNF receptor (TNFR1), TRAIL, and Fas receptors. The *Teucrium chamaedrys* aerial flowering part extract initiated an excessive expression of Fas in SW480 cells [170]. The Fas ligand–receptor junction is inhibited by nucleolin, which is a protein that protects against apoptotic death [175]. *Orthosiphon stamineus* leaf extract treatment significantly decreased the nucleolin level in MCF-7 cells [168]. The attachment of a Fas to a specific receptor triggers the formation of specific death-inducing signaling complex (DISC) possessing a Fas-associated death domain (FADD); this complex can recruit an adaptor protein and then activate initiator caspase-8 and caspase-10. Caspase-8 induction was found to induce apoptosis in MCF-7 and HCT-116 cells following *Micromeria fruticose* aerial part extract administration [144], as well as treatment with *Vitex rotundifolia* leaf extract in T-47D cells [159], *Stachys pilifera* leaf extract in the HT-29 cell line [154], and for *Teucrium chamaedrys* aerial flowering part extract in SW480 cells [170]. In addition, it was speculated that *Satureja khuzistanica* extract enriched in rosmarinic acid can induce apoptosis through activation of the extrinsic pathway in MCF-7 cells [151]. Then, the activation of caspase-8 and caspase-10 is followed by the activation effector caspases 3/7, enzymatic cleavage of numerous downstream targets, and cell death [176,177]. The Fas-mediated apoptosis pathway is believed to play a role in *Scutellaria barbata* extract-induced CL1-5 cell cytotoxicity [153].

An important inhibitor of apoptosis is called survivin. This protein is under-expressed in cancer cells and is related to poor clinical outcome through the blockage of apoptosis by caspase inhibition [178]. Significant reductions of survivin levels were observed for *Micromeria fruticosa* aerial part extract in MCF-7 and HCT-116 cell lines [143,144], *Origanum majorana* leaf extract in HT-29 cells [171], and for *Scutellaria barbata* whole plant extract in HT-29 cells [179]. Another key molecule that plays a crucial role in the negative regulation of apoptosis is Her2, belonging to the human epidermal growth factor receptor family. Excessive Her2 expression is related to antiapoptotic signals via the activation of survivin and Bcl2 protein. *Melissa officinalis* extract shows significant potential to reduce Her2 levels in PC-3 cells [166].

Another regulator of apoptosis and autophagy is mammalian target of rapamycin kinase (mTOR), which also demonstrates pleiotropic features [180]. The activation of the mTOR pathway was promoted by *Ocimum basilicum* leaf extract in MCF-7 cells with p70S6K, which is a downstream target kinase [181]. Similar features were shown for *Scutellaria baicalensis* root extract in H358 and H2087 cell lines [165].

5.2.3. The Activity of Plant Extracts from the Lamiaceae Family as Modulators of p53 Signaling

DNA damage occurs due to metabolic processes and environmental factors including ROS and results in an increase in the levels of tumor suppressor protein p53. The protein serves as a key regulator of the cellular response and triggers target genes including CDK and inhibitor p21, taking part in cell cycle arrest, and the proapoptotic protein Bax [182]. p53 expression was dysregulated in WiDr cells by *Coleus amboinicus* leaf extract [167], and the levels of both p53 and p21 increase in Glc-82 after treatment with *Salvia miltiorrhiza* root extract [149] and in MCF-7 cells after treatment with *Plectranthus amboinicus* leaf extract [120]. The level of p21 was induced in cell lines HT-29 and T84 after incubation with *Melissa officinalis* leaf extract [145]. p53 may be regulated by Sirtuin 1 (SIRT1), which is a member of nicotinamide adenine dinucleotide (NAD)-dependent histone deacetylases. The inhibition of SIRT1 was found to enhance apoptosis in CL1-5 cells treated with *Scutellaria barbata* extract [153]. One of the outcomes of p53 activation is cell cycle arrest, and these mechanisms have potent antitumor effects.

5.2.4. The Activity of Plant Extracts from the Lamiaceae Family as Modulators of PI3K/AKT Signaling

Apoptosis and cell cycle progression are mediated by phosphatidylinositol 3-kinase (PI3K) signal transduction. Activated PI3K is responsible for the conversion of phosphatidylinositol (4,5)-phosphate into phosphatidylinositol (3,4,5)-phosphate [183]. PI3K levels were significantly reduced in A549 cells after the administration of *Nepeta cataria* whole plant extract [184]. That PI3K signaling cascade induces protein kinase B, which is also known as PKB or Akt. Akt is a pro-oncogene and enables tumor proliferation. Akt has numerous downstream effects and controls several biological responses, including the phosphorylation of apoptosis signal proteins Bcl-2 and Bcl-xL followed by the suppression of apoptosis and also caspase-9 and p53. *Prunella vulgaris* root extract was found to modulate the PI3K/Akt signaling pathway in MCF-5 cells [150]. Akt may inactivate mammalian target of rapamycin complex 1 (mTORC1), p70S6 kinase, and p21, which are known to stimulate cell growth and proliferation. The levels of Akt, mTOR, and p70S6K were reduced in A549 cells after treatment with *Rosmarinus officinalis* leaf extract [174].

An important suppressor of PI3K is called PTEN: phosphatase and tensin homolog deleted on chromosome 10 [183]. PTEN expression was detected in A549 cells after *Nepeta cataria* whole plant extract [184]. An increased expression of PTEN was also observed in Glc-82 cells after *Salvia miltiorrhiza* root extract treatment, which then resulted in a reduced level of Akt [149]. The levels of phosphorylated Akt were reduced in human prostate cancer PC-3 cells following treatment with *Dracocephalum palmatum* leaf extract [169].

5.2.5. The Activity of Plant Extracts from the Lamiaceae Family as Modulators of NF-κB Signaling

In addition, the stimulation of nuclear factor kappa B (NF-κB) signaling cascade is mainly related to antiapoptotic properties. The NF-κB protein family has five members: p50, p52, p65, RelB, and c-Rel. NF-KB pathways are divided into the canonical and non-canonical. The canonical one is activated by a range of cell stressor molecules such as TNF-α that interact with tumor necrosis factor (TNF) receptors. A first step is the induction of transforming growth factor-β (TGF-β)-activated kinase 1 (TAK1), which promote stimulation of the IkB kinase (IKK) complex composed of IKKγ, IKKα, and IKKβ that phosphorylates IκB, which results in degradation. The remaining NF-κB (p50 and p65) migrate to the nucleus, bind to the DNA, and activate the transcription of numerous genes such as *Bcl-2* and *Bcl-xL*. [185]. Hence, the suppression of NF-κB by *Stachys pilifera* leaf extract is believed to be responsible for the induction of apoptosis in HT-29 cells [154]. The NF-κB signaling cascade also plays a pivotal role in the inflammatory response by activating the transcription of several pro-inflammatory genes such as interleukin *(IL) 1β, IL-8, and* cyclooxygenase-2 *(COX-2)* [186]. Commercial standardized *Thymus vulgaris* extract (thymol 0.3% w/w) was found to downregulate the activity of p65 and modulate the release of IL-1β and IL-8, which play roles part in the inflammatory mechanisms in the H460 human lung cancer cell line [187]. COX-2 plays a part in numerous malignancies, including several human cancers. COX-2 is associated with apoptosis suppression followed by uncontrolled proliferation, metastasis, and angiogenesis as a consequence of tumor growth [188]. COX-2 expression was dysregulated by high concentrations of *Origanum majorana* extract in A549 cells [189].

5.2.6. The Activity of Plant Extracts from the Lamiaceae Family as Modulators of Wnt/β-catenin Signaling

CDK/cyclin complexes control Wnt/β-catenin signaling [190]. *Scutellaria barbata* extract is related to decreased the expression of β-catenin in HT-29 cells [179], which is a component of the Wnt/β-catenin signaling pathway responsible for regulating cell growth. The signaling cascade is triggered by binding Wnt ligands to their receptors called Frizzled (Fz) and LDL receptor-related proteins 5 and 6 (LRP5 and LRP6). In the inactive state, a scaffolding protein Axin ensures β-catenin phosphorylation and promotes its degradation, but during the activation of the pathway, the Wnt ligand binds to Fz receptor, and it also allows β-catenin dephosphorylation and accumulation in the nucleus by Axin inhibition and the transcription of Wnt targeted genes such as c-Myc oncogene [191]. The suppression of Wnt signaling cascades induces apoptosis in SW480 and HCT-116 cells [192]. Additionally, *Scutellaria barbata* extract showed a potency to decrease the expression of the c-Myc in human colon adenocarcinoma HT-29 cells; excessive expression results in rapid cellular growth [193].

5.2.7. The Activity of Plant Extracts from the Lamiaceae Family as Modulators of Autophagy Signaling

Another type of cell death connected with self-degradation is autophagy. That process may be caused by stress signals that originate from extracellular, intracellular, and endoplasmic reticulum such as growth factor deprivation, nutrient starvation, oxidative stress, protein aggregation, and pathogen infection. Upon autophagy, the organelles named autophagosomes capsules other organelles or a portion of cytosol and then fused them into lysosome and breakdown by lysosomal hydrolases. Nucleation of the phagophore is initiated by the activation of the Unc-51-like kinase 1 (ULK1) complex that triggered the phosphorylation the class IIIPI3K (PI3KC3) complex 1. This step is blocked by Bcl-2 proteins by direct association with becyclin-1, which is a component of that complex. The activated

PI3KC complex mediates the production of phospatydyloinositol-3-posphate (PI3P). The first elongation step involves the enrollment of numerous autophagy-related (Atg) proteins by PI3P. The second phase of the elongation step is the formation of autophagosomal membrane-associated protein light chain 3 (LC3)-II from LC3-I via conjugation with phosphatidyl ethanolamine, which revealed the overexpression ratio of LC3-II/LC3-I in H358 and H2087 cells treated with *Scutellaria baicalensis* root extract [165]. Finally, autophagosomes fuse with lysosome and lysosomal enzymes with proteolytic activity degrade its cargo [194,195]. The autophagy is triggered in HT-29 cells by *Origanum majorana* leaf extract [171] and in CL1-5 cells by *Scutellaria barbata* extract [153].

The negative regulator of autophagy is mTOR. mTOR nucleates two distinct multi-protein complexes, mTORC1 and mTORC2. mTORC1 is composed of mTOR, regulatory-associated protein of mTOR (Raptor), mammalian lethal with Sec13 protein 8 (mLST8), proline-rich AKT substrate 40 kDa (PRAS40), and DEP-domain-containing mTOR-interacting protein (Deptor). mTORC1 positively regulates proliferation and cell growth. One of the most important factors involved in the regulation of mTORC1 activity is the tuberous sclerosis complex (TSC1/2). TSC1/2 functions as an activating protein for Rheb (Ras homolog enriched in brain). In turn, Rheb is able to activate mTORC1 [196]. One of the components of the mTOR pathway, Ras small GTPases—Rags, interact with mTORC1 and promote their translocation to a lysosomal membrane where Rheb resides [197].

5.2.8. The Activity of Plant Extracts from the Lamiaceae Family as Modulators of Necrosis Signaling

Necrosis is referred to as accidental cell death. It is frequently detected following harmful physical and chemical conditions, adverse stimuli, or deleterious mutations. The process is mediated by an imbalance of calcium flux, oxidative stress, and PARP. The physiological role of PARP is participation in DNA repair signaling in response to cell injury [198]. Excessive ROS levels, increased intracellular calcium, and the inhibition of PARP result in damage to cell components, degradation of proteins, and DNA damage. Necrosis is characterized by damage of the cell membrane and the release of its components into the extracellular space, resulting in inflammation and damage to the surrounding tissues [199,200]. This pathway is observed to take place in colon adenocarcinoma HT-29 and SW480 cell lines after *Rosmarinus officinalis* extract treatment. Rosemary extract possesses a strong antiproliferative activity, and its mechanism of action suggests the role of excessive intracellular ROS formation [201].

5.2.9. Plant Extracts from the Lamiaceae family and their Impact on Angiogenesis

The critical moment is tumor-induced angiogenesis. *Melissa officinalis* leaf extract halted neovascularization in breast adenocarcinoma MDA-MB-231 cells [202]. Antiangiogenic effects were also exerted by *Prunella vulgaris* root extract in MCF-5 cells [150]. The formation of new blood vessels from pre-existing ones may be regulated by numerous factors. One of them is epidermal growth factor (EGF) and its receptors (EGFR). It was observed that tumor cells demonstrate abnormally high EGFR activity and enhanced sensitivity to their ligands and the progression of tumor [203]. In turn, EGF was found to target vascular endothelial growth factor (VEGF) and induce their activity, whereas VEGF may modulate the EGFR signaling pathway [204]. VEGF demonstrated an ability to increase the permeability of existing blood vessels. The levels of both EGF and VEGF factors were found to be lowered in PC-3 cells and VEGF in DU-145, after *Salvia triloba* extract incubation [205]. *Nepeta cataria* whole plant extract exhibits a preventive effect against A549 cell invasiveness by reducing the level of VEGF [184], whereas *Melissa officinalis* leaf extract acts against PC-3, MCF-7, and A549 cells spread [166]. VEGF may be activated by human telomerase reverse transcriptase (hTERT), specific oncogene, catalytic subunit of the enzyme telomerase essential for chromosome termini replication. hTERT downregulation was observed in PC-3, MCF-7, and A549 cancer cell lines after *Melissa officinalis* leaf extract usage [166].

Other proangiogenic factors are angiogenin (ANG), IL-8 [206], leptin [207], and RANTES (regulated upon activation, normal T-cell expressed and secreted) [208]. ANG is a protein belonging to the RNase A superfamily, whose activity is related to the formation of blood vessels and tumor growth [209], ENA-78 is a chemokine associated with the activation of granulocytic immune cells and vascularity of the tumors, whereas leptin is an endocrine hormone produced by adipocytes. ENA-78 is strongly related to prostate cancer progression [210]. RANTES is an anti-inflammatory chemokine that recruits inflammatory cells and controls the secretion of growth factors included in the angiogenic process [208]. *Salvia triloba* extract was found to have the opposite effect on angiogenesis in PC-3 and DU-145 cells by reducing the levels of VEGF, ANG, ENA-78, IL-8, leptin, and RANTES [205].

5.3. The Anti-Cancer Activity of Plant-Derived Compounds from the Lamiaceae Family

Some of the compounds isolated from selected members of the Lamiaceae family and their cytotoxic effect against cancer cell lines are presented in Table 2. This section discusses the molecular mechanisms of action of these phytochemicals against lung, colon, breast, and prostate cancer cell lines.

Table 2. Cytotoxic properties of isolated pure compounds from the Lamiaceae family against lung, colon, breast, and prostate cancer cells.

Name of The Species	Part of the Plant	Active Compounds/ Class of Compounds	Cancer Cell Lines	Ref.
Caryopteris incana (Thunb.) Miq.,	whole plant	abietane diterpenes: caryopincaolide A, C, D	A549, Calu-1	[211]
Clerodendranthus spicatus (Thunb.) C. Y. Wu	aerial parts	ursane-type triterpenoids: spicatusoids A–E and three known ones and a known oleanane-type triterpenoid	A-549, MCF-7, SW480	[212]
Clerodendrum indicum (L.) Kuntze and *Clerodendrum villosum* Blume	roots	3b-hydroxy-D:B-friedo-olean-5-ene, oleanolic acid 3-acetate, taraxerol, lupeol, betulinic acid, (22E)-stigmasta-4,22,25-trien-3-one, stigmasta-4,25-dien-3-one, stigmasta-4,22-dien-3-one, 22-dehydroclerosterol, clerosterol, stigmasterol, b-sitosterol, pectolinarigenin, hispidulin	SW620, ChaGo-K-1, BT474	[213]
Clerodendrum inerme (L.) Gaertn	leaves	harwickiic acid, Crolerodendrum B-abietane diterpenes, uncinatone, acacetin, kaempferol 3,7,4′-trimethyl ether, 14,15-dihydro-15β-methoxy-3-epi-caryoptin, 5α,8α-epidioxyergosta-6,22-diene-3β-ol	HCT-116	[214]
Clerodendrum kiangsiense Merrill ex H. L. Li	herb	abeo-abietane diterpenoid: 12-methoxy-6,11,14,16-tetrahydroxy-17(15Ñ16)-abeo5,8,11,13-abietatetraen-3,7-dione, cryptojaponol, fortunin E	A549, MCF-7	[215]
Clerodendrum yaundense Gurke	twigs	lupane-type triterpene: (16a)-lupa-12,20(29)-dien-16-ol (clerodendrumol) and, O-Acetylclerodendrumol (16a)-Lupa-12,20(29)-dien-16-yl Ace-tate	MDA-MB-231	[216]
Isodon excisoides (Sun ex C. H. Hu) H. Hara, J. Jap	aerial parts	1α,7α,14β-trihydroxy-20-acetoxy-ent-kaur-15-one, henryin, reniformin C; kamebacetal A	HCT-116, NCI-H1650	[217]
Isodon rubescens (Hemsl.) H. Hara	aerial parts	ent-7,20-epoxy-kaur-16-en-1α,6β,7β,15β-tetrahydroxyl-11-O-β-d-glucopyranoside, ent-7,20-epoxy-kaur-16-en-6β,7β,14β,15β-tetrahydroxyl-1-O-β-d-glucopyranoside, ent-7,20-epoxy-kaur-16-en-6β,7β,15β-trihydroxyl-1-O-β-d-glucopyranoside, andent-7,20-epoxy-kaur-16-en-7β,11β,14α,15β-tetrahydr-oxyl-6-O-β-d-glucopyranoside, sodonterpene II, enmenol-1-β-glucoside, andenmenol	HCT-116	[218]
Isodon phyllostachys (Diels) Kudo	aerial parts	enmein-type diterpenoids enmein-type diterpenoids: 20-episerrin C, serrin C, isodocarpin, serrin B	A549, MCF-7, SW480	[219]
Isodon rubescens (Hemsl.) H.Hara	leaves	diterpenoids: 6-epi-11-O-acetylangustifolin and 11-O-acetylangustifolin	A549	[220]
Isodon wikstroemioides (Hand.–Mazz.) H. Hara	aerial parts	diterpenoids: 11, 20-epoxy-ent- kauranoids, isowikstroemins H–M, along with two known analogues, macrocalyxin B	A549, MCF-7	[221]
Leonurus japonicus Houtt.	fruits	leonuronins A and B	A549	[222]

Table 2. *Cont.*

Name of The Species	Part of the Plant	Active Compounds/ Class of Compounds	Cancer Cell Lines	Ref.
Ocimum basilicum var.thyrsiflorum (L.) Benth	leaves	C-glycosylated derivative of apigenin: 3′′-O-acetylvitexin	HCT-116	[114]
Ocimum sanctum L.	aerial parts	lignans: (-)-rabdosiin	MCF-7, SKBR3, HCT-116	[201]
Orthosiphon stamineus Benth.	aerial parts	7,4′-dimethylkaempferol, 5,7,4′-trimethylkaempferol, 7,3′,4′-trimethylquercetin, 5,7,3′,4′-tetramethylquercetin, 5,7,4′-trimethylquercetin, 3,5,3′,4′-tetramethylquercetin, 5,7,3′,6′-tetramethoxyflavone, 5,7,3′,4′-tetramethoxyflavone, 2*S*-5,6,7,3′,4′-pentamethoxyflavanone, 2*S*-5′-hydroxy-5,7,3′,4′-tetramethoxyflavanone	MCF-7, MDA-MB-231	[223]
Phlomis bruguieri Desf	aerial parts	4′-methoxy-luteolin-7-phosphate	MCF-7	[224]
Phlomoides umbrosa (Turcz.) Kamelin & Makhm	roots	28-noroleanane-derived spirocyclic triterpenoids: phlomisu D, phlomisu E, (2α,3α,17R,18β)-19(18→17)-abeo-28-norolean-12-ene-2,3,18,23,24-pentol, phlomispentaol	MCF-7	[225]
Plectranthus cylindraceus Hoechst. Ex. Benth	aerial parts	sesquiterpene: plectranol A, maaliol, penduletin and chrysosplenol D	MBD-MB-321	[226]
Plectranthus ecklonii Benth.	whole plant	abietane diterpenoid: parvifloron D	MDA-MB-231	[227]
Plectranthus madagascariensis Benth	whole plant	royleanone diterpenes: 7α-formyloxy-6β-hydroxyroyleanon, 7α,6β-dihydroxyroyleanon, 7α-acetoxy-6β-hydroxyroy-leanone	MDA-MB-231, MCF-7, HCT-116, NCI-H460	[228]
Plectranthus scutellarioides (L.) R. Br.	leaves	diterpenoids: spiroscutelones A–C	MCF-7	[229]
Pogostemon auricularius L. Hassk.	aerial parts	meroterpenoids with pyrone-sesquiterpenoid hybrid skeletons: pogostemins A-C	SW480, SK-LU-1	[230]
Pogostemon cablin (Blanco) Benth	aerial parts	phenylethanoid glycosides: verbascoside, pedicularioside G ()	A549, HCT-15	[231]
Premna odorata Blanco	bark	tetrahydrofurofuran lignin: 4β-hydroxyasarinin	HT-29, MCF-7	[232]
Rabdosia serra (Maxim.) Hara	grasses	diterpenoids: rabdosins E–K, serrin B, serrin A, isodocarpin and lushanrubescensin J	A549, NCI–H661	[233]
Salvia ballotiflora Benth	leaves	diterpenoids: 7α-acetoxy-6,7-dihydroicetexone, anastomosine	SK-LU-1	[234]
Salvia ballotiflora Benth.	aerial parts	diterpenes: 19-deoxyicetexone,7,20-dihydroanastomosine, icetexoneand19-deoxyisoicetexone,	A549, MCF-7	[127]
Salvia lachnocalyx Hedge	shoots	(2*Z*,6*Z*,10*Z*,14*E*)-geranylfarnesol and spathulenol	MCF-7, HT-29	[235]

Table 2. *Cont.*

Name of The Species	Part of the Plant	Active Compounds/ Class of Compounds	Cancer Cell Lines	Ref.
Salvia leriifolia Benth.	aerial parts	labdane diterpenoids: 6β,13β-dihydroxylabd-8, 14-diene-19-oic acid, 13-hydroxylabd-8, 14-diene-6β,19-olide, 8,12E,14-labdatrien-6,19-olid	MDA-MB-231, DU 145	[236]
Salvia leucantha Cav	aerial parts	neoclerodane diterpenoids: leucansalvialins FeI (1–4), and one rare 18(4→3)-abeo-abietane diterpenoid, leucansalvialin J	A549, MCF-7, SW480	[237]
Salvia officinalis L.	leaves	diterpene: manool	MCF-7	[238]
Salvia sahendica Boiss. & Buhs	leaves	terpenoid: sclareol	MDA-MB-231	[239]
Salvia santolinifolia Boiss	callus	salvialactomine, 5-Methylflavone	PC-3	[240]
Salvia tebesana Bunge	roots	diterpenoids: tebesinone A (1) and tebesinone B (2), aegyptinone A (3) andaegyptinone B (4)	MCF-7, PC-	[241]
Salvia tiliifolia L.	aerial parts	neo-clerodane diterpenoids: tiliifolins A–E	A549, MCF-7, SW480	[242]
Salvia urmiensis Bunge	aerial parts	triterpenoids: urmiensolide B and urmiensic acid	MCF-7	[243]
Scutellaria barbata D. Don	whole plant	neoclerodane diterpenoids: barbatin F, barbatin G, scutebata A, scutebata B, scutebata C and scutebata P	LoVo, MCF-7, HCT-116	[244]
Scutellaria barbata D. Don	aerial parts	neo-clerodane diterpenoids: 13(R*)-1β,6α-dibenzoyloxy-7β-hydroxy-8β,13-epoxy-3-neo-cleroden-15,16-olide (scutebata C1), 2-oxo-6α-nicotinoyloxy-7β-benzoyloxy-8β-hy-droxy-3,11(E),13-neo-clerodatrien-15,16-olide.(scutebata X), 13(R*)-2-oxo-6α-acetoxy-7β-nicotinoyloxy-8β,13-epoxy-3-neo-cleroden-15,16-olide, (scutebata A1)	MCF-7, A549	[245]
Scutellaria barbata D. Don	aerial parts	neoclerodane diterpenoid: barbatin H, scutebata P, scutebarbatine F, 6-O-nicotinoylscutebarbatine G, scutebata G, scutebata E, scutebata D, barbatin C, scutebarbatine A, scutebartine G, scutebarbatine B, 6,7-Di-O-acetoxybarbatin A, scutebata C, scutebata A, scutebarbatine X, scutebata B	LoVo, MCF-7, HCT-116	[246]
Scutellaria barbata D.Don	whole plant	neo-clerodane diterpenoids: scutebarbatolides A-C, 4-deoxy-11,12-didehydroandrographolide, scutehenanine H, 14β-hydroxyscutolideK	LNCaP, MCF-7	[247]
Scutellaria coleifolia Levl.	aerial parts	neo-clerodane type diterpenoids: scutefolides G1-S	A549, MCF-7	[248]
Scutellaria strigillosa Hemsley, J. Linn. Soc	whole plant	neo-clerodane diterpenoids: scutestrigillosins A-C	MCF-7, HT-29	[249]

Table 2. *Cont.*

Name of The Species	Part of the Plant	Active Compounds/ Class of Compounds	Cancer Cell Lines	Ref.
Teucrium polium L.	aerial parts	saponin glycosides: poliusaposide A, poliusaposide B, poliusaposide C	MDA-MB-468, HCC-2998, COLO 205	[250]
Teucrium ramosissimum Desf.	leaves	sesquiterpene: β-eudesmol	A549, HT-29, Caco-2	[251]
Teucrium viscidum Blum.	whole plants	abietane diterpenoid: teuvisone, a pair of new dimeric abietane diterpenoid stereoisomers: biteuvisones A and B, and three sesquiterpenoid lactones, teuvislactones A–C	teuvisone and biteuvisones B showed cytotoxic effect against NCI-H460, HCT-116	[252]
Thymus alternans Kloko.	aerial parts	triterpenes: 3a-hydroxy-urs-12,15-diene, a-amyrin, b-amyrin, isoursenol, epitaraxerol, and oleanolic acid	MDA-MB-231, HCT-15 HCT-116, U1810	[253]

5.3.1. The Anticancer Activity of Phenolics Compounds from the Lamiaceae Family

Rosmarinic acid (α-o-caffeoyl-3,4-dihydroxyphenyllactic acid; CAS 20283-92-5), an ester of caffeic acid, and 3,4-dihydroxyphenyllactic acid is commonly found in species of the Lamiaceae family. Rosmarinic acids and their derivatives possess a range of antioxidant, anti-inflammatory, antitumor, anti-angiogenic, and antimicrobial activities, among others [254]. Rosmarinic acid extracted from *Salvia glabra* demonstrates antitumor activity against breast cancer stem-like cells (BCSCs); this has been attributed to apoptosis induction by suppressing the expression of Bcl-2 and increasing that of Bax [255].

Wogonin (5,7-dihydroxy-8-methoxyflavone; CAS 632-85-9) is a flavone with numerous antitumor, anti-inflammatory, antiviral, and neuroprotective properties [256]. A natural source of wogonin is Scutellariae radix, which is the dried root of *Scutellaria baicalensis*. It has been shown to promote both autophagy and apoptosis processes in SW48 cells via the upregulation of autophagic factors including LC3II and Beclin 1 proteins and apoptotic factors such as caspase-3, caspase-8, caspase-9, and Bax proteins. The exposure to wogonin results in G2/M cell cycle arrest and the inhibition of PI3K/Akt signaling through attenuating PI3K protein expression [257]. Wogonin has been found to inhibit the invasiveness of MDA-MB-231 cells via suppressing the synthesis of two key factors related to new blood vessel formation: IL-8 and matrix metallopeptidase-9 (MMP-9) [258]. MMP-9 is critical for the progression of a pro-angiogenic outcome and the release of VEGF during carcinogenesis [259]. Scutellarein (5,6,7,4′-tetrahydroxyflavone), a flavone that is particularly present in the genus *Scutellaria*, has been found to be effective for the prevention and treatment of *Helicobacter pylori* infection, Alzheimer's disease, and vascular complications of diabetes; it has also been found to inhibit certain carcinomas [260]. It was found that the exposure of the HCT116 cells to the scutellarein extracted from *Scutellaria barbata* induces apoptosis via ROS-mediated mitochondrial membrane permeability and cytochrome c release, and by downregulating the expression of Bcl-2, increasing Bax and cleaved-caspase-3 activity [261].

Another common flavanone is naringenin (4′,5,7-trihydroxyflavanone; CAS 480-41-1). Naringenin has shown antitumor, antioxidant, anti-inflammatory, antiviral, antibacterial, antiadipogenic, and cardioprotective potential [262]. Abaza et al. studied the effect of naringenin isolated from *Thymus vulgaris* whole plant on HTB26, HTB132, SW1116, and SW837 cells. Its administration was found to increase G1/S and G2/M phases cell cycle arrest and apoptotic cell death through the upregulation of p18, p21, Bak, Bax, activation of caspases 3, 7, 8, and 9, and the downregulation of CDK 4, 6, and Bcl2 in all cancer cell lines. It was also found to decrease cell survival factors including PI3K, Akt, and NFκBp65.

5.3.2. The Anticancer Activity of Terpenoids Compounds from the Lamiaceae Family

Arguably, the most important class of chemicals produced by the Lamiaceae family is the terpenoids; of these, the most numerous subclass of compounds with confirmed anticancer properties is that of the diterpenoids. Many possess pro-apoptotic properties, including 3-acetoxylteuvincenone from *Ajuga ovalifolia* whole plants [263], sahandone and sahandol II from *Salvia chloroleuca* roots [264], acetyl-macrocalin B from *Isodon sylvatica* [265], parvifloron D from *Plectranthu ecklonii* [227], and 7β-acetoxy-20-hydroxy-19,20-epoxyroyleanone from *Salvia corrugate* shoots [266]. 3-acetoxylteuvincenone activates Src homology phosphotyrosine phosphatase 2 (SHP2) and induces extracellular signal-regulated kinase (ERK) 1/2 and Akt pathways in A549 cells [263]. SHP2 controls the activation of Akt by insulin-like growth factor-1 (IGF-1), thus regulating the PI3K/Akt pathway related to the blockage of caspase 3-mediated apoptosis [267]. Moreover, SNP2 has been implicated in the activation of ERK 1/2, a member of mitogen-activated protein kinases (MAPKs) that restored the levels of c-Myc [268]. Sahandone and sahandol II change the ratio of Bax/Bcl-2 apoptotic proteins and activate PARP in the MCF-7, LNCaP, and PC-3 cell lines [264]. Acetyl-macrocalin B induces apoptosis in an ROS-dependent manner in A549 cells and then upregulates the p38 MAPK signaling pathway that mediates caspase-9 release. Additionally, the initiation of G2/M cell cycle delay throughout checkpoint kinase (Chks) Chk 1 and Chk 2 activation and cell division cycle 25C (Cdc25C) phosphatase degradation. Chk 1/2 are expressed during the cell cycle, where they regulate the spread of checkpoint signals and promote G2/M arrest by degrading Cdc25C phosphatase [269]. Cdc25C phosphatase dephosphorylates the cyclin B-CDK1 complex and enables cell entry into mitosis but inactivates it, preventing cell cycle progression [270]. Another diterpenoid, parvifloron D, induces apoptotic morphological changes in MDA-MB-231 cells [227]. 7β-acetoxy-20-hydroxy-19,20-epoxyroyleanone promotes G0/G1 cell cycle delay and ROS activation of ERK1/2 kinase in human breast cancer SKBR-3 and human breast carcinoma BT474 cell lines [266].

An important subgroup of terpenoid compounds is tanshinone diterpenoids, which are produced by *Salvia miltiorrhiza* roots; these are also connected with the induction of apoptosis in cancer cells. Increases in apoptosis were observed in colon cancer cells (human colorectal cancer DLD-1, human colon carcinoma COLO 205, and human colorectal adenocarcinoma Caco-2) exposed to trijuganone C [271], prostate cancer cells (PC3 and LNCaP) treated with tanshinone analog 2-(Glycine [methyl ester]methyl)-naphtho [272], and lung (human non-small cell lung cancer PC9 and A549) and breast cancer (MCF-7) cells administered by tanshinone [273]; these changes were attributed to the upregulation of numerous apoptotic factors including cytochrome c, pro- and antiapoptotic proteins ratio, caspases, PARP, p53, and p38. In addition, MCF-7 cells treated with three tanshinones isolated from the roots of *Perovskia abrotanoides* (cryptotanshinone, tanshinone 2A, and hydroxycryptotanshinone) exhibit high amounts of PARP protein cleavage, which is a hallmark of apoptosis [274].

Another diterpenoid, 11α, 12α-epoxyleukamenin E isolated from whole plants of *Salvia cavaleriei* show anticancer potential against HCT116 and SW480 cell lines [275]; this activity was attributed to suppression of the crucial Wnt signaling pathway, which regulates cell fate and the activation of targeted genes, including c-Myc and survivin. The diterpene clerodermic acid found in aerial parts of four *Salvia* species including *S. spinosa*, *S. santolinifolia*, *S. syriaca*, and *S. nemorosa* was also shown to be effective in suppressing Hypoxia-Inducible Factor (HIF) 1 alpha in A549 cells [276], which correlates with tumor metastasis and angiogenesis. Hypoxia is a common microenvironment in many types of solid tumors, and the HIF-1α pathway is crucial for their survival; therefore, the reduction of its expression may serve as a potential cancer therapy target [277].

It has been reported that phlomisoside F, a diterpene glycoside isolated from *Phlomis younghusbandii* root, promotes G0/G1 cell cycle delay and apoptosis induction, as confirmed by the overexpression of caspase-3, caspase-9, and Bax, and the underexpression of Bcl-2 and COX-2 in A549 cells [278]. 2α, 3α, 23-trihydroxy-13α, 27-cyclours-11-en-28-oic acid, a triterpene acid isolated from the aerial parts of *Glechoma longituba*, is responsible for NCI-H460 cell cycle arrest, the induction of ROS-mediated apoptosis, and the nullification of NF-κB activity [279]. The exposure of human lung cancer cell line SK-LU-1 cells to pogostemin A, a meroterpenoid isolated from the aerial parts of *Pogostemon auricularius*, triggered apoptosis and caspase-3 activation [280].

5.3.3. The Anticancer Activity of Polysaccharides Compounds from the Lamiaceae Family

Biologically active polysaccharides from natural plant sources also act as potent antitumor agents. They are also believed to be nontoxic and more preferred for living organisms [281]. SPS2p, a polysaccharide composed of carbohydrates, uronic acid, and proteins from *Scutellaria barbata* demonstrated pro-apoptotic activity against HT29 cells, probably by suppressing the PI3K/Akt pathway [282]. Whereas SBPW3, a polysaccharide containing rhamnose, arabinose, xylose, mannose, glucose, and galactose isolated from the same species also demonstrated anti-metastatic activity via the suppression of EMT in the same cell line [283].

5.4. The Anticancer Activity of Essential Oils from the Lamiaceae Family

The members of the Lamiaceae are sources of essential oils. Their cytotoxic potency against cancer cell lines are presented in Table 3. This section discusses their mechanisms of action against lung, colon, breast, and prostate cancer cell lines.

Table 3. Cytotoxic properties of selected essential oils from the Lamiaceae family against lung, colon, breast, and prostate cancer cells.

Name of The Species	Part of the Plant	Compounds Identified in Essential Oils	Cancer Cell Lines	Ref.
Anisomeles indica Kuntze.	leaves	The major compounds: farnesyl acetone (10.67%), nootkatone (8.35%), phytol acetate (7.35%), jasmatone (7.81%)	A549	[284]
Ballota undulata, Ballota saxatilis *Ballota nigra* ssp. foetida	aerial parts	*Ballota nigra* ssp. foetida: germacrene D (23.1%), (E)-β-caryophyllene (20.3%) and caryophyllene oxide (6.2%), *Ballota saxatilis*: linalool (11.2%), (E)-β-caryophyllene (8.8%), caryophyllene oxide (6.3%) and (E)-2-hexenal (5.6%), *Ballota undulata*: germacrene D (16.0%), and bicyclogermacrene (10.4%)	MCF-7	[285]
Cantinoa stricta (Benth.) Harley and J.F.B. Pastore (*formely Hyptis stricta* Benth.)	leaves and flowers	The major compounds: caryophyllene oxide (leaf –31.6%; flower –21.7%) and cis-pinane (leaf –15.4%; flower –9.7%), α-pinene (9.4%) and β-pinene (9.1%)	MCF-7, NCI-H460, PC-3	[286]
Cedronella canariensis var. canariensis (L.) Webb and Berthel.	aerial parts	The major compounds: pinocarvone (58.0%) and β-pinene (10.8%)	MDA-MB-231, HCT-116	[287]
Cunila angustifolia Benth.	leaves	The major compounds: pulegone (29.5%), isomenthol (27.0%), menthone (8.6%), neomenthol (7.2%), menthyl acetate (2.5%), and caryophyllene oxide (2.0%)	A-549, MCF-7	[288]
Elsholtzia ciliata (Thunb.) Hylander	aerial parts	The major compounds: dehydroelsholtzia ketone, elsholtzia ketone, sesquiterpenes β-bourbonene, caryophyllene, α-caryophyllene, germacrene D, and α-farnesene	MDA-MB-231	[289]
Lavandula hybrid Rev., *Lavandula latifolia* Medikus., *Lavandula* vera D.C. *and Lavandula angustifolia* Miller.	aerial parts	Terpenes: linalool and linalyl acetate terpenoids: 1,8-cineole	Caco-2	[290]
Leonotis nepetifolia (L.) R.Br.	leaves	The major compounds: 3-octanone (3.75%), (E)-ocimene (15.85%), (Z)-ocimene (7.01%), linalool, caryophillene oxide, and 1-octen-3-ol (42.58%)	HCT-116	[291]
Melissa officinalis L.	leaves	citral (47.2%), caryophyllene oxide (10.2%), citronellal (5.4%), geraniol (6.6%), geranyl acetate (4.1%) and β- caryophyllene (3,8%)	MCF-7, NCI-H460	[292]
Mentha citrate Ehrh.	aerial part	The major compounds: linalool (34.69%), linalyl acetate (35.75%)	HCT-116	[293]

Table 3. *Cont.*

Name of The Species	Part of the Plant	Compounds Identified in Essential Oils	Cancer Cell Lines	Ref.
Mentha spicata L.	aerial parts	The major compounds: carvone (49.5%), limonene (16.1%), 1,8-cineole (8.7%), cis-dihydrocarvone (3.9%), β-caryophyllene (2.7%), germacrene D (2.1%), and β-pinene (1.1%)	HCT-116, MCF-7	[294]
Meriandra dianthera (Konig ex Roxb.) Benth.	aerial parts	camphor (54.3%), 1,8-cineole (12.2%), and camphene (10.4%)	MCF-7, LoVo	[295]
Nepeta menthoides Boiss. and Bohse.	-	The major compounds: 1,8-cineole (70.06%)	MCF-7, T-47D, MDA-MB-231	[296]
Nepeta schiraziana Boiss.	aerial parts	The major compounds: 1,8-cineole (33.67%), germacrene D (11.45%), β-caryophyllene (9.88%), and caryophyllene oxide (7.34%)	MCF-7	[297]
Nepeta sintenisii Bornm.	aerial parts	4aα,7α7aβ nepetalactone (51.74%), β-farnesene (12.26%), 4aα,7α,7aα nepetalactone (8.01%), germacrene-D (5.01%), and 4aα7β,7aα-nepetalactone (3.71%)	LS180, MCF-7	[298]
Ocimum basilicum L., *Mentha spicata* L.	chopped leaves and stems	*Mentha spicata*: carvone (85.4%), limonene (8.4%), and β-Pinene (1.4%) *Ocimum basilicum*: methyl chavicol (74.9%), linalol (18.4%)	MCF-7, Caco2	[299]
Origanum majorana L.	aerial parts	The major compounds: terpinen-4-ol (23.2%), Cis-sabinene hydrate (17.5%), γ-terpinene (10.5%), p-cymene (9%), α-terpineol (5.6%), α-terpinene (4.7%), and trans-sabinene hydrate (4.0%)	HT-29	[300]
Origanum dictamnus (L.) Kostel., *Origanum libanoticum* Boiss., and *Origanum microphyllum* (Bentham) T. Vogel	-	The major compounds: carvacrol, p-cymene, linalool, γ-terpinene, and terpinen-4-ol as	LoVo	[301]
Origanum vulgare L.	leaves	pulegone (77.4%), menthone (4.8%), cis-Isopulegone (2.2%), piperitenone (2.1%), limonene (1.0%), and myrcene (0.6%)	MCF-7, HT-29	[302]
Plectranthus. cylindraceus Hocst. ex Benth., *Plectranthus. asirensis* JRI Wood. and *Plectranthus barbatus* Andrews.	leaves and branches	The major compounds: α-pinene (46.2%), maaliol (42.8%), and β-caryophyllene (13.3%)	HT-29	[303]
Premna microphylla Turcz.	aerial parts	The major compounds: blumenol C (49.7%), β-cedrene (6.1%), limonene (3.8%), α-guaiene (3.3%), cryptone (3.1%), and gurkeα-cyperone (2.7%)	MCF-7	[304]
Rosmarinus officinalis L.	aerial parts	The major compounds: 1,8-cineole (23.56%), camphene (12.78%), camphor (12.55%), and β-pinene (12.3%)	MCF-7	[305]

Table 3. *Cont.*

Name of The Species	Part of the Plant	Compounds Identified in Essential Oils	Cancer Cell Lines	Ref.
Salvia macrosiphon Boiss.	aerial parts	The major compounds: linalool (19%), β-cedrene (14.64%), and β-elemene (13.33%)	MCF-7, MDA-MB-231, T-47D	[306]
Salvia officinalis L.	aerial parts	The major compounds: α-thujone, 1,8-cineole, and camphor	LNCaP, MCF-7	[307]
Salvia officinalis L.	aerial parts	α-thujone (29.39%), 1,8-cineole (eucalyptol 22.8%), and camphor (13.05%)	Caco-2, HT-29, HCT-116	[308]
Salvia ringens Sibth. and Sm.	whole plant	The major compounds: 1.8-cineole (31.99%), cam-phene (17.06%), borneol (11.94%), and α-pinene (11.52%)	HCT-116	[309]
Satureja intermedia C.A.Mey	aerial parts	γ-terpinene (37.1%), thymol (30.2%), p-cymene (16.2%), limonene (3.9%), α-terpinene (3.3), myrcene (2.5%), germacrene B (1.4%), elemicine (1.1%), and carvacrol (0.5%)	MCF-7	[310]
Satureja thymbra L. *and Satureja parnassica* Heldr. and Sart. ex Boiss	aerial parts	The major compounds: carvacrol, thymol, γ-terpinene, and p-cymene	MCF-7, A549	[311]
Stachys annua L. subsp. annua	aerial parts	The major compounds: phytol (9.8%), germacrene D (9.2%), and spathulenol (8.5%)	HCT-116, MDA-MB-231	[312]
Stachys annua L. subsp. *annua*	aerial parts	phytol (9.8%), germacrene D (9.2%), and spathulenol (8.5%)	MDA-MB 231, HCT-116	[312]
Stachys parviflora L.	aerial parts	The major compounds: α-terpenylacetate (23.6%), caryophyllene (16.8%), bicyclogermacrene (9.3%), spathulenol (4.9%), and α-pinene (4.2%)	HCT-116	[313]
Tetradenia riparia (Hochst.) Codd.	leaves	fenchone (6.1%), dronabinol (11.0%), aromadendrene oxide (14.7%), and (E,E)–farnesol (15.0%)	HT-29, MCF-7	[314]
Thymus alternans Klokov.	aerial parts	The major compounds: (E)-nerolidol, neryl acetate, nerol	MDA-MB-231, HCT-15, HCT-116, U1810	[253]
Thymus munbyanus subsp. Coloratus (Boiss. and Reut.) Greuter and Burdet	stems, leaves	borneol (44.8 and 31.2%) Other components occurring in noteworthy levels were camphor (5.7 and 13.6%), camphene (3.6 and 7.5%), 1,8-cineole (6.0 and 4.2%), and germacrene D (5.0 and 3.1%)	MDA-MB-231	[315]
Zataria multiflora Boiss.	aerial parts	-	MCF-7	[316]

Table 3. *Cont.*

Name of The Species	Part of the Plant	Compounds Identified in Essential Oils	Cancer Cell Lines	Ref.
Zataria multiflora Boiss. *Satureja bakhtiarica* Bunge.	leaves	The major compounds: phenol (56.35%, 37.4%), thymol (13.82%, 22.6%), P-cymene (8.79%, 19.3%), γ-terpinene (3.36%, 5.0%), β-myrcene (1.91%, 0.8%), β-caryophyllene (1.28%, 2.2%), α-terpinene (1.21%, 0.9%), caryophyllene oxide (0.47%, 2.0%), and carvacrole (2.88%, 0.2%)	MDA-MB-231	[317]
Zhumeria majdae Rech.f. and Wendelbo.	aerial parts	The major compounds: linalool (24.4–34.6%), camphor (26.1–34.7%), and translinalool oxide (7.6–28.6%)	MCF-7	[318]

Nepeta rtanjensis essential oils rich in trans,cis-nepetalactone induced programmed cell death against A549 and MDA-MB-231 cells [319], as did *Origanum onites* essential oil, which is rich in carvacrol, against Ht-29 cells [320]. *Ocimum viride* essential oils, which have a high content of γ-terpinene, induced apoptosis as a consequence of DNA damage in HT-29 cells [321], while *Thymus revolutus* essential oil with a high content of γ-terpinene and p-cymene induced apoptosis in A549 cells [322]. *Salvia aurea*, *S. judaica*, and *S. viscosa* essential oils containing caryophyllene oxide as a main constituent induced apoptosis triggered by excessive ROS formation in DU-145 cells [323], as did *Zataria multiflora* essential oils in HCT-116 and SW48 cell lines [324].

G2/M cell cycle delay and apoptosis were observed in PC-3 cells after exposure to *Lavandula angustifolia* essential oil, with linalool and linalyl acetate as major components [325]. *Plectranthus amboinicus* essential oil, containing high amounts of carvacrol, dysregulated levels of pro- and antiapoptotic factors and induced caspase-9 and caspase-3 in A549 cells [326].

Patchouli alcohol, isolated from the essential oil of *Pogostemon cablin*, induced mitochondria-mediated apoptosis and caspase-9 and caspase-3 production in A549 cells [327]. The oil may also demonstrate its anticancer activity by dysregulating the MAPK pathway. *Stachys viticina* essential oils, with their main components being endo-borneol, eucalyptol, and epizonarene, inhibit mediators of apoptosis suppression COX-2 in COLO 205 cells [328]. The caspase-8 and caspase-9-dependent apoptosis pathways are triggered in HT-29 cells by treatment with *Origanum majorana* essential oil containing *inter alia* terpinen-4-ol, alpha-terpinol, alpha-pinene, camphene, p-cymol, B-caryophyllene, bicyclogermacrene, and neophytadiene [329]. *Origanum majorana* essential oil induces non-apoptotic cell death including autophagy and necrosis in HT-29 cells [329]; the same is observed in human lung cancer cell line Calu-3 treatment with *Lavandula dentata* essential oils rich in 1,8-cineole [330].

6. Conclusions

Cancer causes the greatest economic burden of any of the top 15 causes of death worldwide, both for the patient and society in general. Therefore, there is a great need to identify new active molecules with anticancer activities. Medicinal plants and their bioactive compounds are widely used in the treatment of numerous diseases. The species of the Lamiaceae are considered important because of their use in traditional medicine throughout the world. The Lamiaceae include a range of secondary metabolites including polyphenols, terpenoids, alkaloids, or essential oils that demonstrate promising cytotoxic activity against lung, breast, prostate, and colorectal cancer cell lines mainly via the apoptosis pathway by the modulation of cell cycle progression, changes in genes expression, and impact on various signaling cascades. These biologically active compounds represent promising candidates for supportive use in anticancer therapy; however, further extensive scientific and clinical investigations are required.

Author Contributions: Conceptualization, P.S.; writing—review and editing, P.S., A.M.-S., and T.K.; supervision, T.Ś., and R.Z. All authors have read and agreed to the published version of the manuscript.

Abbreviations

Akt	Protein Kinase B
ANG	Angiogenin
Apaf	Apoptotic Protease Activating Factor
Atg	Autophagy Related Protein
Cdc25C	Cell Division Cycle 25C Phosphatase
CDKs	Cyclin-Dependent Kinases
COX	Cyclooxygenase

Deptor	DEP-Domain-Containing mTOR-Interacting Protein
DISC	Death-Inducing Signaling Complex
EGF	Epidermal Growth Factor
EGFR	Epidermal Growth Factor Receptor
ERK	Extracellular Signal-Regulated Kinase
FADD	Fas-Associated Death Domain
Fz receptor	Frizzled Receptor
HIF	Hypoxia-Inducible Factor
hTERT	Human Telomerase Reverse Transcriptase
IKK	IkB Kinase
IL	Interleukin
LC3	Autophagosomal Membrane-Associated Protein Light Chain 3
MAPK	Mitogen-Activated Protein Kinase
mLST8	Mammalian Lethal with Sec13 Protein 8
MMP	Matrix Metallopeptidase
mTOR	Mammalian Target of Rapamycin
mTORC1	Mammalian Target of Rapamycin Complex 1
NF-κB	Nuclear Factor Kappa B
PARP	Poly(ADP-ribose) Polymerase
PI3K	Phosphatidylinositol 3-Kinase
PI3KC3	Class IIIPI3K Complex 1
PI3P	Phospatydyloinositol-3-Posphate
PRAS40	Proline-Rich AKT Substrate 40 kDa
PTEN	Phosphatase and Tensin Homolog
RANTES	Regulated Upon Activation, Normal T-cell Expressed and Secreted
Raptor	Regulatory-Associated Protein of mTOR
Rheb	Ras Homolog Enriched in Brain
ROS	Reactive Oxygen Species
SHP2	Src Homology Phosphotyrosine Phosphatase 2
SIRT1	Sirtuin
TAK	TGF-β-Activated Kinase
TNF	Tumor Necrosis Factor
TRAIL	TNF-Related Apoptosis-Inducing Ligand
ULK1	Unc-51-like Kinase 1 Complex
VEGF	Vascular Endothelial Growth Factor

References

1. Cooper, G.M. Cancer. In *The Cell. A Molecular Approach*, 2nd ed.; Sinauer Associates: Sunderland, MA, USA, 2000.
2. Sarkar, S.; Horn, G.; Moulton, K.; Oza, A.; Byler, S.; Kokolus, S.; Longacre, M. Cancer development, progression, and therapy: An epigenetic overview. *Int. J. Mol. Sci.* **2013**, *14*, 21087–21113. [CrossRef] [PubMed]
3. Bray, F.; Ferlay, J.; Soerjomataram, I.; Siegel, R.L.; Torre, L.A.; Jemal, A. Global cancer statistics 2018: GLOBOCAN estimates of incidence and mortality worldwide for 36 cancers in 185 countries. *CA Cancer J. Clin.* **2018**, *68*, 394–424. [CrossRef]
4. WHO. WHO—CancerReport—2020—Global Profile. Available online: https://www.paho.org/hq/index.php?option=com_docman&view=download&category_slug=4-cancer-country-profiles-2020&alias=51561-global-cancer-profile-2020&Itemid=270&lang=fr (accessed on 27 August 2020).
5. Voda, A.I.; Bostan, I. Public Health Care Financing and the Costs of Cancer Care: A Cross-National Analysis. *Cancers* **2018**, *10*, 117. [CrossRef] [PubMed]
6. Pucci, C.; Martinelli, C.; Ciofani, G. Innovative approaches for cancer treatment: Current perspectives and new challenges. *Ecancermedicalscience* **2019**, *13*, 961. [CrossRef]

7. Wang, H.; Khor, T.O.; Shu, L.; Su, Z.; Fuentes, F.; Lee, J.H.; Tony Kong, A.H. Plants Against Cancer: A Review on Natural Phytochemicals in Preventing and Treating Cancers and Their Druggability. *Anticancer Agents Med. Chem.* **2012**, *12*, 1281–1305. [CrossRef] [PubMed]
8. Tiwari, R.; Rana, C.S. Plant secondary metabolites: A review. *Int. J. Eng. Res. Gen. Sci.* **2015**, *3*, 661–670.
9. Iqbal, J.; Abbasi, B.A.; Mahmood, T.; Kanwal, S.; Ali, B.; Shah, S.A.; Khalil, A.T. Plant-derived anticancer agents: A green anticancer approach. *Asian Pac. J. Trop. Biomed.* **2017**, *7*, 1129–1150. [CrossRef]
10. Hassanpour, S.H.; Dehghani, M. Review of cancer from perspective of molecular. *J. Cancer Res. Pract.* **2017**, *4*, 127–129. [CrossRef]
11. Goodman, S.N.; Samet, J. Cause and Cancer Epidemiology. In *Cancer Epidemiology and Prevention*, 2nd ed.; Schottenfeld, D., Fraumeni, J.F., Eds.; Oxford University Press: New York, NY, USA, 2017.
12. Baylin, S.B.; Jones, P.A. Epigenetic Determinants of Cancer. *Cold Spring Harb. Perspect. Biol.* **2016**, *8*, a019505. [CrossRef]
13. Binder, M.; Roberts, C.; Spencer, N.; Antoine, D.; Cartwright, C. On the antiquity of cancer: Evidence for metastatic carcinoma in a young man from ancient Nubia (c. 1200 BC). *PLoS ONE* **2014**, *9*, e90924. [CrossRef]
14. The Global Cancer Observatory. Available online: https://gco.iarc.fr/ (accessed on 27 August 2020).
15. Vineis, P.; Wild, C.P. Global cancer patterns: Causes and prevention. *Lancet* **2014**, *383*, 549–557. [CrossRef]
16. Nagai, H.; Kim, Y.H. Cancer prevention from the perspective of global cancer burden patterns. *J. Thorac. Dis.* **2017**, *9*, 448–451. [CrossRef] [PubMed]
17. Thun, M.J.; DeLancey, J.O.; Center, M.M.; Jemal, A.; Ward, E.M. The global burden of cancer: Priorities for prevention. *Carcinogenesis.* **2010**, *31*, 100–110. [CrossRef]
18. Bray, F.; Møller, B. Predicting the future burden of cancer. *Nat. Rev. Cancer.* **2006**, *6*, 63–74. [CrossRef]
19. Siegel, R.L.; Miller, K.D.; Goding Sauer, A.; Fedewa, S.A.; Butterly, L.F.; Anderson, J.C.; Cercek, A.; Smith, R.A.; Jemal, A. Colorectal cancer statistics, 2020. *CA Cancer J. Clin.* **2020**, *70*, 145–164. [CrossRef] [PubMed]
20. de Groot, P.M.; Wu, C.C.; Carter, B.W.; Munden, R.F. The epidemiology of lung cancer. *Transl. Lung Cancer Res.* **2018**, *7*, 220–233. [CrossRef]
21. Barta, J.A.; Powell, C.A.; Wisnivesky, J.P. Global epidemiology of lung cancer. *Ann. Glob. Health.* **2019**, *85*, 1–16. [CrossRef]
22. Malvezzi, M.; Bosetti, C.; Rosso, T.; Bertuccio, P.; Chatenoud, L.; Levi, F.; Romano, C.; Negri, E.; la Vecchia, C. Lung cancer mortality in European men: Trends and predictions. *Lung Cancer* **2013**, *80*, 138–145. [CrossRef]
23. Kim, C.H.; Lee, Y.C.; Hung, R.J.; Boffetta, P.; Xie, D.; Wampfler, J.A.; Cote, M.L.; Chang, S.C.; Ugolini, D.; Neri, M.; et al. Secondhand Tobacco Smoke Exposure and Lung Adenocarcinoma In Situ/Minimally Invasive Adenocarcinoma (AIS/MIA). *Cancer Epidemiol. Biomarkers Prev.* **2015**, *24*, 1902–1906. [CrossRef]
24. Boffetta, P.; Pershagen, G.; Jöckel, K.H.; Forastiere, F.; Gaborieau, V.; Heinrich, J.; Jahn, I.; Kreuzer, M.; Merletti, F.; Nyberg, F.; et al. Cigar and pipe smoking and lung cancer risk: A multicenter study from Europe. *J. Natl. Cancer Inst.* **1999**, *91*, 697–701. [CrossRef]
25. Schwartz, A.G.; Cote, M.L. Epidemiology of Lung Cancer. *Adv. Exp. Med. Biol.* **2016**, *893*, 21–41. [CrossRef] [PubMed]
26. Carper, M.B.; Claudio, P.P. Clinical potential of gene mutations in lung cancer. *Clin. Transl. Med.* **2015**, *4*, 33. [CrossRef] [PubMed]
27. Zendehdel, M.; Niakan, B.; Keshtkar, A.; Rafiei, E.; Salamat, F. Subtypes of benign breast disease as a risk factor for breast cancer: A systematic review and meta-analysis protocol. *Iran. J. Med. Sci.* **2018**, *43*, 1–8. [PubMed]
28. George, B.P.; Abrahamse, H. A Review on Novel Breast Cancer Therapies: Photodynamic Therapy and Plant Derived Agent Induced Cell Death Mechanisms. *Anticancer Agents Med Chem.* **2016**, *16*, 793–801. [CrossRef]
29. Malone, K.E.; Daling, J.R.; Thompson, J.D.; O'Brien, C.A.; Francisco, L.V.; Ostrander, E.A. BRCA1 Mutations and Breast Cancer in the General Population. *JAMA* **1998**, *279*, 922–929. [CrossRef]
30. Haber, D. Prophylactic oophorectomy to reduce the risk of ovarian and breast cancer in carriers of BRCA mutations. *N. Engl. J. Med.* **2002**, *346*, 1660–1662. [CrossRef]
31. Armstrong, N.; Ryder, S.; Forbes, C.; Ross, J.; Quek, R.G.W. A systematic review of the international prevalence of BRCA mutation in breast cancer. *Clin. Epidemiol.* **2019**, *11*, 543–561. [CrossRef]
32. Yoshida, K.; Miki, Y. Role of BRCA1 and BRCA2 as regulators of DNA repair, transcription, and cell cycle in response to DNA damage. *Cancer Sci.* **2004**, *95*, 11. [CrossRef]

33. Li, X.; Chen, X.; Wen, L.; Wang, Y.; Chen, B.; Xue, Y.; Guo, L.; Liao, N. Impact of TP53 mutations in breast cancer: Clinicopathological features and prognosisImpact of TP53 mutations in breast CA. *Thorac. Cancer* **2020**, *11*, 1861–1868. [CrossRef]
34. Taitt, H.E. Global Trends and Prostate Cancer: A Review of Incidence, Detection, and Mortality as Influenced by Race, Ethnicity, and Geographic Location. *Am. J. Mens Health* **2018**, *12*, 1807–1823. [CrossRef]
35. Rawla, P. Epidemiology of Prostate Cancer. *Med. Nucl.* **2008**, *32*, 2–4. [CrossRef] [PubMed]
36. Cuzick, J.; Thorat, M.A.; Andriole, G.; Brawley, O.W.; Brown, P.W.; Culig, Z.; Eeles, R.A.; Ford, L.G.; Hamdy, F.C.; Holmberg, L.; et al. Prevention and early detection of prostate cancer. *Lancet Oncol.* **2014**, *15*, e484–e492. [CrossRef]
37. Attard, G.; Parker, C.; Eeles, R.A.; Schröder, F.; Tomlins, S.A.; Tannock, I.; Drake, C.G.; de Bono, J.S. Prostate cancer. *Lancet* **2016**, *387*, 70–82. [CrossRef]
38. Bashir, M.N.; Ahmad, M.R.; Malik, A. Risk factors of prostate cancer: A case-control study in Faisalabad, Pakistan. *Asian Pac. J. Cancer Prev.* **2014**, *15*, 10237–10240. [CrossRef]
39. Yao, J.; Chen, Y.; Nguyen, D.T.; Thompson, Z.J.; Eroshkin, A.M.; Nerlakanti, N.; Patel, A.K.; Agarwal, N.; Teer, J.K.; Dhillon, J.; et al. The Homeobox gene, HOXB13, Regulates a Mitotic Protein-Kinase Interaction Network in Metastatic Prostate Cancers. *Sci. Rep.* **2019**, *9*, 9715. [CrossRef]
40. Wallis, C.J.D.; Nam, R.K. Prostate Cancer Genetics: A Review. *EJIFCC* **2015**, *26*, 79–91.
41. Dong, J.T. Prevalent mutations in prostate cancer. *J. Cell. Biochem.* **2006**, *97*, 433–447. [CrossRef]
42. Markowitz, S.D.; Bertagnolli, M.M. Molecular basis of colorectal cancer. *N. Engl. J. Med.* **2009**, *361*, 2449–2460. [CrossRef]
43. Kheirelseid, E.A.H.; Miller, N.; Kerin, M.J. Molecular biology of colorectal cancer: Review of the literature. *Am. J. Mol. Biol.* **2013**, *3*, 72–80. [CrossRef]
44. Benarba, B.; Pandiella, A. Colorectal cancer and medicinal plants: Principle findings from recent studies. *Biomed. Pharmacother.* **2018**, *107*, 408–423. [CrossRef]
45. Watson, A.J.M.; Collins, P.D. Colon cancer: A civilization disorder. *Dig. Dis.* **2011**, *29*, 222–228. [CrossRef] [PubMed]
46. Johnson, C.M.; Wei, C.; Ensor, J.E.; Smolenski, D.J.; Amos, C.I.; Levin, B.; Berry, D.A. Meta-analyses of colorectal cancer risk factors. *Cancer Causes Control* **2013**, *24*, 1207–1222. [CrossRef] [PubMed]
47. Gallagher, E.J.; LeRoith, D. Epidemiology and molecular mechanisms tying obesity, diabetes, and the metabolic syndrome with cancer. *Diabetes Care* **2013**, *36* (Suppl. 2), S233–S239. [CrossRef]
48. Petrovska, B.B. Historical review of medicinal plants' usage. *Pharmacogn. Rev.* **2012**, *6*, 1–5. [CrossRef] [PubMed]
49. Stephenson, W. History of Medicine. *Br. Med. J.* **1957**, *2*, 413. [CrossRef]
50. Koul, B. *Herbs for Cancer Treatment*, 1st ed.; Springer: New York, NY, USA, 2019.
51. Maione, F.; Russo, R.; Khan, H.; Mascolo, N. Medicinal plants with anti-inflammatory activities. *Nat. Prod. Res.* **2016**, *30*, 1243–1352. [CrossRef]
52. Kasote, D.M.; Katyare, S.S.; Hegde, M.V.; Bae, H. Significance of antioxidant potential of plants and its relevance to therapeutic applications. *Int. J. Biol. Sci.* **2015**, *1*, 982–991. [CrossRef]
53. Sitarek, P.; Merecz-Sadowska, A.; Kowalczyk, T.; Wieczfinska, J.; Zajdel, R.; Śliwiński, T. Potential synergistic action of bioactive compounds from plant extracts against skin infecting microorganisms. *Int. J. Mol. Sci.* **2020**, *21*, 5105. [CrossRef]
54. Ben-Shabat, S.; Yarmolinsky, L.; Porat, D.; Dahan, A. Antiviral effect of phytochemicals from medicinal plants: Applications and drug delivery strategies. *Drug Deliv. Transl. Res.* **2020**, *10*, 354–367. [CrossRef]
55. Zielinska-Blizniewska, H.; Sitarek, P.; Merecz-Sadowska, A.; Malinowska, K.; Zajdel, K.; Jablonska, M.; Sliwinski, T.; Zajdel, R. Plant extracts and reactive oxygen species as two counteracting agents with anti- and pro-obesity properties. *Int. J. Mol. Sci.* **2019**, *20*, 4556. [CrossRef]
56. Seca, A.M.L.; Pinto, D.C.G.A. Biological Potential and Medical Use of Secondary Metabolites. *Medicines* **2019**, *6*, 66. [CrossRef] [PubMed]
57. Wink, M. Modes of Action of Herbal Medicines and Plant Secondary Metabolites. *Medicines (Basel)* **2015**, *2*, 251–286. [CrossRef]
58. Wink, M. *Functions and Biotechnology of Plant Secondary Metabolites*, 2nd ed.; Wiley-Blackwell: Oxford, UK, 2010.

59. Rajeswara Rao, B.; Pandu Sastry, K.; Kumar Kothari, S. Cultivation technology for economically important medicinal plants. In *Advances in Medicinal Plants*, 1st ed.; Reddy, K.J., Bahadur, B., Bhadraiah, B., Rao, M.L.N., Eds.; Universities Press: Hyderabad, India, 2007.
60. Seca, A.M.L.; Pinto, D.C.G.A. Plant secondary metabolites as anticancer agents: Successes in clinical trials and therapeutic application. *Int. J. Mol. Sci.* **2018**, *19*, 263. [CrossRef] [PubMed]
61. Greenwell, M.; Rahman, P.K.S.M. Medicinal Plants: Their Use in Anticancer Treatment. *Int. J. Pharm. Sci. Res.* **2015**, *6*, 4103–4112. [CrossRef] [PubMed]
62. Sitarek, P.; Synowiec, E.; Kowalczyk, T.; Śliwiński, T.; Skała, E. An In Vitro Estimation of the Cytotoxicity and Genotoxicity of Root Extract from Leonurus sibiricus L. Overexpressing AtPAP1 against Different Cancer Cell Lines. *Molecules* **2018**, *23*, 2049. [CrossRef] [PubMed]
63. Skała, E.; Sitarek, P.; Toma, M.; Szemraj, J.; Radek, M.; Nieborowska-Skorska, M.; Skorski, T.; Wysokińska, H.; Śliwiński, T. Inhibition of human glioma cell proliferation by altered Bax/Bcl-2-p53 expression and apoptosis induction by Rhaponticum carthamoides extracts from transformed and normal roots. *J. Pharm. Pharmacol.* **2016**, *68*, 1454–1464. [CrossRef]
64. Sitarek, P.; Kowalczyk, T.; Santangelo, S.; Białas, A.J.; Toma, M.; Wieczfinska, J.; Śliwiński, T.; Skała, E. The Extract of Leonurus sibiricus Transgenic Roots with AtPAP1 Transcriptional Factor Induces Apoptosis via DNA Damage and Down Regulation of Selected Epigenetic Factors in Human Cancer Cells. *Neurochem. Res.* **2018**, *43*, 1363–1370. [CrossRef]
65. Kowalczyk, T.; Sitarek, P.; Skała, E.; Toma, M.; Wielanek, M.; Pytel, D.; Wieczfińska, J.; Szemraj, J.; Śliwiński, T. Induction of apoptosis by in vitro and in vivo plant extracts derived from Menyanthes trifoliata L. in human cancer cells. *Cytotechnology* **2019**, *71*, 165–180. [CrossRef]
66. Kowalczyk, T.; Sitarek, P.; Toma, M.; Picot, L.; Wielanek, M.; Skała, E.; Śliwiński, T. An Extract of Transgenic Senna obtusifolia L. hairy roots with Overexpression of PgSS1 Gene in Combination with Chemotherapeutic Agent Induces Apoptosis in the Leukemia Cell Line. *Biomolecules* **2020**, *10*, 510. [CrossRef]
67. Gali-Muhtasib, H.; Hmadi, R.; Kareh, M.; Tohme, R.; Darwiche, N. Cell death mechanisms of plant-derived anticancer drugs: Beyond apoptosis. *Apoptosis* **2015**, *20*, 1531–1562. [CrossRef]
68. Moudi, M.; Go, R.; Yien, C.Y.S.; Nazre, M. Vinca alkaloids. *Int. J. Prev. Med.* **2013**, *4*, 1231–1235. [PubMed]
69. Cragg, G.M.; Newman, D.J. Natural products: A continuing source of novel drug leads. *Biochim. Biophys. Acta.* **2013**, *1830*, 3670–3695. [CrossRef] [PubMed]
70. Pan, L.; Chai, H.B.; Kinghorn, A.D. Discovery of new anticancer agents from higher plants. *Front. Biosci. (Schol Ed.)* **2012**, *4*, 142–156. [CrossRef] [PubMed]
71. Lichota, A.; Gwozdzinski, K. Anticancer activity of natural compounds from plant and marine environment. *Int. J. Mol. Sci.* **2018**, *19*, 3533. [CrossRef] [PubMed]
72. Uritu, C.M.; Mihai, C.T.; Stanciu, G.D.; Dodi, G.; Alexa-Stratulat, T.; Luca, A.; Leon-Constantin, M.M.; Stefanescu, R.; Bild, V.; Melnic, S.; et al. Medicinal plants of the family Lamiaceae in pain therapy: A review. *Pain Res. Manag.* **2018**. [CrossRef] [PubMed]
73. Carović-Stanko, K.; Petek, M.; Grdiša, M.; Pintar, J.; Bedeković, D.; Ćustić, M.H.; Satovic, Z. Medicinal plants of the family Lamiaceae as functional foods-A review. *Czech J. Food Sci.* **2016**, *34*, 377–390. [CrossRef]
74. Bekut, M.; Brkić, S.; Kladar, N.; Dragović, G.; Gavarić, N.; Božin, B.B. Potential of selected Lamiaceae plants in anti(retro) viral therapy. *Pharmacol. Res.* **2018**, *133*, 301–314. [CrossRef]
75. Stankovic, M. *Lamiaceae Species*, 1st ed.; MDPI: Basel, Switzerland, 2020.
76. Ganesan, K.; Xu, B. A critical review on polyphenols and health benefits of black soybeans. *Nutrients* **2017**, *9*, 455. [CrossRef]
77. Rasouli, H.; Farzaei, M.H.; Khodarahmi, R. Polyphenols and their benefits: A review. *Int. J. Food Prop.* **2017**, *20*, 1700–1741. [CrossRef]
78. Alam, M.N.; Almoyad, M.; Huq, F. Polyphenols in Colorectal Cancer: Current State of Knowledge including Clinical Trials and Molecular Mechanism of Action. *Biomed. Res. Int.* **2018**, *2018*, 4154185. [CrossRef]
79. Luo, J.; Wei, Z.; Zhang, S.; Peng, X.; Huang, Y.; Zhang, Y.; Lu, J. Phenolic Fractions from Muscadine Grape "Noble" Pomace can Inhibit Breast Cancer Cell MDA-MB-231 Better than those from European Grape "Cabernet Sauvignon" and Induce S-Phase Arrest and Apoptosis. *J. Food Sci.* **2017**, *82*, 1254–1263. [CrossRef] [PubMed]

80. Omodanisi, E.I.; Aboua, Y.G.; Oguntibeju, O.O. Assessment of the anti-hyperglycaemic, anti-inflammatory and antioxidant activities of the methanol extract of moringa oleifera in diabetes-induced nephrotoxic male wistar rats. *Molecules* **2017**, *22*, 439. [CrossRef] [PubMed]
81. González-Sarrías, A.; Núñez-Sánchez, M.Á.; Tomás-Barberán, F.A.; Espín, J.C. Neuroprotective effects of bioavailable polyphenol-derived metabolites against oxidative stress-induced cytotoxicity in human neuroblastoma SH-SY5Y cells. *J. Agric. Food Chem.* **2017**, *65*, 752–758. [CrossRef]
82. Franceschelli, S.; Pesce, M.; Ferrone, A.; Gatta, D.M.P.; Patruno, A.; De Lutiis, M.A.; Quiles, J.L.; Grilli, A.; Felaco, M.; Speranza, L. Biological effect of licochalcone C on the regulation of PI3K/Akt/eNOS and NF-κB/iNOS/NO signaling pathways in H9c2 cells in response to LPS stimulation. *Int. J. Mol. Sci.* **2017**, *18*, 690. [CrossRef] [PubMed]
83. Alam, P.; Parvez, M.K.; Arbab, A.H.; Al-Dosari, M.S. Quantitative analysis of rutin, quercetin, naringenin, and gallic acid by validated RP- and NP-HPTLC methods for quality control of anti-HBV active extract of Guiera senegalensis. *Pharm. Biol.* **2017**, *55*, 1317–1323. [CrossRef]
84. Ayub, M.A.; Hussain, A.I.; Hanif, M.A.; Chatha, S.A.S.; Kamal, G.M.; Shahid, M.; Janneh, O. Variation in Phenolic Profile, β-Carotene and Flavonoid Contents, Biological Activities of Two Tagetes Species from Pakistani Flora. *Chem. Biodivers.* **2017**, *14*, e1600463. [CrossRef]
85. Miyamoto, T.; Zhang, X.; Ueyama, Y.; Apisada, K.; Nakayama, M.; Suzuki, Y.; Ozawa, T.; Mitani, A.; Shigemune, N.; Shimatani, K.; et al. Development of novel monoclonal antibodies directed against catechins for investigation of antibacterial mechanism of catechins. *J. Microbiol. Methods* **2017**, *137*, 6–13. [CrossRef]
86. D'Archivio, M.; Santangelo, C.; Scazzocchio, B.; Varì, R.; Filesi, C.; Masella, R.; Giovannini, C. Modulatory effects of polyphenols on apoptosis induction: Relevance for cancer prevention. *Int. J. Mol. Sci.* **2008**, *9*, 213–228. [CrossRef]
87. Thomas-Charles, C.; Fennell, H. Anti-Prostate Cancer Activity of Plant-Derived Bioactive Compounds: A Review. *Curr. Mol. Biol. Rep.* **2019**, *5*, 140–151. [CrossRef]
88. Perveen, S. Introductory Chapter: Terpenes and Terpenoids. In *Terpenes and Terpenoids*, 1st ed.; IntechOpen: London, UK, 2018.
89. Hanson, J.R. Diterpenoids of terrestrial origin. *Nat. Prod. Rep.* **2016**, *33*, 1227–1238. [CrossRef]
90. Hanson, J.R.; Nichols, T.; Mukhrish, Y.; Bagley, M.C. Diterpenoids of terrestrial origin. *Nat. Prod. Rep.* **2019**, *36*, 1499–1512. [CrossRef] [PubMed]
91. Topçu, G.; Yücer, R.; Şenol, H. Bioactive constituents of Anatolian Salvia species. In *Salvia Biotechnology*, 1st ed.; Georgiev, V., Atanas, P., Eds.; Springer: New York, NY, USA, 2018.
92. Bisio, A.; Pedrelli, F.; D'Ambola, M.; Labanca, F.; Schito, A.M.; Govaerts, R.; De Tommasi, N.; Milella, L. Quinone diterpenes from Salvia species: Chemistry, botany, and biological activity. *Phytochem. Rev.* **2019**, *18*, 665–842. [CrossRef]
93. Demetzos, C.; Dimas, K.S. Labdane-type diterpenes: Chemistry and biological activity. *Stud. Nat. Prod. Chem.* **2001**, *25*, 235–292. [CrossRef]
94. Banerjee, A.; Laya, M.; Mora, H.; Cabrera, E. The Chemistry of Bioactive Diterpenes. *Curr. Org. Chem.* **2008**, *12*, 1050–1070. [CrossRef]
95. Khattak, S.; Khan, H. Anti-cancer Potential of Phyto-alkaloids: A Prospective Review. *Curr. Cancer Ther. Rev.* **2016**, *12*, 66–75. [CrossRef]
96. Debnath, B.; Singh, W.S.; Das, M.; Goswami, S.; Singh, M.K.; Maiti, D.; Manna, K. Role of plant alkaloids on human health: A review of biological activities. *Mater. Today Chem.* **2018**, *9*, 56–72. [CrossRef]
97. Aniszewski, T. *Alkaloids–Secrets of Life: Alkaloid Chemistry, Biological Significance, Applications and Ecological Role*, 1st ed.; Elsevier Science: Amsterdam, The Netherlands, 2007.
98. Burnet, M.W.; Goldmann, A.; Message, B.; Drong, R.; El Amrani, A.; Loreau, O.; Slightom, J.; Tepfer, D. The stachydrine catabolism region in Sinorhizobium meliloti encodes a multi-enzyme complex similar to the xenobiotic degrading systems in other bacteria. *Gene* **2000**, *244*, 151–161. [CrossRef]
99. Dhifi, W.; Bellili, S.; Jazi, S.; Bahloul, N.; Mnif, W. Essential Oils' Chemical Characterization and Investigation of Some Biological Activities: A Critical Review. *Medicines* **2016**, *3*, 25. [CrossRef]
100. Bhalla, Y.; Gupta, V.K.; Jaitak, V. Anticancer activity of essential oils: A review. *J. Sci. Food Agric.* **2013**, *93*, 3643–3653. [CrossRef]

101. Sharifi-Rad, J.; Sureda, A.; Tenore, G.C.; Daglia, M.; Sharifi-Rad, M.; Valussi, M.; Tundis, R.; Sharifi-Rad, M.; Loizzo, M.R.; Oluwaseun Ademiluyi, A.; et al. Biological activities of essential oils: From plant chemoecology to traditional healing systems. *Molecules* **2017**, *22*, 70. [CrossRef]
102. Sitarek, P.; Rijo, P.; Garcia, C.; Skała, E.; Kalemba, D.; Białas, A.J.; Szemraj, J.; Pytel, D.; Toma, M.; Wysokińska, H.; et al. Antibacterial, Anti-Inflammatory, Antioxidant, and Antiproliferative Properties of Essential Oils from Hairy and Normal Roots of Leonurus sibiricus L. and Their Chemical Composition. *Oxid. Med. Cell Longev.* **2017**, *2017*, 7384061. [CrossRef]
103. Yousef, I.; Oran, S.; Bustanji, Y.; Al Eisawi, D.; Irmaileh, B.A. Cytotoxic Effect of Selected Wild Medicinal Plant Species from Jordan on Two Different Breast Cancer Cell Lines, MCF7 and T47D. *Biol. Med.* **2018**, *10*, 4. [CrossRef]
104. Özdemir, A.; Yildiz, M.; Senol, F.S.; Şimay, Y.D.; Ibişoglu, B.; Gokbulut, A.; Orhan, I.E.; Ark, M. Promising anticancer activity of Cyclotrichium niveum L. extracts through induction of both apoptosis and necrosis. *Food Chem. Toxicol.* **2017**, *109*, 898–909. [CrossRef] [PubMed]
105. Asnaashari, S.; Delazar, A.; Asgharian, P.; Lotfipour, F.; Moghaddam, S.B.; Afshar, F.H. In-vitro bioactivity and phytochemical screening of extracts from rhizomes of eremostachys azerbaijanica rech. F. Growing in Iran. *Iran. J. Pharm. Res.* **2017**, *16*, 306–314.
106. Hoshyar, R.; Mostafavinia, S.E.; Zarban, A.; Hassanpour, M.; Partovfari, M.; Taheri, A.; Pouyan, M. Correlation of Anticancer Effects of 12 Iranian Herbs on Human breast Adenocarcinoma cells with antioxidant Properties. *Free Radic. Antioxid.* **2015**, *5*, 65–73. [CrossRef]
107. Amalina, N.D.; Suzery, M.; Cahyono, B. Cytotoxic Activity of Hyptis Pectinate Extracts on MCF-7 Human Breast Cancer Cells. *Indones. J. Cancer Chemoprevent.* **2020**, *11*, 1–6. [CrossRef]
108. Santana, F.R.; Luna-Dulcey, L.; Antunes, V.U.; Tormena, C.F.; Cominetti, M.R.; Duarte, M.C.; da Silva, J.A. Evaluation of the cytotoxicity on breast cancer cell of extracts and compounds isolated from Hyptis pectinata (L.) poit. *Nat. Prod. Res.* **2020**, *34*, 102–109. [CrossRef]
109. Al-Sheddi, E.S. Cytotoxic potential of Petroleum ether, ethyl acetate, chloroform, and ethanol extracts of Lavandula Coronopifolia against human breast carcinoma cell line (MDA-MB-321). *Asian Pac. J. Cancer Prev.* **2019**, *20*, 2943–2949. [CrossRef] [PubMed]
110. Yusufoglu, H.; Foudah, A.I.; Alqarni, M.; Alam, A.; Salkini, A.; Ahmed, E.O. Phenolic contents, cytotoxicity and antimicrobial activity of five medicinal plants of the lamiaceae family obtained from Saudi Arabia local markets. *Indo Am. J. Pharm. Sci.* **2019**, *06*, 14418–14425. [CrossRef]
111. Jahanban-Esfahlan, A.; Modaeinama, S.; Abasi, M.; Abbasi, M.M.; Jahanban-Esfahlan, R. Anti proliferative properties of Melissa officinalis in different human cancer cells. *Asian Pac. J. Cancer Prev.* **2015**, *16*, 5703–5707. [CrossRef] [PubMed]
112. Magalhães, D.B.; Castro, I.; Lopes-Rodrigues, V.; Pereira, J.M.; Barros, L.; Ferreira, I.C.F.R.; Xavier, C.P.R.; Vasconcelos, M.H. Melissa officinalis L. ethanolic extract inhibits the growth of a lung cancer cell line by interfering with the cell cycle and inducing apoptosis. *Food Funct.* **2018**, *9*, 3134–3142. [CrossRef]
113. Zengin, G.; Ferrante, C.; Gnapi, D.E.; Sinan, K.I.; Orlando, G.; Recinella, L.; Diuzheva, A.; Jekő, J.; Cziáky, Z.; Chiavaroli, A.; et al. Comprehensive approaches on the chemical constituents and pharmacological properties of flowers and leaves of American basil (Ocimum americanum L). *Food Res. Int.* **2019**, *125*, 108610. [CrossRef] [PubMed]
114. Abdelhady, M.I.S.; Motaal, A.A. A cytotoxic C-glycosylated derivative of apigenin from the leaves of Ocimum basilicum var. *thyrsiflorum. Braz. J. Pharmacogn.* **2016**, *26*, 763–766. [CrossRef]
115. Makrane, H.; El Messaoudi, M.; Melhaoui, A.; El Mzibri, M.; Benbacer, L.; Aziz, M. Cytotoxicity of the Aqueous Extract and Organic Fractions from Origanum majorana on Human Breast Cell Line MDA-MB-231 and Human Colon Cell Line HT-29. *Adv. Pharmacol. Sci.* **2018**, *2018*, 3297193. [CrossRef] [PubMed]
116. Aldisi, S.S.; Jaganjac, M.; Eid, A.H.; Goktepe, I. Evaluation of Apoptotic, Antiproliferative, and Antimigratory Activity of Origanum syriacum against Metastatic Colon Cancer Cells. *J. Herbs Spices Med. Plants* **2019**, *25*, 202–217. [CrossRef]
117. Pobba, R.; Rama Kotaiah, M.; Chandra Sekar, K.B. Evaluation of antioxidant and anticancer activities of Orthosiphon aristatus (Blume). *Int. J. Res. Pharm. Sci.* **2015**, *6*, 193–198.
118. Singh, M.K.; Dhongade, H.; Tripathi, D.K. Orthosiphon pallidus, a potential treatment for patients with breast cancer. *J. Pharmacopunct.* **2017**, *20*, 265–273. [CrossRef]

119. Yarmolinsky, L.; Budovsky, A.; Ben-Shabat, S.; Khalfin, B.; Gorelick, J.; Bishitz, Y.; Miloslavski, R.; Yarmolinsky, L. Recent Updates on the Phytochemistry and Pharmacological Properties of Phlomis viscosa Poiret. *Rejuvenation Res.* **2019**, *22*, 282–288. [CrossRef]
120. Yulianto, W.; Andarwulan, N.; Giriwono, P.E.; Pamungkas, J. HPLC-based metabolomics to identify cytotoxic compounds from Plectranthus amboinicus (Lour.) Spreng against human breast cancer MCF-7Cells. *J. Chromatogr.* **2016**, *1039*, 28–34. [CrossRef]
121. Rai, V.; Pai, V.R.; Kedilaya, P. A preliminary evaluation of anticancer and antioxidant potential of two traditional medicinal plants from lamiaceae-pogostemon heyneanus and plectranthus amboinicus. *J. Appl. Pharm. Sci.* **2016**, *6*, 73–78. [CrossRef]
122. Borrás-Linares, I.; Pérez-Sánchez, A.; Lozano-Sánchez, J.; Barrajón-Catalán, E.; Arráez-Román, D.; Cifuentes, A.; Micol, V.; Carretero, A.S. A bioguided identification of the active compounds that contribute to the antiproliferative/cytotoxic effects of rosemary extract on colon cancer cells. *Food Chem. Toxicol.* **2015**, *80*, 215–222. [CrossRef]
123. El-burai, H.R. Cytotoxic and Antiproliferative Effects of Four Natural Plants Extracts on Colon Cancer Caco-2 Cell Line. Master's Thesis, The Islamic University, Gaza, Palestine, 2017.
124. Marrelli, M.; Cristaldi, B.; Menichini, F.; Conforti, F. Inhibitory effects of wild dietary plants on lipid peroxidation and on the proliferation of human cancer cells. *Food Chem. Toxicol.* **2015**, *86*, 16–24. [CrossRef] [PubMed]
125. Shen, Y.; Han, J.; Zheng, X.; Ai, B.; Yang, Y.; Xiao, D.; Zheng, L.; Sheng, Z. Rosemary leaf extract inhibits glycation, breast cancer proliferation, and diabetes risks. *Appl. Sci.* **2020**, *10*, 2249. [CrossRef]
126. Tundis, R.; Iacopetta, D.; Sinicropi, M.S.; Bonesi, M.; Leporini, M.; Passalacqua, N.G.; Ceramella, J.; Menichini, F.; Loizzo, M.R. Assessment of antioxidant, antitumor and pro-apoptotic effects of Salvia fruticosa Mill. subsp. thomasii (Lacaita) Brullo, Guglielmo, Pavone & Terrasi (Lamiaceae). *Food Chem. Toxicol.* **2017**, *106*, 155–164. [CrossRef] [PubMed]
127. Campos-Xolalpa, N.; Alonso-Castro, Á.J.; Sánchez-Mendoza, E.; Zavala-Sánchez, M.Á.; Pérez-Gutiérrez, S. Cytotoxic activity of the chloroform extract and four diterpenes isolated from Salvia ballotiflora. *Braz. J. Pharmacogn.* **2017**, *27*, 302–305. [CrossRef]
128. Eltawaty, S.I.; Yagoub, S.O.; Shouman, S.A.; Ahmed, A.; Omer, F.A. Anticancer Effects of Methanol Extract of Libyan Salvia Fruticosa Mill on Mcf7, T47D and (Mda-Mb-468) Breast Cells Lines. *Eur. J. Pharm. Med. Res.* **2020**, *7*, 165–169.
129. Altay, A.; Kılıc Suloglu, A.; Sagdıcoglu Celep, G.; Selmanoglu, G.; Bozoglu, F. Anatolıan sage Salvıa frutıcosa ınhıbıts cytosolic glutathione-s-transferase activity and colon cancer cell prolıferatıon. *J. Food Meas. Charact.* **2019**, *13*, 1390–1399. [CrossRef]
130. Güzel, S.; Ülger, M.; Özay, Y. Antimicrobial and Antiproliferative Activities of Chia (Salvia hispanica L.) Seeds. *Int. J. Second. Metab.* **2020**, *7*, 174–180. [CrossRef]
131. Kumar, D.G.; Perumal, P.C.; Kumar, K.; Muthusami, S.; Gopalakrishnan, V.K. Dietary evaluation, antioxidant and cytotoxic activity of crude extract from chia seeds (Salvia hispanica L.) against human prostate cancer cell line (PC-3). *Int. J. Pharmacogn. Phytochem. Res.* **2016**, *8*, 1358–1362.
132. Garcia, C.S.C.; Menti, C.; Lambert, A.P.F.; Barcellos, T.; Moura, S.; Calloni, C.; Branco, C.S.; Salvador, M.; Roesch-Ely, M.; Henriques, J.A.P. Pharmacological perspectives from Brazilian Salvia officinalis (Lamiaceae): Antioxidant, and antitumor in mammalian cells. *An. Acad. Bras. Cienc.* **2016**, *88*, 281–292. [CrossRef]
133. Darwish, A.; Hamad, G.; Sohaimy, S. Nutrients and Constituents Relevant to Antioxidant, Antimicrobial and Anti-Breast Cancer Properties of *Salvia officinalis* L. *Int. J. Biochem. Res. Rev.* **2018**, *23*, 1–13. [CrossRef]
134. Yumrutaş, Ö.; Pehlivan, M.; Güven, C.; Bozgeyik, İ.; Bozgeyik, E.; Temiz, E.; Yumrutaş, P.; Üçkardeş, F. Investigation of Cytotoxic Effect of Salvia pilifera Extracts and Synthetic Chlorogenic and Caffeic Acids on DU145 Prostate Cancer Cells Line. *KSU J. Agric Nat.* **2018**, *21*, 141–147. [CrossRef]
135. Güzel, S.; Kahraman, A.; Ülger, M.; Özay, Y.; Bozgeyik, İ.; Sarikaya, Ö. Morphology, myxocarpy, mineral content and in vitro antimicrobial and antiproliferative activities of mericarps of the vulnerable Turkish endemic Salvia pilifera. *J. Res. Pharm.* **2019**, *23*, 729–739. [CrossRef]
136. Al-Zereini, W.A. Ononis natrix and Salvia verbenaca: Two Jordanian Medicinal Plants with Cytotoxic and Antibacterial Activities. *J. Herbs Spices Med. Plants.* **2017**, *23*, 18–25. [CrossRef]

137. Yfanti, P.; Batistatou, A.; Manos, G.; Lekka, M.E. The Aromatic Plant Satureja horvatii ssp. macrophylla Induces Apoptosis and Cell Death to the A549 Cancer Cell Line. *Am. J. Plant Sci.* **2015**, *6*, 2092–2103. [CrossRef]
138. Demirelma, H.; Gelinci, E. Determination of the cytotoxic effect on human colon cancer and phe nolic substance cont ent of the endemic species sideritis ozturkii Aytaç & Aksoy. *Appl. Ecol. Environ. Res.* **2019**, *17*, 7407–7419. [CrossRef]
139. Yumrutas, O.; Oztuzcu, S.; Pehlivan, M.; Ozturk, N.; Eroz Poyraz, I.; Iğci, Y.Z.; Cevik, M.O.; Bozgeyik, I.; Aksoy, A.F.; Bagis, H.; et al. Cell viability, anti-proliferation and antioxidant activities of Sideritis syriaca, Tanacetum argenteum sub sp. argenteum and Achillea aleppica subsp. zederbaueri on human breast cancer cell line (MCF-7). *J. Appl. Pharm. Sci.* **2015**, *5*, 1–5. [CrossRef]
140. Calderón-Montaño, J.M.; Martínez-Sánchez, S.M.; Burgos-Morón, E.; Guillén-Mancina, E.; Jiménez-Alonso, J.J.; García, F.; Aparicio, A.; López-Lázaro, M. Screening for Selective Anticancer Activity of 65 Extracts of Plants Collected in Western Andalusia, Spain. *Preprints* **2018**, 2018060177. [CrossRef]
141. Sadeghisamani, F.; Sazgar, H.; Ghasemi Pirbalouti, A. Investigation Cytotoxic Effect of Hydroalcholic Extract from Combination of Kelussia odaratissma Mozaff and Thymus daenesis Celak on MCF-7 Cancer Cells Line. *J. Jahrom Univ. Med Sci.* **2016**, *14*, 59–67. [CrossRef]
142. Garbi, M.I.; Osman, E.E.; Kabbashi, A.S.; Saleh, M.S.; Yuosof, Y.S.; Mahmoud, S.A.; Salam, H.A.A. Cytotoxicity of Vitex trifolia leaf extracts on MCF-7 and Vero cell lines. *J. Sci. Innov. Res.* **2015**, *4*, 89–93.
143. Abu-Gharbieh, E.; El-Huneidi, W.; Shehab, N.G.; Bajbouj, K.; Vinod, A.; El-Serafi, A.; Malhab, L.B.; Abdel-Rahman, W.M. Anti-tumor activity of the ethanolic extract of Micromeria fruticosa on human breast and colon cancer cells. *FASEB J.* **2020**, 34. [CrossRef]
144. El-Huneidi, W.; Shehab, N.G.; Bajbouj, K.; Vinod, A.; El-serafi, A.; Shafarin, J.; Boumalhab, L.J.; Abdel-rahman, W.M.; Abu-gharbieh, E. Micromeriafruticosa induces cell cycle arrest and apoptosis in breast and colorectal cancer cells. *Pharmaceuticals* **2020**, *13*, 115. [CrossRef] [PubMed]
145. Weidner, C.; Rousseau, M.; Plauth, A.; Wowro, S.J.; Fischer, C.; Abdel-Aziz, H.; Sauer, S. Melissa officinalis extract induces apoptosis and inhibits proliferation in colon cancer cells through formation of reactive oxygen species. *Phytomedicine* **2015**, *22*, 262–270. [CrossRef] [PubMed]
146. Song, H.M.; Park, G.H.; Park, S.B.; Kim, H.S.; Son, H.J.; Um, Y.; Jeong, J.B. Vitex rotundifolia Fruit Suppresses the Proliferation of Human Colorectal Cancer Cells through Down-regulation of Cyclin D1 and CDK4 via Proteasomal-Dependent Degradation and Transcriptional Inhibition. *Am. J. Chin. Med.* **2018**, *46*, 191–207. [CrossRef] [PubMed]
147. Chen, J. The cell-cycle arrest and apoptotic functions of p53 in tumor initiation and progression. *Cold Spring Harb. Perspect. Med.* **2016**, *6*, a026104. [CrossRef]
148. Elansary, H.O.; Mahmoud, E.A. In vitro antioxidant and antiproliferative activities of six international basil cultivars. *Nat. Prod. Res.* **2015**, *29*, 2149–2154. [CrossRef]
149. Ye, Y.T.; Zhong, W.; Sun, P.; Wang, D.; Wang, C.; Hu, L.M.; Qian, J.Q. Apoptosis induced by the methanol extract of Salvia miltiorrhiza Bunge in non-small cell lung cancer through PTEN-mediated inhibition of PI3K/Akt pathway. *J. Ethnopharmacol.* **2017**, *200*, 107–116. [CrossRef]
150. Gao, W.; Xu, H.L.Y.L.Y.L.Y. Root extract of Prunella vulgaris inhibits in vitro and in vivo carcinogenesis in MCF-5 human breast carcinoma via suppression of angiogenesis, induction of apoptosis, cell cycle arrest and modulation of PI3K/AKT signalling pathway. *J. BUON* **2019**, *24*, 549–554.
151. Khojasteh, A.; Metón, I.; Camino, S.; Cusido, R.M.; Eibl, R.; Palazon, J. In Vitro Study of the Anticancer Effects of Biotechnological Extracts of the Endangered Plant Species Satureja Khuzistanica. *Int. J. Mol. Sci.* **2019**, *20*, 2400. [CrossRef]
152. Sridevi, M.; Bright, J.; Yamini, K. Anti-cancer effect of ocimum-sanctum ethanolic extract in non-small cell lung carcinoma cell line. *Int. J. Pharm. Pharm. Sci.* **2016**, *8*, 8–20.
153. Chen, C.C.; Kao, C.P.; Chiu, M.M.; Wang, S.H. The anti-cancer effects and mechanisms of Scutellaria barbata D. Don on CL1-5 lung cancer cells. *Oncotarget* **2017**, *8*, 109340–109357. [CrossRef] [PubMed]
154. Kokhdan, E.P.; Sadeghi, H.; Ghafoori, H.; Sadeghi, H.; Danaei, N.; Javadian, H.; Aghamaali, M.R. Cytotoxic effect of methanolic extract, alkaloid and terpenoid fractions of Stachys pilifera against HT-29 cell line. *Res. Pharm. Sci.* **2018**, *13*, 404–412. [CrossRef] [PubMed]
155. Sicora, O.; Naghi, M.A.; Soos, I.; Sicora, C. The ethanolic stem extract of Caryopteris x Clandonensis posseses antiproliferative potential by blocking breast cancer cells in mitosis. *Farmacia* **2019**, *67*, 1077–1082. [CrossRef]

156. Panicker, N.G.; Balhamar, S.O.M.S.; Akhlaq, S.; Qureshi, M.M.; Rizvi, T.S.; AlHarrasi, A.; Hussain, J.; Mustafa, F. Identification and Characterization of the Caspase-Mediated Apoptotic Activity of Teucrium mascatense and an Isolated Compound in Human Cancer Cells. *Molecules* **2019**, *24*, 977. [CrossRef] [PubMed]
157. Fadok, V.A.; Bratton, D.L.; Frasch, S.C.; Warner, M.L.; Henson, P.M. The role of phosphatidylserine in recognition of apoptotic cells by phagocytes. *Cell Death Differ.* **1998**, *5*, 551–562. [CrossRef] [PubMed]
158. Grujičić, D.; Marković, A.; Vukajlović, J.T.; Stanković, M.; Jakovljević, M.R.; Ćirić, A.; Djordjević, K.; Planojević, N.; Milutinović, M.; Milošević-Djordjević, O. Genotoxic and cytotoxic properties of two medical plants (Teucrium arduini L.and Teucrium flavum L.) in relation to their polyphenolic contents. *Mutat. Res.* **2020**, *852*, 503168. [CrossRef] [PubMed]
159. Chaudhry, G.E.S.; Jan, R.; Mohamad, H.; Tengku Muhammad, T. Vitex rotundifolia fractions induce apoptosis in human breast cancer cell line, MCF-7, via extrinsic and intrinsic pathways. *Res. Pharm. Sci.* **2019**, *14*, 273–285. [CrossRef] [PubMed]
160. Dhandayuthapani, S.; Azad, H.; Rathinavelu, A. Apoptosis Induction by Ocimum sanctum Extract in LNCaP Prostate Cancer Cells. *J. Med. Food.* **2015**, *18*, 776–785. [CrossRef]
161. Geryani, M.A.; Mahdian, D.; Mousavi, S.H.; Hosseini, A. Ctotoxic and apoptogenic effects of Perovskia abrotanoides flower extract on MCF-7 and HeLa cell lines. *Avicenna J. Phytomed.* **2016**, *6*, 410–417.
162. Golshan, A.; Amini, E.; Emami, S.A.; Asili, J.; Jalali, Z.; Sabouri-Rad, S.; Sanjar-Mousavi, N.; Tayarani-Najaran, Z. Cytotoxic evaluation of different fractions of Salvia chorassanica Bunge on MCF-7 and du 145 cell lines. *Res. Pharm. Sci.* **2016**, *11*, 73–80.
163. Tarhan, L.; Nakipoğlu, M.; Kavakcıoğlu, B.; Tongul, B.; Nalbantsoy, A. The Induction of Growth Inhibition and Apoptosis in HeLa and MCF-7 Cells by Teucrium sandrasicum, Having Effective Antioxidant Properties. *Appl. Biochem. Biotechnol.* **2016**, *178*, 1028–1041. [CrossRef] [PubMed]
164. Mohammed, H.; Arab, F. Antiproliferative activity of Origanum compactum extract on lung cancer and hepatoma cells. *Arab. J. Med. Aromat. Plants.* **2015**, *1*, 44–56. [CrossRef]
165. Kim, H.I.; Hong, S.H.; Ku, J.M.; Lim, Y.S.; Lee, S.J.; Song, J.; Kim, T.Y.; Cheon, C.; Ko, S.G. Scutellaria radix promotes apoptosis in non-small cell lung cancer cells via induction of AMPK-dependent autophagy. *Am. J. Chin. Med.* **2019**, *47*, 691–705. [CrossRef] [PubMed]
166. Jahanban-Esfahlan, R.; Seidi, K.; Monfaredan, A.; Shafie-Irannejad, V.; Abbasi, M.M.; Karimian, A.; Yousefi, B. The herbal medicine Melissa officinalis extract effects on gene expression of p53, Bcl-2, Her2, VEGF-A and hTERT in human lung, breast and prostate cancer cell lines. *Gene* **2017**, *613*, 14–19. [CrossRef] [PubMed]
167. Laila, F.; Fardiaz, D.; Yuliana, N.D.; Damanik, M.R.M.; Nur Annisa Dewi, F. Methanol Extract of Coleus amboinicus (Lour) Exhibited Antiproliferative Activity and Induced Programmed Cell Death in Colon Cancer Cell WiDr. *Int. J. Food Sci.* **2020**. [CrossRef]
168. Saravanan, R.; Pemaiah, B.; Sridharan, S.; Narayanan, M.; Ramalingam, S. Enhanced cytotoxic potential of Orthosiphon stamineus extract in MCF-7 cells through suppression of nucleolin and BCL2. *Bangladesh J. Pharmacol.* **2017**, *12*, 268–275. [CrossRef]
169. Lee, M.J.; Lee, S.; Choi, N.R.; Jo, S.H.; Cho, S. Dracocephalum palmatum Stephan on human-derived prostate cancer cell death. *Kor. J. Herbology.* **2018**, *33*, 69–76. [CrossRef]
170. Milutinović, M.G.; Maksimović, V.M.; Cvetković, D.M.; Nikodijević, D.D.; Stanković, M.S.; Pešić, M.; Marković, S.D. Potential of Teucrium chamaedrys L. to modulate apoptosis and biotransformation in colorectal carcinoma cells. *J. Ethnopharmacol.* **2019**, *240*, 111951. [CrossRef]
171. Benhalilou, N.; Alsamri, H.; Alneyadi, A.; Athamneh, K.; Alrashedi, A.; Altamimi, N.; Dhaheri, Y.A.; Eid, A.H.; Iratni, R. Origanum majorana ethanolic extract promotes colorectal cancer cell death by triggering abortive autophagy and activation of the extrinsic apoptotic pathway. *Front. Oncol.* **2019**, *9*, 795. [CrossRef]
172. Emami, S.A.; Asili, J.; HosseinNia, S.; Yazdian-Robati, R.; Sahranavard, M.; Tayarani-Najaran, Z. Growth inhibition and apoptosis induction of essential oils and extracts of Nepeta cataria L. on human prostatic and breast cancer cell lines. *Asian Pac. J. Cancer Prev.* **2016**, *17*, 125–130. [CrossRef]
173. Boulares, A.H.; Yakovlev, A.G.; Ivanova, V.; Stoica, B.A.; Wang, G.; Iyer, S.; Smulson, M. Role of Poly(ADP-ribose) Polymerase (PARP) Cleavage in Apoptosis. *J. Biol. Chem.* **1999**, *274*, 22932–22940. [CrossRef] [PubMed]
174. Moore, J.; Megaly, M.; MacNeil, A.J.; Klentrou, P.; Tsiani, E. Rosemary extract reduces Akt/mTOR/p70S6K activation and inhibits proliferation and survival of A549 human lung cancer cells. *Biomed. Pharmacother.* **2016**, *83*, 725–732. [CrossRef]

175. Wise, J.F.; Berkova, Z.; Mathur, R.; Zhu, H.; Braun, F.K.; Tao, R.H.; Sabichi, A.L.; Ao, X.; Maeng, H.; Samaniego, F. Nucleolin inhibits Fas ligand binding and suppresses Fas-mediated apoptosis in vivo via a surface nucleolin-Fas complex. *Blood* **2013**, *121*, 4729–4739. [CrossRef] [PubMed]
176. Wattanathamsan, O.; Hayakawa, Y.; Pongrakhananon, V. Molecular mechanisms of natural compounds in cell death induction and sensitization to chemotherapeutic drugs in lung cancer. *Phyther. Res.* **2019**, *33*, 2531–2547. [CrossRef]
177. Jan, R.; Chaudhry, G.e.S. Understanding apoptosis and apoptotic pathways targeted cancer therapeutics. *Adv. Pharm. Bull.* **2019**, *9*, 205–218. [CrossRef]
178. Jaiswal, P.K.; Goel, A.; Mittal, R.D. Survivin: A molecular biomarker in cancer. *Indian J. Med. Res.* **2015**, *141*, 389–397. [CrossRef]
179. Wei, L.H.; Lin, J.M.; Chu, J.F.; Chen, H.W.; Li, Q.Y.; Peng, J. Scutellaria barbata D. Don inhibits colorectal cancer growth via suppression of Wnt/β-catenin signaling pathway. *Chin. J. Integr. Med.* **2017**, *23*, 858–863. [CrossRef]
180. Castedo, M.; Ferri, K.F.; Kroemer, G. Mammalian Target of Rapamycin (mTOR): Pro- and Anti-Apoptotic. *Cell Death Differ.* **2002**, *9*, 99–100. [CrossRef]
181. Torres, R.G.; Casanova, L.; Carvalho, J.; Marcondes, M.C.; Costa, S.S.; Sola-Penna, M.; Zancan, P. Ocimum basilicum but not Ocimum gratissimum present cytotoxic effects on human breast cancer cell line MCF-7, inducing apoptosis and triggering mTOR/Akt/p70S6K pathway. *J. Bioenerg. Biomembr.* **2018**, *50*, 93–105. [CrossRef]
182. Aubrey, B.J.; Kelly, G.L.; Janic, A.; Herold, M.J.; Strasser, A. How does p53 induce apoptosis and how does this relate to p53-mediated tumour suppression? *Cell Death Differ.* **2018**, *25*, 104–113. [CrossRef]
183. Chang, F.; Lee, J.T.; Navolanic, P.M.; Steelman, L.S.; Shelton, J.G.; Blalock, W.L.; Franklin, R.A.; McCubrey, J.A. Involvement of PI3K/Akt pathway in cell cycle progression, apoptosis, and neoplastic transformation: A target for cancer chemotherapy. *Leukemia* **2003**, *17*, 590–603. [CrossRef] [PubMed]
184. Fan, J.; Bao, Y.; Meng, X.; Wang, S.; Li, T.; Chang, X.; Yang, G.; Bo, T. Mechanism of modulation through PI3K-AKT pathway about Nepeta cataria L.'s extract in non-small cell lung cancer. *Oncotarget* **2017**, *8*, 31395–31405. [CrossRef] [PubMed]
185. Lin, Y.; Bai, L.; Chen, W.; Xu, S. The NF-κB activation pathways, emerging molecular targets for cancer prevention and therapy. *Expert Opin. Ther. Targets.* **2010**, *14*, 45–55. [CrossRef] [PubMed]
186. Liu, T.; Zhang, L.; Joo, D.; Sun, S.C. NF-κB signaling in inflammation. *Signal Transduct. Target. Ther.* **2017**, *2*, 17023. [CrossRef] [PubMed]
187. Oliviero, M.; Romilde, I.; Beatrice, M.M.; Matteo, V.; Giovanna, N.; Consuelo, A.; Claudio, C.; Giorgio, S.; Maggi, F.; Massimo, N. Evaluations of thyme extract effects in human normal bronchial and tracheal epithelial cell lines and in human lung cancer cell line. *Chem. Biol. Interact.* **2016**, *256*, 125–133. [CrossRef]
188. Bakhle, Y.S.; Botting, R.M. Cyclooxygenase-2 and its regulation in inflammation. *Mediators Inflamm.* **1996**, *5*, 305–323. [CrossRef]
189. Uzunhisarcikli, E.; Gürbüz, P.; Yerer, M.B. Investigation of Antiinflamatory Effects of Origanum majorana L. Extract in LPS-Induced Beas-2b and A549 Cells. *Proceedings* **2019**, *40*, 8. [CrossRef]
190. Lim, S.; Kaldis, P. Cdks, cyclins and CKIs: Roles beyond cell cycle regulation. *Development* **2013**, *140*, 3079–3093. [CrossRef]
191. MacDonald, B.T.; Tamai, K.; He, X. Wnt/beta-catenin signaling: Components, mechanisms, and diseases. *Dev. Cell.* **2009**, *17*, 9–26. [CrossRef]
192. He, B.; Reguart, N.; You, L.; Mazieres, J.; Xu, Z.; Lee, A.Y.; Mikami, I.; McCormick, F.; Jablons, D.M. Blockade of Wnt-1 signaling induces apoptosis in human colorectal cancer cells containing downstream mutations. *Oncogene.* **2005**, *24*, 3054–3058. [CrossRef]
193. Miller, D.M.; Thomas, S.D.; Islam, A.; Muench, D.; Sedoris, K. c-Myc and cancer metabolism. *Clin. Cancer Res.* **2012**, *18*, 5546–5553. [CrossRef] [PubMed]
194. Yu, L.; Chen, Y.; Tooze, S.A. Autophagy pathway: Cellular and molecular mechanisms. *Autophagy* **2018**, *14*, 207–215. [CrossRef] [PubMed]
195. Parzych, K.R.; Klionsky, D.J. An overview of autophagy: Morphology, mechanism, and regulation. *Antioxid. Redox Signal.* **2014**, *20*, 460–473. [CrossRef] [PubMed]
196. Laplante, M.; Sabatini, D.M. mTOR signaling at a glance. *J. Cell Sci.* **2009**, *122*, 3589–3594. [CrossRef]

197. Saxton, R.A.; Sabatini, D.M. mTOR Signaling in Growth, Metabolism, and Disease. *Cell* **2017**, *168*, 960–976. [CrossRef]
198. Morales, J.C.; Li, L.; Fattah, F.J.; Dong, Y.; Bey, E.A.; Patel, M.; Gao, J.; Boothman, D.A. Review of poly (ADP-ribose) polymerase (PARP) mechanisms of action and rationale for targeting in cancer and other diseases. *Crit. Rev. Eukaryot. Gene Expr.* **2014**, *21*, 15–28. [CrossRef]
199. Zong, W.X.; Thompson, C.B. Necrotic death as a cell fate. *Genes Dev.* **2006**, *20*, 1–15. [CrossRef]
200. Henriquez, M.; Armisen, R.; Stutzin, A.; Quest, A.F.G. Cell Death by Necrosis, a Regulated Way to go. *Curr. Mol. Med.* **2008**, *8*, 187–206. [CrossRef]
201. Pérez-Sánchez, A.; Barrajón-Catalán, E.; Ruiz-Torres, V.; Agulló-Chazarra, L.; Herranz-López, M.; Valdés, A.; Cifuentes, A.; Micol, V. Rosemary (Rosmarinus officinalis) extract causes ROS-induced necrotic cell death and inhibits tumor growth in vivo. *Sci. Rep.* **2019**, *9*, 808. [CrossRef]
202. Ghiulai, R.; Avram, S.; Stoian, D.; Pavel, I.Z.; Coricovac, D.; Oprean, C.; Vlase, L.; Farcas, C.; Mioc, M.; Minda, D.; et al. Lemon Balm Extracts Prevent Breast Cancer Progression in Vitro and in Ovo on Chorioallantoic Membrane Assay. *Evid. Based Complement. Altern. Med.* **2020**, *2020*, 6489159. [CrossRef]
203. Van Cruijsen, H.; Giaccone, G.; Hoekman, K. Epidermal growth factor receptor and angiogenesis: Opportunities for combined anticancer strategies. *Int. J. Cancer.* **2005**, *117*, 883–888. [CrossRef] [PubMed]
204. Folkman, J. Tumor Angiogenesis: From Bench to Bedside. In *Tumor Angiogenesis: Basic Mechanisms and Cancer Therapy*, 1st ed.; Marmé, D., Fusenig, N., Eds.; Springer: New York, NY, USA, 2008; pp. 3–28.
205. Atmaca, H.; Bozkurt, E. Apoptotic and anti-angiogenic effects of Salvia triloba extract in prostate cancer cell lines. *Tumor Biol.* **2016**, *37*, 3639–3646. [CrossRef] [PubMed]
206. Li, A.; Dubey, S.; Varney, M.L.; Dave, B.J.; Singh, R.K. IL-8 Directly Enhanced Endothelial Cell Survival, Proliferation, and Matrix Metalloproteinases Production and Regulated Angiogenesis. *J. Immunol.* **2003**, *170*, 3369–3376. [CrossRef] [PubMed]
207. Tahergorabi, Z.; Khazaei, M. Leptin and its cardiovascular effects: Focus on angiogenesis. *Adv. Biomed. Res.* **2015**, *4*, 79. [CrossRef]
208. Suffee, N.; Richard, B.; Hlawaty, H.; Oudar, O.; Charnaux, N.; Sutton, A. Angiogenic properties of the chemokine RANTES/CCL5. *Biochem. Soc. Trans.* **2011**, *39*, 1649–1653. [CrossRef]
209. Shestenko, O.P.; Nikonov, S.D.; Mertvetsov, N.P. Angiogenin and its functions in angiogenesis. *Mol. Biol.* **2001**, *35*, 294–314. [CrossRef]
210. Begley, L.A.; Kasina, S.; Mehra, R.; Adsule, S.; Admon, A.J.; Lonigro, R.J.; Chinnaiyan, A.M.; Macoska, J.A. CXCL5 promotes prostate cancer progression. *Neoplasia* **2008**, *10*, 244–254. [CrossRef]
211. Zhao, S.M.; Chou, G.X.; Yang, Q.S.; Wang, W.; Zhou, J.L. Abietane diterpenoids from Caryopteris incana (Thunb.) Miq. *Org. Biomol. Chem.* **2016**, *14*, 3510–3520. [CrossRef]
212. Luo, Y.; Cheng, L.Z.; Luo, Q.; Yan, Y.M.; Wang, S.M.; Sun, Q.; Cheng, Y.X. New ursane-type triterpenoids from Clerodendranthus spicatus. *Fitoterapia* **2017**, *119*, 69–74. [CrossRef]
213. Somwong, P.; Suttisri, R. Cytotoxic activity of the chemical constituents of Clerodendrum indicum and Clerodendrum villosum roots. *J. Integr. Med.* **2018**, *16*, 57–61. [CrossRef]
214. Ba Vinh, L.; Thi Minh Nguyet, N.; Young Yang, S.; Hoon Kim, J.; Thi Vien, L.; Thi Thanh Huong, P.; Van Thanh, N.; Xuan Cuong, N.; Hoai Nam, N.; Van Minh, C.; et al. A new rearranged abietane diterpene from Clerodendrum inerme with antioxidant and cytotoxic activities. *Nat. Prod. Res.* **2018**, *32*, 2002–2007. [CrossRef] [PubMed]
215. Xu, M.; Wang, S.; Jia, O.; Zhu, Q.; Shi, L. Bioactive diterpenoids from clerodendrum kiangsiense. *Molecules* **2016**, *21*, 86. [CrossRef] [PubMed]
216. Awouafack, M.D.; Aimaiti, S.; Tane, P.; Morita, H. Clerodendrumol, a new triterpenoid from Clerodendrum yaundense Gürke (Lamiaceae). *Helv. Chim. Acta* **2016**, *99*, 161–164. [CrossRef]
217. Dai, L.P.; Li, C.; Yang, H.Z.; Lu, Y.Q.; Yu, H.Y.; Gao, H.M.; Wang, Z.M. Three new cytotoxic ent-kaurane diterpenes from isodon excisoides. *Molecules* **2015**, *20*, 17544–17556. [CrossRef]
218. Liu, Y.L.; Zhang, L.X.; Wu, H.; Chen, S.Q.; Li, J.; Dai, L.P.; Wang, Z.M. Four New ent-Kaurane Diterpene Glycosides from Isodon henryi. *Molecules* **2019**, *24*, 2736. [CrossRef]
219. Yang, J.; Wang, W.G.; Wu, H.Y.; Du, X.; Li, X.N.; Li, Y.; Pu, J.X.; Sun, H.D. Bioactive Enmein-Type ent-Kaurane Diterpenoids from Isodon phyllostachys. *J. Nat. Prod.* **2016**, *79*, 132–140. [CrossRef]
220. Luo, G.Y.; Deng, R.; Zhang, J.J.; Ye, J.H.; Pan, L.T. Two cytotoxic 6,7-seco-spiro-lacton-ent-kauranoids from Isodon rubescens. *J. Asian Nat. Prod. Res.* **2018**, *20*, 227–233. [CrossRef]

221. Wu, H.Y.; Wang, W.G.; Du, X.; Yang, J.; Pu, J.X.; Sun, H.D. Six new cytotoxic and anti-inflammatory 11, 20-epoxy-ent-kaurane diterpenoids from Iso Isodon wikstroemioides. *Chin. J. Nat. Med.* **2015**, *13*, 383–389. [CrossRef]
222. Peng, W.; Huo, G.; Zheng, L.; Xiong, Z.; Shi, X.; Peng, D. Two new oleanane derivatives from the fruits of Leonurus japonicus and their cytotoxic activities. *J. Nat. Med.* **2019**, *73*, 252–256. [CrossRef]
223. To, D.C.; Hoang, D.T.; Tran, M.H.; Pham, M.Q.; Huynh, N.T.; Nguyen, P.H. PTP1B Inhibitory Flavonoids From Orthosiphon stamineus Benth. and Their Growth Inhibition on Human Breast Cancer Cells. *Nat. Prod. Commun.* **2020**, *15*, 1934578X19899517. [CrossRef]
224. Sajjadi, S.; Delazari, Z.; Aghaei, M.; Ghannadian, M. Flavone constituents of *Phlomis bruguieri* Desf. with cytotoxic activity against MCF-7 breast cancer cells. *Res. Pharm. Sci.* **2018**, *13*, 422–429. [PubMed]
225. Le, D.D.; Nguyen, D.H.; Zhao, B.T.; Kim, J.A.; Kim, S.K.; Min, B.S.; Choi, J.S.; Woo, M.H. 28-Noroleanane-derived spirocyclic triterpenoids and iridoid glucosides from the roots of Phlomoides umbrosa (Turcz.) Kamelin & Makhm with their cytotoxic effects. *Phytochemistry* **2018**, *153*, 138–146. [CrossRef] [PubMed]
226. Amina, M.; Alam, P.; Parvez, M.K.; Al-Musayeib, N.M.; Al-Hwaity, S.A.; Al-Rashidi, N.S.; Al-Dosari, M.S. Isolation and validated HPTLC analysis of four cytotoxic compounds, including a new sesquiterpene from aerial parts of Plectranthus cylindraceus. *Nat. Prod. Res.* **2018**, *32*, 804–809. [CrossRef] [PubMed]
227. Saraiva, N.; Costa, J.G.; Reis, C.; Almeida, N.; Rijo, P.; Fernandes, A.S. Anti-migratory and pro-apoptotic properties of parvifloron D on triple-negative breast cancer cells. *Biomolecules* **2020**, *10*, 158. [CrossRef]
228. Matias, D.; Nicolai, M.; Saraiva, L.; Pinheiro, R.; Faustino, C.; Diaz Lanza, A.; Pinto Reis, C.; Stankovic, T.; Dinic, J.; Pesic, M.; et al. Cytotoxic Activity of Royleanone Diterpenes from Plectranthus madagascariensis Benth. *ACS Omega* **2019**, *4*, 8094–8103. [CrossRef]
229. Ito, T.; Rakainsa, S.K.; Nisa, K.; Morita, H. Three new abietane-type diterpenoids from the leaves of Indonesian Plectranthus scutellarioides. *Fitoterapia* **2018**, *127*, 146–150. [CrossRef]
230. Nguyen, H.T.; Tran, L.T.T.; Ho, D.V.; Le, D.V.; Raal, A.; Morita, H. Pogostemins A-C, three new cytotoxic meroterpenoids from Pogostemon auricularius. *Fitoterapia* **2018**, *130*, 100–104. [CrossRef]
231. Kim, K.H.; Beemelmanns, C.; Clardy, J.; Cao, S. A new antibacterial octaketide and cytotoxic phenylethanoid glycosides from Pogostemon cablin (Blanco) Benth. *Bioorg. Med. Chem. Lett.* **2015**, *25*, 2834–2836. [CrossRef]
232. Elmaidomy, A.H.; Mohammed, R.; Hassan, H.M.; Owis, A.I.; Rateb, M.E.; Khanfar, M.A.; Krischke, M.; Mueller, M.J.; Abdelmohsen, U.R. Metabolomic profiling and cytotoxic tetrahydrofurofuran lignans investigations from Premna odorata Blanco. *Metabolites* **2019**, *9*, 223. [CrossRef]
233. Wang, W.Q.; Xuan, L.J. Ent-6,7-Secokaurane diterpenoids from Rabdosia serra and their cytotoxic activities. *Phytochemistry* **2016**, *122*, 119–125. [CrossRef]
234. Esquivel, B.; Bustos-Brito, C.; Sánchez-Castellanos, M.; Nieto-Camacho, A.; Ramírez-Apan, T.; Joseph-Nathan, P.; Quijano, L. Structure, absolute configuration, & antiproliferative activity of abietane & icetexane diterpenoids from salvia ballotiflora. *Molecules* **2017**, *22*, 1690. [CrossRef]
235. Mirzaei, H.H.; Firuzi, O.; Baldwin, I.T.; Jassbi, A.R. Cytotoxic activities of different iranian solanaceae and lamiaceae plants and bioassay-guided study of an active extract from salvia lachnocalyx. *Nat. Prod. Commun.* **2017**, *12*, 1563–1566. [CrossRef]
236. Farimani, M.M.; Taleghani, A.; Aliabadi, A.; Aliahmadi, A.; Esmaeili, M.A.; Sarvestani, N.N.; Khavasi, H.R.; Smieško, M.; Hamburger, M.; Ebrahimi, S.N. Labdane diterpenoids from Salvia leriifolia: Absolute configuration, antimicrobial and cytotoxic activities. *Planta Med.* **2016**, *82*, 1279–1285. [CrossRef] [PubMed]
237. Li, L.W.; Qi, Y.Y.; Liu, S.X.; Wu, X.D.; Zhao, Q.S. Neo-clerodane and abietane diterpenoids with neurotrophic activities from the aerial parts of Salvia leucantha Cav. *Fitoterapia* **2018**, *127*, 367–374. [CrossRef]
238. de Oliveira, P.F.; Munari, C.C.; Nicolella, H.D.; Veneziani, R.C.S.; Tavares, D.C. Manool, a Salvia officinalis diterpene, induces selective cytotoxicity in cancer cells. *Cytotechnology* **2016**, *68*, 2139–2143. [CrossRef] [PubMed]
239. Mofidi Tabatabaei, S.; Salehi, P.; Moridi Farimani, M.; Neuburger, M.; De Mieri, M.; Hamburger, M.; Nejad-Ebrahimi, S. A nor-diterpene from Salvia sahendica leaves. *Nat. Prod. Res.* **2017**, *31*, 1758–1765. [CrossRef] [PubMed]
240. Jan, T.; Qadri, R.; Naqvi, B.; Adhikari, A.; Nadeem, S.; Muhammad, A. A novel Salvialactomine from the callus culture of Salvia santolinifolia Boiss. *Nat. Prod. Res.* **2018**, *32*, 749–754. [CrossRef]

241. Eghbaliferiz, S.; Emami, S.A.; Tayarani-Najaran, Z.; Iranshahi, M.; Shakeri, A.; Hohmann, J.; Asili, J. Cytotoxic diterpene quinones from Salvia tebesana Bunge. *Fitoterapia* **2018**, *128*, 97–101. [CrossRef]
242. Fan, M.; Bao, Y.; Zhang, Z.J.; Zhang, H.B.; Zhao, Q.S. New neo-clerodane diterpenoids with neurotrophic activity from the aerial parts of Salvia tiliifolia. *Fitoterapia* **2017**, *123*, 44–50. [CrossRef]
243. Farimani, M.M.; Bahadori, M.B.; Koulaei, S.A.; Salehi, P.; Ebrahimi, S.N.; Khavasi, H.R.; Hamburger, M. New ursane triterpenoids from Salvia urmiensis Bunge: Absolute configuration and anti-proliferative activity. *Fitoterapia* **2015**, *106*, 1–6. [CrossRef]
244. Wang, M.; Chen, Y.; Hu, P.; Ji, J.; Li, X.; Chen, J. Neoclerodane diterpenoids from Scutellaria barbata with cytotoxic activities. *Nat. Prod. Res.* **2020**, *34*, 1345–1351. [CrossRef] [PubMed]
245. Yang, G.C.; Hu, J.H.; Li, B.L.; Liu, H.; Wang, J.Y.; Sun, L.X. Six New neo -Clerodane Diterpenoids from Aerial Parts of Scutellaria barbata and Their Cytotoxic Activities. *Planta Med.* **2018**, *84*, 1292–1299. [CrossRef] [PubMed]
246. Wang, M.; Ma, C.; Chen, Y.; Li, X.; Chen, J. Cytotoxic Neo-Clerodane Diterpenoids from Scutellaria barbata D.Don. *Chem. Biodivers.* **2019**, *16*, e1800499. [CrossRef]
247. Hanh, T.T.H.; Anh, D.H.; Quang, T.H.; Trung, N.Q.; Thao, D.T.; Cuong, N.T.; An, N.T.; Cuong, N.X.; Nam, N.H.; Van Kiem, P.; et al. Scutebarbatolides A-C, new neo-clerodane diterpenoids from Scutellaria barbata D. Don with cytotoxic activity. *Phytochem. Lett.* **2019**, *29*, 65–69. [CrossRef]
248. Kurimoto, S.I.; Pu, J.X.; Sun, H.D.; Shibata, H.; Takaishi, Y.; Kashiwada, Y. Acylated neo-clerodane type diterpenoids from the aerial parts of Scutellaria coleifolia Levl. (Lamiaceae). *J. Nat. Med.* **2016**, *70*, 241–252. [CrossRef] [PubMed]
249. Dai, S.J.; Zhang, L.; Xiao, K.; Han, Q.T. New cytotoxic neo-clerodane diterpenoids from Scutellaria strigillosa. *Bioorg. Med. Chem. Lett.* **2016**, *26*, 1750–1753. [CrossRef] [PubMed]
250. Elmasri, W.A.; Hegazy, M.E.F.; Mechref, Y.; Paré, P.W. Cytotoxic saponin poliusaposide from Teucrium polium. *RSC Adv.* **2015**, *5*, 27126–27133. [CrossRef]
251. Ben Sghaier, M.; Mousslim, M.; Pagano, A.; Ammari, Y.; Luis, J.; Kovacic, H. β-eudesmol, a sesquiterpene from Teucrium ramosissimum, inhibits superoxide production, proliferation, adhesion and migration of human tumor cell. *Environ. Toxicol. Pharmacol.* **2016**, *46*, 227–233. [CrossRef]
252. Gao, C.; Han, L.; Zheng, D.; Jin, H.; Gai, C.; Wang, J.; Zhang, H.; Zhang, L.; Fu, H. Dimeric abietane diterpenoids and sesquiterpenoid lactones from Teucrium viscidum. *J. Nat. Prod.* **2015**, *78*, 630–638. [CrossRef]
253. Dall'Acqua, S.; Peron, G.; Ferrari, S.; Gandin, V.; Bramucci, M.; Quassinti, L.; Mártonfi, P.; Maggi, F. Phytochemical investigations and antiproliferative secondary metabolites from Thymus alternans growing in Slovakia. *Pharm. Biol.* **2017**, *55*, 1162–1170. [CrossRef]
254. Kim, G.D.; Park, Y.S.; Jin, Y.H.; Park, C.S. Production and applications of rosmarinic acid and structurally related compounds. *Appl. Microbiol. Biotechnol.* **2015**, *99*, 2083–2092. [CrossRef] [PubMed]
255. Li, H.; Zhang, Y.; Chen, H.-H.; Huang, E.; Zhuang, H.; Li, D.; Ni, F. Rosmarinic acid inhibits stem-like breast cancer through hedgehog and Bcl-2/Bax signaling pathways. *Pharmacogn. Mag.* **2019**, *15*, 600–606. [CrossRef]
256. Tai, M.C.; Tsang, S.Y.; Chang, L.Y.F.; Xue, H. Therapeutic potential of wogonin: A naturally occurring flavonoid. *CNS Drug Rev.* **2005**, *11*, 141–150. [CrossRef] [PubMed]
257. Tan, H.; Li, X.; Yang, W.H.; Yong, K. A flavone, Wogonin from Scutellaria baicalensis inhibits the proliferation of human colorectal cancer cells by inducing of autophagy, apoptosis and G2/M cell cycle arrest via modulating the PI3K/AKT and STAT3 signalling pathways. *J. BUON* **2019**, *24*, 1143–1149. [PubMed]
258. Ji-Hyun, G.O.; Wei, J.D.; Park, J.I.; Ahn, K.S.; Kim, J.H. Wogonin suppresses the LPS-enhanced invasiveness of MDA-MB-231 breast cancer cells by inhibiting the 5-LO/BLT2 cascade. *Int. J. Mol. Med.* **2018**, *42*, 1899–1908. [CrossRef]
259. Bergers, G.; Brekken, R.; McMahon, G.; Vu, T.H.; Itoh, T.; Tamaki, K.; Tanzawa, K.; Thorpe, P.; Itohara, S.; Werb, Z.; et al. Matrix metalloproteinase-9 triggers the angiogenic switch during carcinogenesis. *Nat. Cell Biol.* **2000**, *2*, 737–744. [CrossRef]
260. Chledzik, S.; Strawa, J.; Matuszek, K.; Nazaruk, J. Pharmacological Effects of Scutellarin, An Active Component of Genus Scutellaria and Erigeron: A Systematic Review. *Am. J. Chin. Med.* **2018**, *46*, 319–337. [CrossRef]

261. Guo, F.; Yang, F.; Zhu, Y.H. Scutellarein from Scutellaria barbata induces apoptosis of human colon cancer HCT116 cells through the ROS-mediated mitochondria-dependent pathway. *Nat. Prod. Res.* **2019**, *33*, 2372–2375. [CrossRef]
262. Salehi, B.; Fokou, P.V.T.; Sharifi-Rad, M.; Zucca, P.; Pezzani, R.; Martins, N.; Sharifi-Rad, J. The therapeutic potential of naringenin: A review of clinical trials. *Pharmaceuticals* **2019**, *12*, 11. [CrossRef]
263. Liu, D.M.; Cao, Z.X.; Yan, H.L.; Li, W.; Yang, F.; Zhao, W.J.; Diao, Q.C.; Tan, Y. zhu A new abietane diterpenoid from Ajuga ovalifolia var. calantha induces human lung epithelial A549 cell apoptosis by inhibiting SHP2. *Fitoterapia* **2020**, *141*, 104484. [CrossRef]
264. Shakeri, A.; Delavari, S.; Ebrahimi, S.N.; Asili, J.; Emami, S.A.; Tayarani-Najaran, Z. A new tricyclic abietane diterpenoid from Salvia chloroleuca and evaluation of cytotoxic and apoptotic activities. *Braz. J. Pharmacogn.* **2019**, *29*, 30–35. [CrossRef]
265. Wang, J.N.; Zhang, Z.R.; Che, Y.; Yuan, Z.Y.; Lu, Z.L.; Li, Y.; Li, N.; Wan, J.; Sun, H.D.; Sun, N.; et al. Acetyl-macrocalin B, an ent-kaurane diterpenoid, initiates apoptosis through the ROS-p38-caspase 9-dependent pathway and induces G2/M phase arrest via the Chk1/2-Cdc25C-Cdc2/cyclin B axis in non-small cell lung cancer. *Cancer Biol. Ther.* **2018**, *19*, 609–621. [CrossRef]
266. Cortese, K.; Marconi, S.; D'Alesio, C.; Calzia, D.; Panfoli, I.; Tavella, S.; Aiello, C.; Pedrelli, F.; Bisio, A.; Castagnola, P. The novel diterpene 7β-acetoxy-20-hydroxy-19,20-epoxyroyleanone from Salvia corrugata shows complex cytotoxic activities against human breast epithelial cells. *Life Sci.* **2019**, *232*, 116610. [CrossRef] [PubMed]
267. Zito, C.I.; Kontaridis, M.I.; Fornaro, M.; Feng, G.S.; Bennett, A.M. SHP-2 Regulates the Phosphatidylinositide 3′-Kinase/Akt Pathway and Suppresses Caspase 3-Mediated Apoptosis. *J. Cell. Physiol.* **2004**, *199*, 227–236. [CrossRef] [PubMed]
268. Cagnol, S.; Chambard, J.C. ERK and cell death: Mechanisms of ERK-induced cell death—Apoptosis, autophagy and senescence. *FEBS J.* **2010**, *277*, 2–21. [CrossRef]
269. Bartek, J.; Lukas, J. Chk1 and Chk2 kinases in checkpoint control and cancer. *Cancer Cell.* **2003**, *3*, 421–429. [CrossRef]
270. Cho, Y.C.; Park, J.E.; Park, B.C.; Kim, J.H.; Jeong, D.G.; Park, S.G.; Cho, S. Cell cycle-dependent Cdc25C phosphatase determines cell survival by regulating apoptosis signal-regulating kinase 1. *Cell Death Differ.* **2015**, *22*, 1605–1617. [CrossRef]
271. Uto, T.; Tung, N.H.; Ohta, T.; Juengsanguanpornsuk, W.; Hung, L.Q.; Hai, N.T.; Long, D.D.; Thuong, P.T.; Okubo, S.; Hirata, S.; et al. Antiproliferative activity and apoptosis induction by trijuganone C isolated from the root of Salvia miltiorrhiza Bunge (Danshen). *Phyther. Res.* **2018**, *32*, 657–666. [CrossRef]
272. Wang, M.; Zeng, X.; Li, S.; Sun, Z.; Yu, J.; Chen, C.; Shen, X.; Pan, W.; Luo, H. A novel tanshinone analog exerts anti-cancer effects in prostate cancer by inducing cell apoptosis, arresting cell cycle at G2 phase and blocking metastatic ability. *Int. J. Mol. Sci.* **2019**, *20*, 4459. [CrossRef]
273. Shen, L.; Lou, Z.; Zhang, G.; Xu, G.; Zhang, G. Diterpenoid Tanshinones, the extract from Danshen (Radix Salviae Miltiorrhizae) induced apoptosis in nine human cancer cell lines. *J. Tradit. Chin. Med.* **2016**, *36*, 514–521. [CrossRef]
274. Zaker, A.; Asili, J.; Abrishamchi, P.; Tayarani-Najaran, Z.; Mousavi, S.H. Cytotoxic and apoptotic effects of root extract and tanshinones isolated from Perovskia abrotanoides kar. *Iran. J. Basic Med. Sci.* **2017**, *20*, 1377–1384. [CrossRef] [PubMed]
275. Ye, Q.; Yao, G.; Zhang, M.; Guo, G.; Hu, Y.; Jiang, J.; Cheng, L.; Shi, J.; Li, H.; Zhang, Y.; et al. A novel ent-kaurane diterpenoid executes antitumor function in colorectal cancer cells by inhibiting Wnt/β-catenin signaling. *Carcinogenesis* **2014**, *36*, 318–326. [CrossRef] [PubMed]
276. Bahadori, M.B.; Eskandani, M.; De Mieri, M.; Hamburger, M.; Nazemiyeh, H. Anti-proliferative activity-guided isolation of clerodermic acid from Salvia nemorosa L.: Geno/cytotoxicity and hypoxia-mediated mechanism of action. *Food Chem. Toxicol.* **2018**, *120*, 155–163. [CrossRef] [PubMed]
277. Masoud, G.N.; Li, W. HIF-1α pathway: Role, regulation and intervention for cancer therapy. *Acta Pharm. Sin. B.* **2015**, *5*, 378–389. [CrossRef] [PubMed]
278. Lu, X.X.; Ji, X.X.; Bao, J.; Li, Q.Q.; Ji, D.D.; Luo, L. Inhibition of proliferation, migration and invasion of human non-small cell lung cancer cell line a549 by phlomisoside f from phlomis younghusbandii mukerjee. *Trop. J. Pharm. Res.* **2016**, *15*, 1413–1421. [CrossRef]

279. Ouyang, X.L.; Qin, F.; Huang, R.Z.; Liang, D.; Wang, C.G.; Wang, H.S.; Liao, Z.X. NF-κB inhibitory and cytotoxic activities of hexacyclic triterpene acid constituents from Glechoma longituba. *Phytomedicine* **2019**, *63*, 153037. [CrossRef] [PubMed]
280. Tran, L.T.T.; Ho, D.V.; Le, D.V.; Van Phan, K.; Nguyen, H.T.; Raal, A. Apoptosis-Inducing Effect of Pogostemin A Isolated from the Aerial Parts of Pogostemon auricularius Against the Human Lung Cancer Cells. *J. Biol. Act. Prod. from Nat.* **2019**, *9*, 320–327. [CrossRef]
281. Ullah, S.; Khalil, A.A.; Shaukat, F.; Song, Y. Sources, extraction and biomedical properties of polysaccharides. *Foods* **2019**, *8*, 304. [CrossRef]
282. Sun, P.; Sun, D.; Wang, X. Effects of Scutellaria barbata polysaccharide on the proliferation, apoptosis and EMT of human colon cancer HT29 Cells. *Carbohydr. Polym.* **2017**, *167*, 90–96. [CrossRef]
283. Li, H.; Su, J.; Jiang, J.; Li, Y.; Gan, Z.; Ding, Y.; Li, Y.; Liu, J.; Wang, S.; Ke, Y. Characterization of polysaccharide from Scutellaria barbata and its antagonistic effect on the migration and invasion of HT-29 colorectal cancer cells induced by TGF-β1. *Int. J. Biol. Macromol.* **2019**, *131*, 886–895. [CrossRef]
284. Basappa, G.; Kumar, V.; Sarojini, B.K.; Poornima, D.V.; Gajula, H.; Sannabommaji, T.K.; Rajashekar, J. Chemical composition, biological properties of Anisomeles indica Kuntze essential oil. *Ind. Crops Prod.* **2015**, *77*, 89–96. [CrossRef]
285. Rigano, D.; Marrelli, M.; Formisano, C.; Menichini, F.; Senatore, F.; Bruno, M.; Conforti, F. Phytochemical profile of three Ballota species essential oils and evaluation of the effects on human cancer cells. *Nat. Prod. Res.* **2017**, *31*, 436–444. [CrossRef] [PubMed]
286. Scharf, D.R.; Simionatto, E.L.; Carvalho, J.E.; Salvador, M.J.; Santos, É.P.; Stefanello, M.É.A. Chemical composition and cytotoxic activity of the essential oils of Cantinoa stricta (Benth.) Harley & J.F.B. Pastore (Lamiaceae). *Rec. Nat. Prod.* **2015**, *10*, 257–261.
287. Zorzetto, C.; Sánchez-Mateo, C.C.; Rabanal, R.M.; Lupidi, G.; Bramucci, M.; Quassinti, L.; Iannarelli, R.; Papa, F.; Maggi, F. Antioxidant activity and cytotoxicity on tumour cells of the essential oil from Cedronella canariensis var. canariensis (L.) Webb & Berthel. (Lamiaceae). *Nat. Prod. Res.* **2015**, *29*, 1641–1649. [CrossRef] [PubMed]
288. de Sousa, M.H.O.; Morgan, J.M.S.; Cesca, K.; Flach, A.; de Moura, N.F. Cytotoxic Activity of Cunila angustifolia Essential Oil. *Chem. Biodivers.* **2020**, *17*, e1900656. [CrossRef] [PubMed]
289. Pudziuvelyte, L.; Stankevicius, M.; Maruska, A.; Petrikaite, V.; Ragazinskiene, O.; Draksiene, G.; Bernatoniene, J. Chemical composition and anticancer activity of Elsholtzia ciliata essential oils and extracts prepared by different methods. *Ind. Crops Prod.* **2017**, *107*, 90–96. [CrossRef]
290. Donadu, M.G.; Usai, D.; Mazzarello, V.; Molicotti, P.; Cannas, S.; Bellardi, M.G.; Zanotti, S. Change in Caco-2 cells following treatment with various lavender essential oils. *Nat. Prod. Res.* **2017**, *31*, 2203–2206. [CrossRef]
291. Damasceno, L.M.O.; Silva, A.L.N.; dos Santos, R.F.; Feitosa, T.A.; Viana, L.G.F.; de Oliveira, R.G.; e Silva, M.G.; Rolim, L.A.; Araújo, C.S.; Araújo, E.C.C.; et al. Cytotoxic activity of chemical constituents and essential oil from the leaves of leonotis nepetifolia (Lamiaceae). *Rev. Virtual Quim.* **2019**, *11*, 517–528. [CrossRef]
292. Nikšić, H.; Durić, K.; Sijamić, I.; Korić, E.; Kusturica, J.; Omeragić, E.; Muratovic, S. In vitro antiproliferative activity of Melissa officinalis L. (Lamiaceae) leaves essential oil. *Bol. Latinoam. Caribe Plantas Med. Aromat.* **2019**, *18*, 480–491. [CrossRef]
293. Ouakouak, H.; Benchikha, N.; Hassani, A.; Ashour, M.L. Chemical composition and biological activity of Mentha citrata Ehrh., essential oils growing in southern Algeria. *J. Food Sci. Technol.* **2019**, *56*, 5346–5353. [CrossRef]
294. Bardaweel, S.K.; Bakchiche, B.; ALSalamat, H.A.; Rezzoug, M.; Gherib, A.; Flamini, G. Chemical composition, antioxidant, antimicrobial and Antiproliferative activities of essential oil of Mentha spicata L. (Lamiaceae) from Algerian Saharan atlas. *BMC Complement. Altern. Med.* **2018**, *18*, 201. [CrossRef] [PubMed]
295. Mothana, R.A.; Nasr, F.A.; Khaled, J.M.; AL-Zharani, M.; Noman, O.M.; Abutaha, N.; Al-Rehaily, A.J.; Almarfadi, O.M.; Kumar, A.; Kurkcuoglu, M. Analysis of chemical composition and assessment of cytotoxic, antimicrobial, and antioxidant activities of the essential oil of meriandra dianthera growing in Saudi Arabia. *Molecules* **2019**, *24*, 2647. [CrossRef]
296. Kahkeshani, N.; Hadjiakhoondi, A.; Navidpour, L.; Akbarzadeh, T.; Safavi, M.; Karimpour-Razkenari, E.; Khanavi, M. Chemodiversity of Nepeta menthoides Boiss. & Bohse. essential oil from Iran and antimicrobial, acetylcholinesterase inhibitory and cytotoxic properties of 1,8-cineole chemotype. *Nat. Prod. Res.* **2018**, *32*, 2745–2748. [CrossRef] [PubMed]

297. Sharifi-Rad, J.; Ayatollahi, S.A.; Varoni, E.M.; Salehi, B.; Kobarfard, F.; Sharifi-Rad, M.; Iriti, M.; Sharifi-Rad, M. Chemical composition and functional properties of essential oils from Nepeta schiraziana Boiss. *Farmacia* **2017**, *65*, 802–812.
298. Shakeri, A.; Khakdan, F.; Soheili, V.; Sahebkar, A.; Shaddel, R.; Asili, J. Volatile composition, antimicrobial, cytotoxic and antioxidant evaluation of the essential oil from Nepeta sintenisii Bornm. *Ind. Crops Prod.* **2016**, *84*, 224–229. [CrossRef]
299. Fitsiou, E.; Mitropoulou, G.; Spyridopoulou, K.; Tiptiri-Kourpeti, A.; Vamvakias, M.; Bardouki, H.; Panayiotidis, M.I.; Galanis, A.; Kourkoutas, Y.; Chlichlia, K.; et al. Phytochemical profile and evaluation of the biological activities of essential oils derived from the greek aromatic plant species Ocimum basilicum, Mentha spicata, Pimpinella anisum and Fortunella margarita. *Molecules* **2016**, *21*, 1069. [CrossRef]
300. Hajlaoui, H.; Mighri, H.; Aouni, M.; Gharsallah, N.; Kadri, A. Chemical composition and in vitro evaluation of antioxidant, antimicrobial, cytotoxicity and anti-acetylcholinesterase properties of Tunisian Origanum majorana L. essential oil. *Microb. Pathog.* **2016**, *95*, 86–94. [CrossRef]
301. Marrelli, M.; Conforti, F.; Formisano, C.; Rigano, D.; Arnold, N.A.; Menichini, F.; Senatore, F. Composition, antibacterial, antioxidant and antiproliferative activities of essential oils from three Origanum species growing wild in Lebanon and Greece. *Nat. Prod. Res.* **2016**, *30*, 735–739. [CrossRef]
302. Elansary, H.O.; Abdelgaleil, S.A.M.; Mahmoud, E.A.; Yessoufou, K.; Elhindi, K.; El-Hendawy, S. Effective antioxidant, antimicrobial and anticancer activities of essential oils of horticultural aromatic crops in northern Egypt. *BMC Complement. Altern. Med.* **2018**, *18*, 214. [CrossRef]
303. Mothana, R.A.; Khaled, J.M.; Noman, O.M.; Kumar, A.; Alajmi, M.F.; Al-Rehaily, A.J.; Kurkcuoglu, M. Phytochemical analysis and evaluation of the cytotoxic, antimicrobial and antioxidant activities of essential oils from three Plectranthus species grown in Saudi Arabia. *BMC Complement. Altern. Med.* **2018**, *18*, 237. [CrossRef]
304. Zhang, H.Y.; Gao, Y.; Lai, P.X. Chemical composition, antioxidant, antimicrobial and cytotoxic activities of essential oil from premna microphylla turczaninow. *Molecules* **2017**, *22*, 381. [CrossRef] [PubMed]
305. Jardak, M.; Elloumi-Mseddi, J.; Aifa, S.; Mnif, S. Chemical composition, anti-biofilm activity and potential cytotoxic effect on cancer cells of Rosmarinus officinalis L. essential oil from Tunisia. *Lipids Health Dis.* **2017**, *16*, 190. [CrossRef] [PubMed]
306. Eftekhari, M.; Ardekani, M.R.S.; Amini, M.; Akbarzadeh, T.; Safavi, M.; Razkenari, E.K.; Khanavi, M. Biological activities of the essential oil and total extract of Salvia macrosiphon Boiss. *J. Basic Clin. Pharm.* **2017**, *8*, 82–86.
307. Privitera, G.; Luca, T.; Castorina, S.; Passanisi, R.; Ruberto, G.; Napoli, E. Anticancer activity of Salvia officinalis essential oil and its principal constituents against hormone-dependent tumour cells. *Asian Pac. J. Trop. Biomed.* **2019**, *9*, 24–28. [CrossRef]
308. Luca, T.; Napoli, E.; Privitera, G.; Musso, N.; Ruberto, G.; Castorina, S. Antiproliferative Effect and Cell Cycle Alterations Induced by Salvia officinalis Essential Oil and Its Three Main Components in Human Colon Cancer Cell Lines. *Chem. Biodivers.* **2020**, *17*, e2000309. [CrossRef] [PubMed]
309. Alimpić, A.; Pljevljakušić, D.; Šavikin, K.; Knežević, A.; Ćurčić, M.; Veličković, D.; Stević, T.; Petrović, G.; Matevski, V.; Vukojević, J.; et al. Composition and biological effects of Salvia ringens (Lamiaceae) essential oil and extracts. *Ind. Crops Prod.* **2015**, *76*, 702–709. [CrossRef]
310. Sharifi-Rad, J.; Sharifi-Rad, M.; Hoseini-Alfatemi, S.M.; Iriti, M.; Sharifi-Rad, M.; Sharifi-Rad, M. Composition, cytotoxic and antimicrobial activities of Satureja intermedia CA Mey essential oil. *Int. J. Mol. Sci.* **2015**, *16*, 17812–17825. [CrossRef]
311. Fitsiou, E.; Anestopoulos, I.; Chlichlia, K.; Galanis, A.; Kourkoutas, I.; Panayiotidis, M.I.; Pappa, A. Antioxidant and antiproliferative properties of the essential oils of Satureja thymbra and Satureja parnassica and their major constituents. *Anticancer Res.* **2016**, *36*, 5757–5763. [CrossRef]
312. Venditti, A.; Bianco, A.; Quassinti, L.; Bramucci, M.; Lupidi, G.; Damiano, S.; Papa, F.; Vittori, S.; Maleci Bini, L.; Giuliani, C.; et al. Phytochemical analysis, biological activity, and secretory structures of Stachys annua (L.) L. subsp. annua (Lamiaceae) from central Italy. *Chem. Biodivers.* **2015**, *12*, 1172–1183. [CrossRef]
313. Shakeri, A.; D'Urso, G.; Taghizadeh, S.F.; Piacente, S.; Norouzi, S.; Soheili, V.; Asili, J.; Salarbashi, D. LC-ESI/LTQOrbitrap/MS/MS and GC–MS profiling of Stachys parviflora L. and evaluation of its biological activities. *J. Pharm. Biomed. Anal.* **2019**, *168*, 209–216. [CrossRef]

314. de Oliveira, P.F.; Alves, J.M.; Damasceno, J.L.; Oliveira, R.A.M.; Júnior Dias, H.; Crotti, A.E.M.; Tavares, D.C. Cytotoxicity screening of essential oils in cancer cell lines. *Rev. Bras. Farmacogn.* **2015**, *25*, 183–188. [CrossRef]
315. Bendif, H.; Boudjeniba, M.; Miara, M.D.; Biqiku, L.; Bramucci, M.; Lupidi, G.; Quassinti, L.; Vitali, L.A.; Maggi, F. Essential Oil of Thymus munbyanus subsp. coloratus from Algeria: Chemotypification and in vitro Biological Activities. *Chem. Biodivers.* **2017**, *14*, e1600299. [CrossRef] [PubMed]
316. Janitermi, M.; Nemati, F. Cytotoxic effect of Zataria multiflora on breast cancer cell line (MCF-7) and normal fibroblast cell. *Sci. J.* **2015**, *36*, 1895–1904.
317. Mohammadpour, G.; Tahmasbpour, R.; Noureini, S.K.; Tahmasbpour, E.; Bagherpour, G. In vitro Antimicrobial and Cytotoxicity Assays of Satureja bakhtiarica and Zataria multiflora Essential Oils. *Am. J. Phytomed. Clin. Ther.* **2015**, *3*, 502–511.
318. Saeidi, M.; Asili, J.; Emami, S.A.; Moshtaghi, N.; Malekzadeh-Shafaroudi, S. Comparative volatile composition, antioxidant and cytotoxic evaluation of the essential oil of Zhumeria majdae from south of Iran. *Iran. J. Basic Med. Sci.* **2019**, *22*, 80–85. [CrossRef]
319. Skorić, M.; Gligorijević, N.; Čavić, M.; Todorović, S.; Janković, R.; Ristić, M.; Mišić, D.; Radulović, S. Cytotoxic activity of Nepeta rtanjensis Diklić & Milojević essential oil and its mode of action. *Ind. Crops Prod.* **2017**, *100*, 163–170. [CrossRef]
320. Spyridopoulou, K.; Fitsiou, E.; Bouloukosta, E.; Tiptiri-Kourpeti, A.; Vamvakias, M.; Oreopoulou, A.; Papavassilopoulou, E.; Pappa, A.; Chlichlia, K. Extraction, Chemical Composition, and Anticancer Potential of Origanum onites L. Essential Oil. *Molecules* **2019**, *24*, 2612. [CrossRef]
321. Bhagat, M.; Sangral, M.; Arya, K.; Rather, R. Chemical characterization, biological assessment and molecular docking studies of essential oil of Ocimum viride for potential antimicrobial and anticancer activities. *bioRxiv.* **2018**, 390906. [CrossRef]
322. Özkan, A.; Erdoğan, A. Evaluation of cytotoxic, membrane, and DNA damaging effects of Thymus revolutus célak essential oil on different cancer cells. *Turk. J. Med. Sci.* **2017**, *47*, 702–714. [CrossRef]
323. Russo, A.; Cardile, V.; Graziano, A.C.E.; Avola, R.; Bruno, M.; Rigano, D. Involvement of Bax and Bcl-2 in induction of apoptosis by essential oils of three Lebanese Salvia species in human prostate cancer cells. *Int. J. Mol. Sci.* **2018**, *19*, 292. [CrossRef]
324. Ahani, N.; Sangtarash, M.H.; Alipour Eskanda-Ni, M.; Houshmand, M. Zataria multiflora boiss. Essential oil induce apoptosis in two human colon cancer cell lines (HCT116 & SW48). *Iran. J. Public Health* **2020**, *49*, 753–762. [PubMed]
325. Zhao, Y.; Chen, R.; Wang, Y.; Qing, C.; Wang, W.; Yang, Y. In Vitro and in Vivo Efficacy Studies of Lavender angustifolia Essential Oil and Its Active Constituents on the Proliferation of Human Prostate Cancer. *Integr. Cancer Ther.* **2017**, *16*, 215–226. [CrossRef] [PubMed]
326. Lipin Dev, M.S.; Menon, D.B. Essential Oil Extracted from Plectranthus amboinicus Induces Apoptosis in the Lung Cancer Cells via Mitochondrial Pathway. *Int. J. Pharm. Sci. Drug Res.* **2017**, *9*, 83–89. [CrossRef]
327. Lu, X.; Yang, L.; Lu, C.; Xu, Z.; Qiu, H.; Wu, J.; Wang, J.; Tong, J.; Zhu, Y.; Shen, J. Molecular Role of EGFR-MAPK Pathway in Patchouli Alcohol-Induced Apoptosis and Cell Cycle Arrest on A549 Cells in Vitro and in Vivo. *BioMed Res. Int.* **2016**, *2016*, 4567580. [CrossRef] [PubMed]
328. Jaradat, N.; Al-Maharik, N. Fingerprinting, antimicrobial, antioxidant, anticancer, cyclooxygenase and metabolic enzymes inhibitory characteristic evaluations of Stachys viticina Boiss. essential oil. *Molecules* **2019**, *24*, 3880. [CrossRef]
329. Athamneh, K.; Alneyadi, A.; Alsamri, H.; Alrashedi, A.; Palakott, A.; El-Tarabily, K.A.; Eid, A.H.; Dhaheri, Y.A.; Iratni, R. Origanum majorana essential oil triggers p38 mapk-mediated protective autophagy, apoptosis, and caspase-dependent cleavage of P70S6K in colorectal cancer cells. *Biomolecules* **2020**, *10*, 412. [CrossRef]
330. Justus, B.; Kanunfre, C.C.; Budel, J.M.; de Faria, M.F.; Raman, V.; de Paula, J.P.; Farago, P.V. New insights into the mechanisms of French lavender essential oil on non-small-cell lung cancer cell growth. *Ind. Crops Prod.* **2019**, *136*, 28–36. [CrossRef]

2

Bioactive Composition, Antioxidant Activity and Anticancer Potential of Freeze-Dried Extracts from Defatted Gac (*Momordica cochinchinensis* Spreng) Seeds

Anh V. Le [1,2,*], Tien T. Huynh [3], Sophie E. Parks [1,4], Minh H. Nguyen [1,5] and Paul D. Roach [1]

[1] School of Environmental and Life Sciences, University of Newcastle, Ourimbah, NSW 2258, Australia; sophie.parks@dpi.nsw.gov.au (S.E.P.); Minh.Nguyen@newcastle.edu.au (M.H.N.); Paul.Roach@newcastle.edu.au (P.D.R.)

[2] Faculty of Bio-Food Technology and Environment, University of Technology (HUTECH), Ho Chi Minh City 700000, Vietnam

[3] School of Science, RMIT University, Bundoora, VIC 3083, Australia; tien.huynh@rmit.edu.au

[4] Central Coast Primary Industries Centre, NSW Department of Primary Industries, Ourimbah, NSW 2258, Australia

[5] School of Science and Health, Western Sydney University, Penrith, NSW 2751, Australia

[*] Correspondence: vananh.le@uon.edu.au

Abstract: Background: Gac (*Momordica cochinchinensis* Spreng) seeds have long been used in traditional medicine as a remedy for numerous conditions due to a range of bioactive compounds. This study investigated the solvent extraction of compounds that could be responsible for antioxidant activity and anticancer potential. **Methods:** Defatted Gac seed kernel powder was extracted with different solvents: 100% water, 50% methanol:water, 70% ethanol:water, water saturated butanol, 100% methanol, and 100% ethanol. Trypsin inhibitors, saponins, phenolics, and antioxidant activity using the 2,2′-azino-bis(3-ethylbenzothiazoline-6-sulfonic acid) diammonium salt (ABTS), the 2,2-diphenyl-1-picrylhydrazyl (DPPH) and the ferric reducing antioxidant power (FRAP) assays; and anticancer potential against two melanoma cancer cell lines (MM418C1 and D24) were analysed to determine the best extraction solvents. **Results:** Water was best for extracting trypsin inhibitors (581.4 ± 18.5 mg trypsin/mg) and reducing the viability of MM418C1 and D24 melanoma cells (75.5 ± 1.3 and $66.9 \pm 2.2\%$, respectively); the anticancer potential against the MM418C1 cells was highly correlated with trypsin inhibitors ($r = 0.92$, $p < 0.05$), but there was no correlation between anticancer potential and antioxidant activity. The water saturated butanol had the highest saponins (71.8 ± 4.31 mg aescin equivalents/g), phenolic compounds (20.4 ± 0.86 mg gallic acid equivalents/g), and antioxidant activity, but these measures were not related to anticancer potential. **Conclusions:** Water yielded a Gac seed extract, rich in trypsin inhibitors, which had high anticancer potential against two melanoma cell lines.

Keywords: *Momordica cochinchinensis*; Gac; seeds; saponins; trypsin inhibitors; phenolics; anticancer; antioxidant; extraction; freeze dried extract

1. Introduction

Momordica cochinchinensis Spreng, commonly called Gac, is a plant species of the family *Cucurbitaceae*, which is also known as red melon, baby jackfruit, spiny bitter gourd, sweet gourd, and cochinchin gourd. It is native to Southeast Asia and is commonly grown as a food crop in Vietnam, Thailand, Laos, Myanmar, and Cambodia [1,2]. From the food and commercial perspectives, the most commonly used part of the mature fruit is the red flesh surrounding the seeds, called the aril, which is traditionally used as a colourant in rice or, more recently, as a material that is processed into functional food ingredients or supplements [3].

The seeds are not eaten; they are removed from the aril and are mostly considered as waste [3,4]. However, in traditional medicine, Gac seeds are purported to have an array of therapeutic effects on a variety of conditions, such as fluxes, liver and spleen disorders, haemorrhoids, wounds, bruises, swelling, and pus [2,5]. In modern research, several constituents have been identified, which could be involved in the putative medicinal properties of Gac seeds, including trypsin inhibitors (e.g., MCoTI-I, MCoTI-II and MCoTI-III) [6–8], saponins (e.g., Momordica Saponin I and Momordica Saponin II) [9,10], and phenolic compounds (e.g., gallic acid and *p*-hydroxybenzoic acid) [11]. Gac seed extracts have been linked with many medicinal properties, such as gastroprotective [12–14], anti-inflammatory [15,16], anticancer [17], and antitumor [18] activities. Most of these properties are linked to the seed's saponins [12,13,15,16]. Furthermore, karounidiol, a triterpenoid compound, likely a saponin, present in Gac seeds [19], possess cytotoxic activity against human cancer cell lines [20]. Protease inhibitors, like the trypsin inhibitors in Gac seeds [7,8,21], have diverse biochemical functions [4,22], including acting as anticancer agents by inhibiting the growth of transformed cells [23–26]. Some trypsin inhibitors, such as those from *Cajanus cajan* and *Phaseolus limensis*, possess antioxidant, anti-inflammatory, and anti-bacterial activity [27].

There is limited information on how to best recover the bioactive compounds from Gac seeds, particularly to optimise anticancer potential. Efficient extraction and preservation methods are important for their immediate and long-term use. For any given plant bioactive, extractable yield depends on the extraction solvent, the chemical nature of the targeted component, and the characteristics of the extraction procedure. When other factors are kept constant, the extraction solvent plays a key role in obtaining the desired quality and quantity of the target constituents [28,29]. The choice of solvent is mainly based on the chemical properties of the targeted compounds, such as their polarity or hydrophobicity.

Due to the hydrophilic or amphiphilic nature of the trypsin inhibitors, phenolics, and saponins in Gac seeds, aqueous solvents and the low alcohols are likely to be the best extraction solvents for these bioactive compounds. They are also the safest and the most environmentally-friendly solvents for the extraction of bioactive compounds from plant materials [30,31]. For drying after solvent extractions, numerous methods have been developed; however, freeze drying is considered to be superior for preserving the medicinal qualities of botanical extracts and it is therefore widely used [32]. Additionally, to make it easier for the extraction of trypsin inhibitors [33] and to avoid interference of sticky oil during the freeze-drying procedure, the Gac seeds need to be defatted before they are extracted with solvents.

Thus, this study aimed to investigate the effectiveness of different solvents (water, alcohols, and mixtures) to extract the bioactive compounds of interest (trypsin inhibitors, saponins, and phenolics) from defatted Gac seed kernel powder. The relationships between the extracted compounds and the antioxidant activity and the anticancer potential of the extracts were also investigated.

2. Materials and Methods

2.1. Materials

2.1.1. Solvents, Reagents, and Chemicals

Solvents (ethanol, methanol and butanol) and chemicals (vanillin, sulphuric acid and potassium persulfate) were purchased from Merck (Bayswater, VIC, Australia). Folin-ciocalteu's phenol reagent, anhydrous sodium carbonate, sodium nitrile, ferric chloride, gallic acid, catechin, 2,4,6-tris(2-pyridyl)-s-triazine, (±)-6-hydroxy-2,5,7,8-tetramethylchromane-2-carboxylic acid (trolox), aescin, 2,2-diphenyl-1-picrylhydrazyl (DPPH), 2,2′-azino-bis(3-ethylbenzothiazoline-6-sulfonic acid) diammonium salt (ABTS), trypsin (type I) from bovine pancreas, benzyl-DL-arginine-para-nitroanilide

(BAPNA), Tris, and dimethylsulfoxide (DMSO) were purchased from Sigma-Aldrich Co. (Castle Hill, NSW, Australia). Sodium acetate trihydrate was purchased from Government Stores Department (Sydney, NSW, Australia). Aluminium chloride was a product of J. T. Baker Chem. Co. (Thermo Fisher Scientific, North Ryde, NSW, Australia). Acetic acid was a product of BDH Laboratory Supplies (Bio-Strategy, Tingalpa, QLD, Australia). Sodium hydroxide was a product of Ajax FineChem (Thermo Fisher Scientific, North Ryde, NSW, Australia) and hydrochloride acid a product of Lab-Scan Ltd. (Bacto, Mt Pritchard, NSW, Australia).

Human melanoma MM418C1 (mutated BRAF oncogene), referred to as C1 melanoma cells, and D24 (wild type BRAF oncogene) and human keratinocyte (HaCat) cell lines were provided by the School of Health and Biomedical Sciences, RMIT University (Bundoora, VIC, Australia). RPMI-1640 media, streptomycin, and penicillin were Gibco products (Thermo Fisher Scientific, North Ryde, NSW, Australia). Fetal bovine serum (FBS) was from Serana (Melbourne, VIC, Australia).

2.1.2. Gac Seeds

Gac seeds, from accession VS7 as classified by Wimalasiri et al. [1], were collected from 450 kg of fresh Gac fruit. These fruits were bought at Gac fruit fields in Dong Nai province, Ho Chi Minh City, Vietnam (Latitude: 10.757410; Longitude: 106.673439). After their separation from the fresh fruit, the seeds were vacuum dried at 40 °C for 24 h to reduce moisture and increase the crispness of the shell, which facilitated shell removal. The dried seeds were de-coated to get the kernels, which were then packaged in vacuum-sealed aluminium bags and stored at −18 °C until used.

Preparation of Defatted Gac Seed Kernel Powder

Defatted Gac seed kernel powder was prepared as described by Le et al. [34]. Briefly, the Gac seed kernels were ground in an electric grinder (100 g ST-02A Mulry Disintegrator, Taiwan Machinary, Sydney, NSW, Australia) to a powder that could pass through a sieve of 1.4 mm. The powder was then freeze-dried using a Dynavac FD3 Freeze Dryer (Dynapumps, Seven Hills, NSW, Australia) for 48 h, at −45 °C under vacuum at a pressure loading of 10^{-2} mbar (1 Pa), to reduce the moisture content to $1.21 \pm 0.02\%$. The powder was then defatted using three 30-min extractions with hexane at a powder to hexane ratio of 1:5 w/v. The resulting slurry was suction filtered and the residue (defatted meal) was air-dried for 12 h and stored in a desiccator at ambient room temperature until used. The moisture content of the defatted powder, measured using a Shimadzu MOC63u moisture analyser (Rydalmere, NSW, Australia), was $8.61 \pm 0.15\%$.

2.2. *Methods*

2.2.1. Extraction

Based on a previous study [34], six solvents (deionised water, 100% methanol, 50% methanol in water, 100% ethanol, 70% ethanol in water, and 90% *n*-butanol in water), were used for the extraction of bioactive compounds from the defatted and dried Gac seed kernel powder. Twenty grams of the powder were added to 400 mL of each solvent and the suspension was kept under constant magnetic stirring for 30 min at 40 ± 1 °C. Following extraction, the mixtures were filtered through two layers of cheese cloth and then through a Whatman No. 1 filter paper (Thermo Fisher Scientific, North Ryde, NSW, Australia), and the clear filtrates were collected in 500 mL evaporating flasks. Triplicate extractions were done for each solvent.

2.2.2. Freeze Drying Extracts

The filtrates collected from the extractions were freeze-dried into powders as summarized in Figure 1. First, the liquid extracts were concentrated using a rotary evaporator (Buchi Rotavapor B480, Buchi Australia, Noble Park, VIC, Australia) at 40 °C under vacuum until thick but not completely dried in the 500 mL evaporating flasks. Then, to transfer the extracts into pre-weighed 100 mL evaporating flasks, three different solvents were used. For each of the butanol, methanol, and 50% methanol extracts, 50 mL of 50% methanol in water was used, for each of the ethanol and 70% ethanol extracts, 50 mL of 50% ethanol in water was used, and for the water extract, 30 mL of water was used. The suspensions were mixed well, and the evaporation resumed until around 20 mL of the concentrated extracts were left. The concentrates were then frozen using liquid nitrogen before freeze drying with a BenchTop Pro freeze dryer (Scitek, Lane Cove, NSW, Australia) at −60 °C and 30 mbar for 48 h. The flasks with residue were placed in a desiccator and quickly weighed. The difference in weight between the flasks with residue and the empty flasks was taken to be the mass recovered for each extract. These freeze dried (FD) crude extracts were then stored in air-tight containers at −20 °C for use within 3 months.

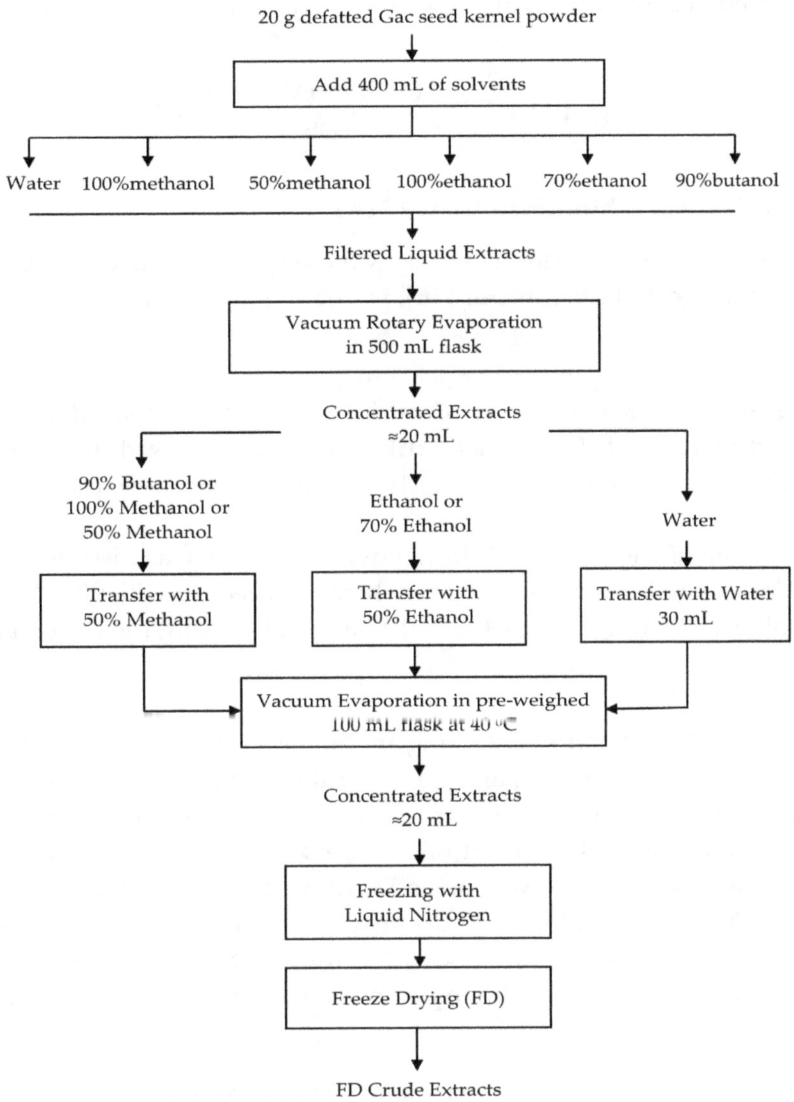

Figure 1. Procedure for producing freeze dried (FD) crude extracts from defatted Gac seed kernel powder.

2.2.3. Determination of Extractable Yield

To determine the extractable yield, 10 mL of each filtered liquid extract, resulting from Section 2.2.1, was transferred into a tared flat-bottomed glass vial and then dried at 105 °C with a vacuum pressure of 60 kPa for 24 h in a vacuum oven (Thermoline, Wetherill Park, NSW, Australia) until a constant weight was achieved. These vials were cooled in a desiccator for 30 min and weighed. The extractable yield was calculated, in g dried extract per 100 g of dried defatted Gac seed kernel powder, using Equation (1), where EY was the extractable yield, DE (g) was the mass of dried extract after the vacuum oven drying,

40 was the ratio of the 10 mL used for the vacuum oven drying to the 400 mL originally used for the extract, and DS (g) was the mass of dried defatted Gac seed kernel powder used for the extraction.

$$\text{EY (g/100 g)} = \frac{\text{DE} \times 40}{\text{DS}} \times 100 \quad (1)$$

2.2.4. Determination of Dry Mass Yield

Dry mass yield was defined as the amount (g) of FD crude extract, produced as described in Section 2.2.2, per 100 g of dried defatted Gac seed kernel powder. Equation (2) was used to calculate the dry mass yield (DM), in which FD (g) was the weight of the FD crude extract, DS (g) was the mass of dried defatted Gac seed kernel powder used for the extraction, and V was the volume of the filtrate collected after extraction.

$$\text{DM (g/100 g)} = \frac{\text{FD} \times \text{V}/(\text{V} - 10)}{\text{DS}} \times 100 \quad (2)$$

2.2.5. Determination of Trypsin Inhibitor Activity (TIA)

The TIA assay was performed as described by Makkar et al. [35] except that the absorbance was measured at 385 nm, as suggested by Stauffer [36], instead of at 410 nm.

Reagent Preparation

Substrate solution: A substrate solution of 92 mM BAPNA was prepared as follows. First, 40.0 mg BAPNA was dissolved in 1.00 mL DMSO and diluted to 100 mL with 0.05 M Tris-buffer (pH 8.2) containing 0.02 M $CaCl_2$ pre-warmed to 37 °C. This solution was prepared daily and kept at 37 °C while in use.

Trypsin solution: 20.0 mg of trypsin (type I) from bovine pancreas was dissolved in 1 mM HCl to make 1 L and stored at 4 °C for use within a week. In the analytical procedure with 92 mM BAPNA, this solution gave an absorbance value in the range of 0.900 ± 0.010 after subtracting the reagent blank at 385 nm.

Determination of TIA

Each FD crude extract from Section 2.2.2 (Figure 1) was dissolved in water at a concentration to give an inhibition of Trypsin between 40% and 60% and the assay was setup as shown in Table 1 with four test tubes prepared for each FD crude extract. All the prepared test tubes were kept in a water bath at 37 °C for 10 min to promote the formation of an enzyme–inhibitor complex and then 5.0 mL of BAPNA solution, pre-warmed to 37 °C, was added into each tube and the tubes were incubated in a water bath at 37 °C for 10 min. One mL of 30% acetic acid solution was added to each tube to stop the reaction. Then, 2.0 mL of trypsin solution was added into each reagent and sample blank (Table 1). After thorough mixing, the absorbance of the reaction mixture due to the release of *p*–nitroaniline was measured at 385 nm.

Table 1. The trypsin inhibitor activity assay setup.

Component	Reagent Blank (a)	Standard (b)	Sample Blank (c)	Sample (d)
Deionised water (mL)	2	2	1	1
Trypsin solution (mL)	-	2	-	2
Diluted extract (mL)	-	-	1	1
BAPNA (mL)	5	5	5	5
Acetic acid (mL)	1	1	1	1
Trypsin solution after reaction inactivation (mL)	2	-	2	-

BAPNA (benzyl-DL-arginine-para-nitroanilide) was added to start the reaction and acetic acid for inactivation.

Calculation

The change in absorbance (A_I) due to the trypsin inhibitor per mL of diluted extract was $(A_b - A_a) - (A_d - A_c)$, where the subscripts referred to tubes (a) to (d) in Table 1. Since 1 µg of trypsin gave an absorbance of 0.0190, the weight of trypsin inhibited per mL of extract was $A_I/0.019$ µg. From this value, The TIA of the FD crude extracts was calculated using Equation (3) and expressed as mg of pure trypsin inhibited per mg of FD crude extract.

$$\text{TIA} = \frac{A_I}{0.019 \times S \times \left(1 - \frac{m\%}{100}\right)} \quad (3)$$

where,

A_I: Change in absorbance due to inhibition per 1 mL of extract;
$A_I = (A_b - A_a) - (A_d - A_c)$, subscripts as per Table 1;
S: Weight (mg) of the FD crude extract dissolved in 1 mL;
m%: Moisture content of the FD crude extract powder.

2.2.6. Determination of Total Saponin Content (TSC)

The FD crude extracts from Section 2.2.2 were dissolved in water at a concentration of 2 mg/mL and vortexed before the TSC was determined according to Tan et al. [37] with some modifications. Briefly, 0.25 mL of each extract was mixed with 0.25 mL of 8% (*w*/*v*) vanillin solution and 2.5 mL of 72% (*v*/*v*) sulphuric acid. The mixture was vortexed and incubated in a water bath at 60 °C for 15 min and then cooled on ice for 10 min. The absorption of the mixture was measured at 560 nm using a Cary 60 UV-Vis spectrophotometer (Agilent Technologies, Mulgrave, VIC, Australia). Aecsin was used as a standard and the results were expressed as milligram aecsin equivalents (AE) per gram of the FD crude extract powder (mg AE/g).

2.2.7. Determination of Total Phenolic Content (TPC)

The FD crude extracts from Section 2.2.2 were dissolved in water at a concentration of 2 mg/mL and vortexed before the TPC was determined according to the method of Tan et al. [38] with some modifications. Briefly, 0.5 mL of each extract was mixed with 2.5 mL of 10% (*v*/*v*) Folin–Ciocalteu reagent in water and incubated at room temperature for 2 min to equilibrate. Then, 2 mL of 7.5% (*w*/*v*) sodium carbonate solution in water was added and the mixture was incubated at ambient temperature for 1 h. The absorption of the reaction mixture was measured at 765 nm using a Cary 60 UV-Vis spectrophotometer. Gallic acid was used as a standard and the results were expressed as milligram gallic acid equivalents (GAE) per gram dry weight of the FD crude extract powder (mg GAE/g).

2.2.8. Determination of Antioxidant Capacity

The FD crude extracts from Section 2.2.2 were dissolved in water at the concentration of 2 mg/mL and mixed before analysing antioxidant capacity using three assays: the 2,2′-azino-bis(3-ethylbenzothiazoline-6-sulfonic acid) diammonium salt (ABTS), the 2,2-diphenyl-1-picrylhydrazyl (DPPH) and the ferric reducing antioxidant power (FRAP).

DPPH

The DPPH assay measures the total free radical scavenging capacity of the extracts. The assay was performed as described by Tan et al. [38]. A stock solution of 0.6 M DPPH in methanol was prepared and kept at −20 °C until use. The working solution was prepared by mixing 10 mL of stock solution with 45 mL of methanol to obtain an absorbance of 1.1 ± 0.02 units at 515 nm using a spectrophotometer. Each extract (0.15 mL) was mixed with 2.85 mL of the working solution and the mixture was allowed to stand for 3 h, after which the absorption was measured at 515 nm using a

Cary 60 UV-Vis spectrophotometer. Trolox was used as a standard and the results were expressed as milligram Trolox equivalents (TE) per gram of the FD crude extract powder (mg TE/g).

ABTS

The ABTS assay measures the total free radical scavenging capacity of the extracts. The assay was performed as described by Tan et al. [38] with slight modifications. Stock solutions of 7.4 mM ABTS and 2.6 mM potassium persulfate were freshly prepared or kept at 4 °C in a dark bottle for use within a month, respectively. A fresh working solution was prepared for each assay by mixing equal quantities of the two stock solutions and incubated for 15 h to 16 h in the dark at ambient temperature. Then, 1 mL of the working solution was diluted with approximately 30 mL of methanol to obtain an absorbance of 1.1 ± 0.02 units at 734 nm using a Cary 60 UV-Vis spectrophotometer. Each extract (0.15 mL) was mixed with 2.85 mL of the working solution and the mixture was incubated for 2 h in the dark at ambient temperature. The absorption of the reaction mixture was measured at 734 nm using a Cary 60 UV-Vis spectrophotometer. Trolox was used as a standard and the results were expressed as milligram Trolox equivalents (TE) per gram of the FD crude extract powder (mg TE/g).

FRAP

The FRAP assay measures the ferric reducing power. The assay was performed following the method of Thaipong et al. [39], based on the increase in absorbance at 593 nm. A fresh FRAP working solution was initially prepared by mixing 300 mM acetate buffer (pH 3.6), 10 mM iron reagent (TPTZ) in 40 mM HCl, and 20 mM $FeCl_3{\bullet}6H_2O$ in the ratio of 10:1:1 (*v*/*v*/*v*). The fresh working solution was warmed to 37 °C before using. Each extract (0.15 mL) was mixed with 2.85 mL of the working FRAP solution and the mixture was incubated at ambient temperature in the dark for 30 min before its absorbance was measured at 593 nm using a Cary 60 UV-Vis spectrophotometer. Trolox was used as a standard and the antioxidant capacity of each sample, based on its ability to reduce ferric ions, was expressed as milligram Trolox equivalents (TE) per gram of the FD crude extract powder (mg TE/g).

2.2.9. Determination of Cytotoxicity

Cell Lines and Culture

The human melanoma MM418C1 (C1, wild type BRAF oncogene) and D24 (mutated BRAF oncogene) cell lines were maintained in RPMI-1640 media supplemented with 10% (*v*/*v*) FBS, 1% (*v*/*v*) streptomycin and penicillin at 37 °C in 5% CO_2. HaCat keratinocytes were used as normal untransformed cells and grown in the same media.

In Vitro Cytotoxicity Assay

All cells were seeded in 96 well plates (Greiner Bio-One, Labfriend, Sydney, NSW, Australia), 5000 cells/well along with 100 μL of fresh media. The FD crude extracts from Section 2.2.2 were dissolved in RPMI-1640 cell culture media at a concentration of 2 mg/mL and UV-sterilised for 10 min in a laminar flow hood before use on cells. The cells were allowed to attach for 4 h before being treated with 10 μL of the extract and incubated for 48 h.

The effect of the extracts on cell growth was determined using the CCK-8 (Cell Counting Kit-8) assay (Sigma-Aldrich, St Louis, MO, USA). The assay measured cytotoxicity based on the conversion of a water-soluble tetrazolium salt, 2-(2-methoxy-4-nitrophenyl)-3-(4-nitrophenyl)-5-(2,4-disulfophenyl)-2*H*-tetrazolium, monosodium salt (WST-8), to a water-soluble formazan dye upon reduction by dehydrogenases in the presence of an electron carrier [40].

To determine cell viability, 10 μL of CCK-8 solution was added to each well of the 96-well plate containing treated and control samples. The plates were incubated at 37 °C for 2 h and the absorbance was measured spectrophotometrically at 450 nm using a CLARIOstar® High Performance Monochromator Multimode Microplate Reader (BMG LABTECH, Mornington, NSW, Australia) and the results were analysed using the MARS data analysis software (version 3.00R2, BMG LABTECH, Mornington, NSW, Australia). The data were presented as a proportional viability (%) by comparing the treated cells with the untreated cells (control) using Equation (4):

$$\text{Cell viability} = \frac{At - Ab}{Ac - Ab} \times 100 \quad (4)$$

where At was the absorbance value of the treated cells, Ab was the absorbance of CCK-8 only, and Ac was the negative control which included cells and CCK-8 only. Two types of controls were used: the media control consisted of cultured cells in 10% (v/v) FBS containing medium alone and the vehicle control consisted of cells in 10% (v/v) FBS containing medium, to which 10 μL of RPMI-1640 media without FBS was added. However, as both controls did not cause cytotoxicity, the media control was used to calculate cell viability.

Cell morphology was analysed at 48 h using a Nikon Eclipse TS100 (Nikon, Tokyo, Japan) phase contrast inverted microscope and the images were captured using a Nikon DS-Fi1digital camera.

2.2.10. Statistical Analyses

Extractions were performed in triplicate and means ± standard deviation (SD) were assessed with the one-way Analysis of Variance (ANOVA) and Tukey's *Post Hoc* Multiple Comparisons test using the IBM SPSS Statistics 24 program (IBM Corp., Armonk, NY, USA). Differences in means were considered statistically significant at $p < 0.05$. Correlations and their significance were determined using the Microsoft Excel 2016 (Microsoft Corp., Seattle, WA, USA) and Principle Component Analysis (Minitab 17.1.0, Sydney, NSW, Australia).

3. Results

3.1. Effect of Solvent on the Extractable Yield and the Dry Mass Yield

Extractable yield and dry mass yield were calculated for each extract. The extractable yields ranged from 4.4 g/100 g for the ethanol extract to 15.5 g/100 g for the aqueous extract while the dry mass yield ranged from 3.7 g/100 g for the ethanol extract to 13.1 g/100 g for the aqueous extract (Table 2). For both the extractable yield and the dry mass yield, the values were substantially higher for the aqueous extracts than for the organic solvents, whether they were mixed with water or not. Furthermore, the extractable yield (before drying) was higher than the dry mass yield (after freeze drying) for all extracts. The observed loss during the drying process was highest for the 70% ethanol extract (−31%) followed by the methanol extract (−28%) and the butanol extract (−20%). The aqueous and ethanol extracts had the same loss (−15%), while the lowest lost was for the 50% methanol extract (−11%).

Table 2. Effect of solvent on the extractable yield (EY) and the dry mass yield (DM).

Solvent	EY (g/100 g)	DM (g/100 g)	Original Volume (mL)	Collected Volume (mL)	Yield Loss (%)
Water	15.5 ± 0.1^{a}	13.1 ± 0.1^{b}	400 ± 3	355 ± 0	15.3 ± 0.1^{d}
50% Methanol	10.2 ± 0.0^{c}	9.1 ± 0.3^{d}	400 ± 3	348 ± 3	10.9 ± 0.2^{f}
70% Ethanol	10.2 ± 0.0^{c}	7.1 ± 0.4^{e}	400 ± 3	340 ± 5	30.6 ± 0.3^{a}
90% Butanol	6.9 ± 0.1^{e}	5.5 ± 0.1^{f}	400 ± 3	350 ± 0	19.9 ± 0.1^{c}
Methanol	6.7 ± 0.2^{e}	4.8 ± 0.2^{g}	400 ± 3	330 ± 0	27.8 ± 0.2^{b}
Ethanol	4.4 ± 0.0^{g}	3.7 ± 0.0^{h}	400 ± 3	345 ± 0	14.9 ± 0.0^{e}

The values were the means ± SD of three replicate extractions for each solvent. All the values for EY and DM were compared to each other, the values for yield loss were compared separately and the values not sharing the same superscript letter for EY and DM, and separately for yield loss, were significantly different at $p < 0.05$.

3.2. *Effect of Solvents on the Content of Bioactive Compounds*

3.2.1. Trypsin Inhibitors

The yield of trypsin inhibitors was measured as the trypsin inhibitor activity (TIA) of the FD crude extracts (Figure 2). The water extract had the highest TIA (581.4 mg/mg) and the yield decreased relative to the concentration of water in the water and low alcohol mixtures: −40% for the 50% methanol (≈50% water) extract, −54% for the 70% ethanol (≈30% water) extract and −97% for the water-saturated butanol (≈10% water) extract. The 100% methanol and 100% ethanol extracts had much lower TIA values than the water extract, −96% and −95%, respectively (Figure 2). Therefore, water was the best solvent for extracting trypsin inhibitors from the defatted Gac seed kernel powder.

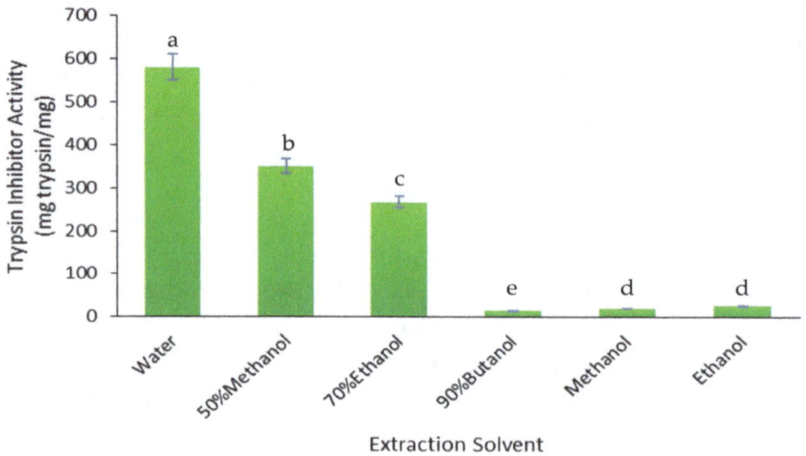

Figure 2. Effect of solvent on the trypsin inhibitor activity (TIA) of the FD crude extracts. The values are the means ± SD of three replicate extractions for each solvent. Columns not sharing the same letter are significantly different at $p < 0.05$.

3.2.2. Saponins

The yield of saponins was measured as the total saponin content (TSC) of the FD crude extracts (Figure 3). The highest TSC was found in the butanol and methanol extracts, which were 24% higher than the TSC in the 50% methanol and 70% ethanol extracts, 48% higher than the ethanol extract, and 53% higher than the water extract. Therefore, butanol and methanol were the best solvents for extracting the saponins from the defatted Gac seed kernel powder.

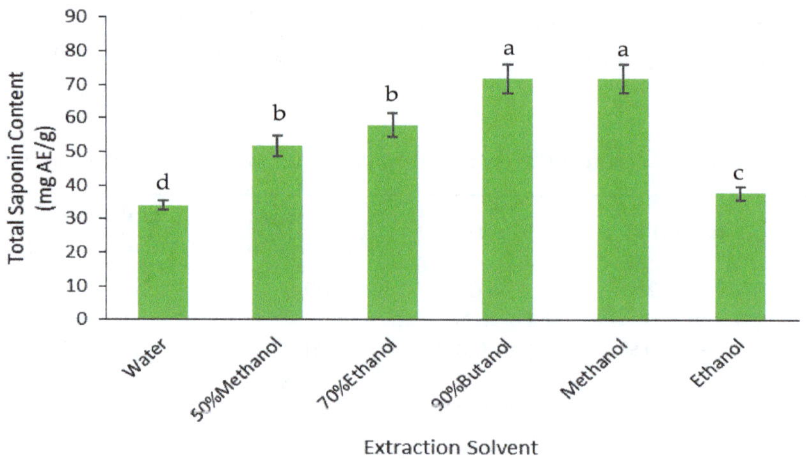

Figure 3. Effect of solvent on the total saponin content (TSC) extraction from Gac seed. The values were the means ± SD of three replicate extractions for each solvent. Columns not sharing the same letter were significantly different at $p < 0.05$.

3.2.3. Phenolics

The yield of phenolics was measured as the total phenolic content (TPC) of the FD crude extracts (Figure 4). The highest TPC was found in the butanol extract; the TPC in this extract was 13% higher than the water extract, 29% higher than the 50% methanol and 70% ethanol extracts, 35% higher than the methanol extract, and 63% higher than the ethanol extract. Therefore, butanol extracted the highest phenolics from the defatted Gac seed kernel powder.

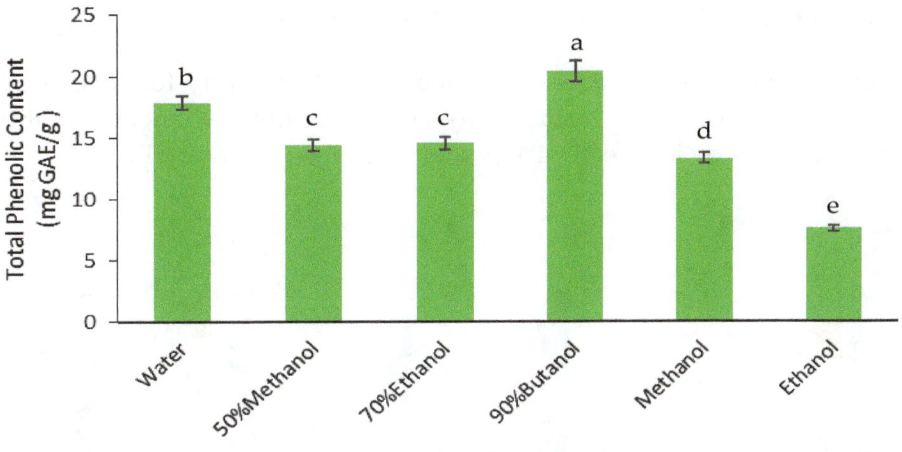

Figure 4. Effect of solvent on the total phenolic content (TPC) of the FD Gac seed crude extracts. The values were the means ± SD of three replicate extractions for each solvent. Columns not sharing the same letter were significantly different at $p < 0.05$. GAE, Gallic acid equivalents.

3.3. *Effect of Solvents on Antioxidant Activity*

The antioxidant activity of the extracts was measured using three assays: DPPH, ABTS, and FRAP. The butanol extract gave the highest values for ABTS and DPPH assays and the ethanol extract gave the highest value for FRAP assay (Figure 5). These two extracts produced significantly higher antioxidant activity based on the ABTS, DPPH, and FRAP assays (Figure 5).

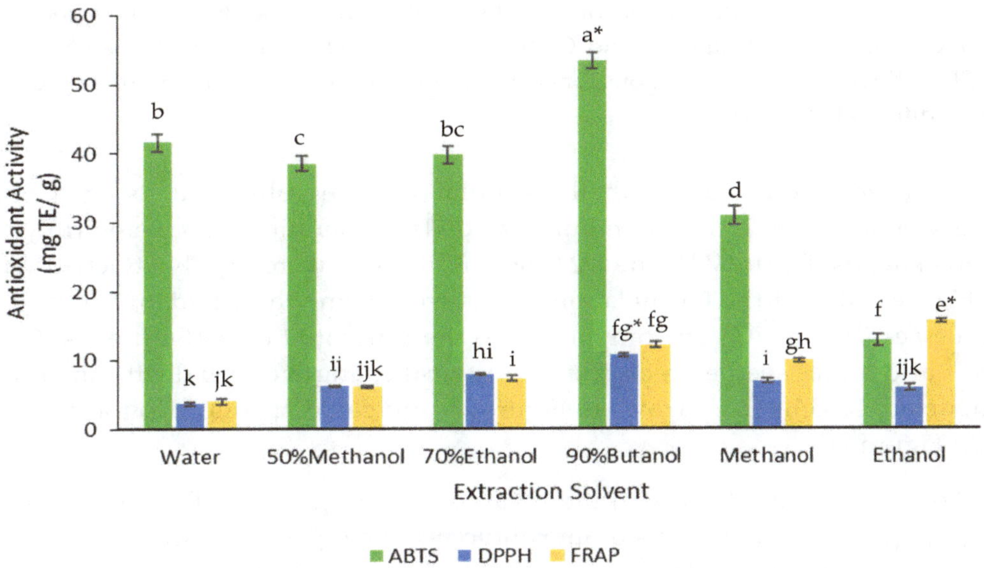

Figure 5. Effect of solvent on the antioxidant capacity of the FD crude extracts. The values were the means ± SD of three replicate extractions for each solvent. Columns not sharing the same superscript letter were significantly different at $p < 0.05$. * indicated the highest antioxidant activity. TE, Trolox equivalents.

3.4. *Effect of Extraction Solvent on Cancer Cell Viability*

The FD crude extracts were tested for cell toxicity using two melanoma cell lines (D24 and C1) and a normal keratinocyte line (HaCat). The water extract was the most cytotoxic towards both cancer cell lines compared to the other extracts (Figure 6); the extract decreased the cell viability by 67% for D24 and 75% for C1 melanoma cells. The 70% ethanol and 50% methanol extracts also showed cytotoxic activity towards the C1 melanoma cells, decreasing their viability by 69% and 46%, respectively, while the butanol, methanol, and ethanol extracts had no effect. Besides the water extract, no other FD crude extract had any effect on the viability of the D24 melanoma cells.

In contrast, all the FD crude extracts decreased the cell viability for the normal keratinocytes (HaCat). Except for the ethanol extract, which only decreased the HaCat cell viability by 24%, all the extracts reduced the viability by between 64% (water) and 75% (methanol).

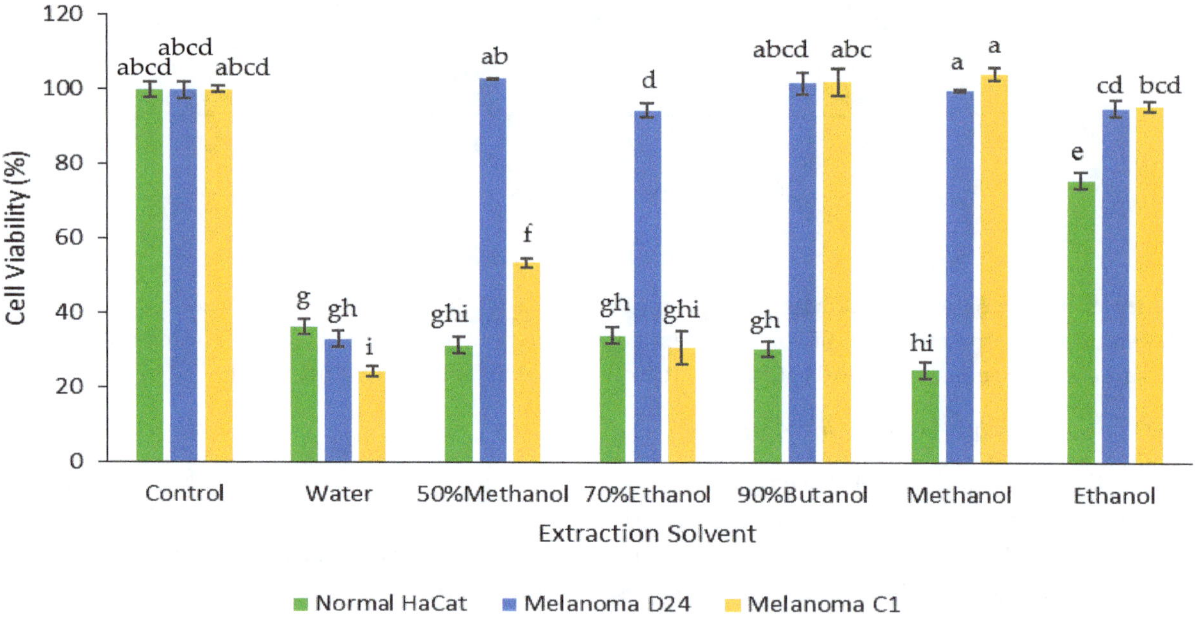

Figure 6. Effect of the FD crude extracts prepared with the different solvents on the cell viability of normal (HaCat) and melanoma (D24 and C1) cell lines after 48 h treatment. The values were the means ± SD of three replicate extractions for each solvent. Columns not sharing the same letter were significantly different at $p < 0.05$.

These results were consistent with the cellular changes observed using a phase contrast microscope. As seen in Figure 7, the control untreated HaCat keratinocytes were firmly attached with flattened oblong shapes (Figure 7A), the D24 melanoma cells were lightly attached with advanced elongations (Figure 7B), and the C1 melanoma cells were firmly attached and tightly packed with elongated processes (Figure 7C). In comparison to the untreated cells (Figure 7A–C), exposure of the cells to the various Gac seed extracts induced typical changes of cell death, such as cytoplasmic condensation, detached cells (red arrows in Figure 7), and cell disruption, to form apoptotic bodies (blue arrows in Figure 7).

The cellular changes observed with the water extract (Figure 7D–F) were consistent with the viability results (Figure 6) in that signs of morphological changes were seen for all three cell types. The 50% methanol and 70% ethanol extracts also caused substantial morphological changes to the C1 melanoma cells (Figure 7I,L) and HaCat cells (Figure 7G,J). The butanol and methanol extracts also caused substantial morphological changes to the HaCat cells (Figure 7M,P). In contrast, the ethanol extract had the least effect on the morphology of all three cells (Figure 7S–U) akin to controls.

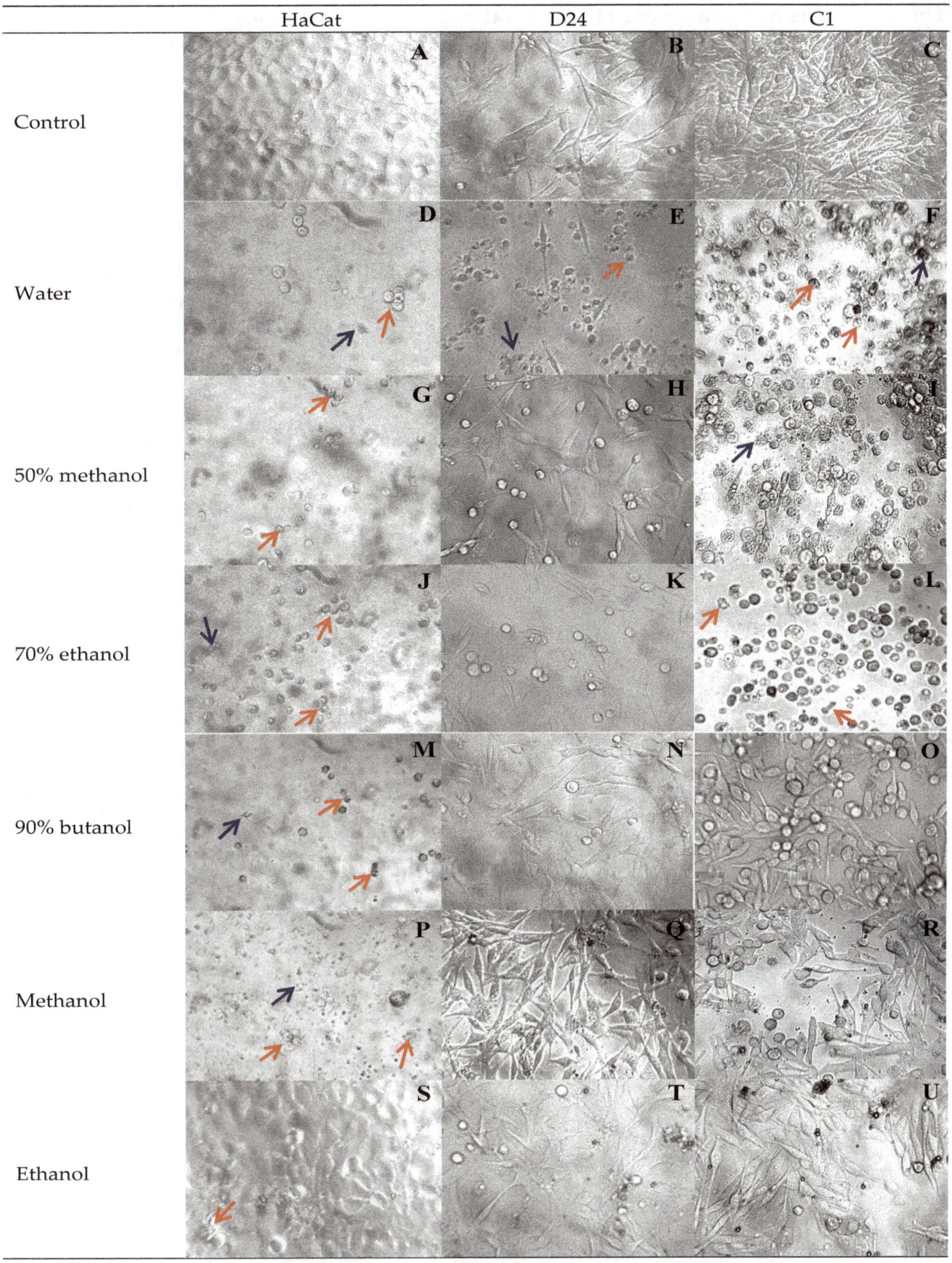

Figure 7. Morphological effects of different extraction solvents of Gac seed on HaCat (control) and melanoma D24 and C1 cell lines observed under a phase contrast microscope after 48 h treatment. Cytotoxicity is indicated by red arrows pointed to condensation and detached cells; blue arrows pointed to apoptotic bodies. Magnification: 100×.

The most sensitive cells were HaCat keratinocytes, while the least sensitive were the D24 melanoma cells, which had the least morphological changes when treated with all the solvent extracts, except for the water extract (Figure 7).

3.5. Correlations between Extract Yields, Bioactive Compounds, Antioxidant Activity, and Cancer Cell Viability across the FD Crude Extracts

TIA of the extracts was strongly and positively correlated with the extractable yield and the dry mass yield (Table 3, Figure 8). Essentially, the more material extracted, the higher the TIA, with the water extract having the highest values for both. TIA and extracted yields were also negatively correlated with the FRAP antioxidant activity and the viability of the C1 melanoma cells (Table 3, Figure 8). For example, almost 85% (r^2) of the variability in the C1 cell viability could be explained by variability in the TIA. In contrast, the C1 cell viability was positively correlated with the FRAP antioxidant activity. Therefore, the negative effect of the water extract on the C1 cell viability may be related to its high TIA but not FRAP activity.

Table 3. Coefficient of correlations (r) between yields, bioactive compounds, antioxidant activity, and cell viability across the Gac seed crude extracts.

	Yield		Bioactive Compound			Antioxidant Activity			Cell Viability		
	EY	DMY	TIA	TSC	TPC	ABTS	DPPH	FRAP	HaCat	D24	C1
EY	1.00										
DMY	0.98 †	1.00									
TIA	0.96 ‡	0.97 ‡	1.00								
TSC	−0.42	−0.50	−0.61	1.00							
TPC	0.51	0.49	0.31	0.36	1.00						
ABTS	0.48	0.43	0.29	0.44	0.97 †	1.00					
DPPH	−0.52	−0.58	−0.66	0.81 §	0.37	0.46	1.00				
FRAP	−0.93 ‡	−0.89 §	−0.88 §	0.19	−0.48	−0.50	0.44	1.00			
HaCat	−0.42	−0.35	−0.22	−0.63	−0.73	−0.78	−0.28	0.63	1.00		
D24	−0.79	−0.80	−0.77	0.65	−0.28	−0.13	0.69	0.56	−0.01	1.00	
C1	−0.88 §	−0.83 §	−0.92 §	0.53	−0.23	−0.26	0.50	0.83 §	0.18	0.61	1.00

† $p < 0.001$, ‡ $p < 0.01$, § $p < 0.05$, EY: Extraction yield; DMY: Dry mass yield; TIA: Trypsin inhibitor activity; TSC: Total saponin content; TPC: Total phenolic content; ABTS: 2,2′-Azino-bis(3-ethylbenzothiazoline-6-sulfonic acid) assay; DPPH: 2,2-diphenyl-1-picrylhydrazyl assay; FRAP: ferric reducing antioxidant power assay.

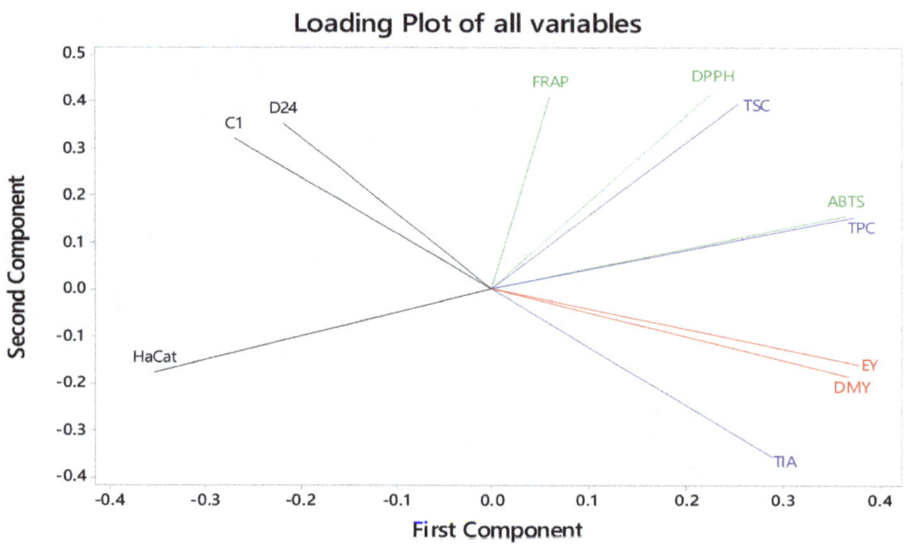

Figure 8. Correlations between extraction yields (red lines), bioactive compounds (blue lines), antioxidant activity (green lines), and cell viability (black lines) from Gac seed crude extracts.

There were positive correlations between the TSC with DPPH antioxidant activity, and TPC with ABTS antioxidant activity (Table 3, Figure 8). However, there were no significant correlations between these bioactive compounds and any other variables, including the effects of the extracts on cytotoxicity for both C1 and D24 cancer cells (Table 3, Figure 8). Furthermore, there were no other significant correlations between any of the other measured parameters.

4. Discussion

Gac seeds have long been used in traditional medicine as a remedy for numerous conditions. Several bioactive constituents have been identified in Gac seeds, such as trypsin inhibitors, saponins, and phenolics. In this study, the extraction of these bioactive constituents with different solvents was investigated and their relationships with antioxidant activity and anticancer potential were explored. The results revealed that the water extract had the highest anticancer potential, which may be related to its high content of trypsin inhibitors but not to its antioxidant activity.

The water extract from defatted Gac seeds had the highest anticancer potential, reducing the growth of the melanoma cells compared to the control. This is consistent with the finding that a water extract from Gac seeds was the best extract for supressing the migration and invasion of a breast cancer cell line [18]. Water extracts from Gac aril have also been shown to suppress the viability of colon, liver [17], and melanoma [41] cancer cell lines. Compared to the previous study [17], where the Gac aril water extract at 1.24 mg/mL inhibited colon and liver cancer cells by 38 and 45%, respectively, in the present study, the water extract at the much lower concentration of 0.2 mg/mL had a significantly higher anticancer activity of 67% and 75% for the D24 and C1 melanoma cells, respectively. This suggests that water is not only safe and inexpensive, but it is also a highly efficient solvent for extracting compounds with anticancer potential from Gac, especially Gac seeds. The use of water as the extraction solvent also means that the methodology is widely accessible to more people, particularly in rural and underdeveloped countries that do not have access to organic solvents and processing facilities.

The water extract also had the highest TIA value, which was likely due to the presence of trypsin inhibitor proteins because Gac seeds are known to contain trypsin inhibitor peptides that are soluble in buffered aqueous solvents [31,33,42]. The strong inverse correlation between TIA and the viability of the C1 melanoma cells also suggests that trypsin inhibitors were involved in the water extract's anticancer potential against these cells. The known Gac seed trypsin inhibitors have a low molecular weight of 3–4 kDa with a compact cyclic conformation [6,21], which can make it easy for them to penetrate into cancer cells and illicit cytotoxicity [43]. However, this is also consistent with the known anticancer potential of bigger proteins from Gac aril (35 kDa) [17] and other seeds, such as soybeans [44], which has been studied extensively [26,45–47].

However, although the water extract was the only extract to decrease the viability of the D24 melanoma cells, an inverse correlation between TIA and the viability of the D24 cells was not seen ($p = 0.07$) mainly because the 50% methanol and the 70% ethanol extracts had no activity against this cell line while they had activity against the C1 melanoma cell line. This could be due to the D24 cells, which have a mutated BRAF oncogene, being more resistant [48] to the presence of trypsin inhibitors, and therefore, they could only be killed when the trypsin inhibitors reach a high enough concentration, for example, in the water extract compared to the lower concentrations in the other extracts. However, it could also be that the D24 cells, and maybe also the C1 cells, were affected by other water soluble constituents of the Gac seeds, for example cyclotides which do not have trypsin inhibition activity [6]. For example, although many Gac seed trypsin inhibitors are cyclotides, MCoCC-1, a 3.3 kDa cyclotide unique to Gac seeds, which does not have trypsin inhibitor activity, has been shown to exhibit high cytotoxicity against the human melanoma MM96L cell line [6]; cell survival was decreased 43% in the presence of 2 μM MCoCC-1. The TIA is a measure of trypsin inhibitors, which may be cyclotides because they are found in Gac seeds [21], but other cyclotides are also present in Gac seeds that are purported to have anticancer potential [6,22]; however, these may not have antitrypsin activity and therefore would not be measured by the TIA.

The higher antioxidant activity of the butanol extract was likely due to its high content of saponin and phenolic compounds; this solvent had the highest TSC and TPC values among the extracts. There were strong positive correlations between saponins with DPPH antioxidant activity and phenolics with ABTS antioxidant activity, but neither saponins nor phenolic compounds were related to the FRAP antioxidant activity. Therefore, the extracted Gac seed saponins and phenolic compounds acted as antioxidants through the mechanism of scavenging the free radicals produced by DPPH and ABTS [39] rather than the reduction of oxidised intermediates in the FRAP chain reaction or through chelation [39]. A similar correlation was also reported by Chan et al. [49] for saponins and phenolic compounds extracted from defatted kenaf seeds. In that study, butanol was the most effective solvent for the extraction of saponins and phenolics. This solvent was non-polar enough to dissolve the saponin aglycones [50] and the phenolic rings [11], yet polar enough to also interact with the carbohydrate end of the saponin molecules and the carboxyl groups of gallic acid and p-hydroxybenzoic acid, which are reported to be present in Gac seeds [11]. Because butanol is classified by the FDA as a Class 3 solvent [51] with no known human hazards and approved for pharmaceutical applications, the use of it as an extraction solvent is regarded as less toxic and of low risk to human health.

Despite the high saponins, phenolics, and antioxidant activity of the butanol extract, it did not exhibit any anticancer potential against the two melanoma cell lines. This observation was not consistent with previous findings, which showed that one of the triterpenoid compounds found in Gac seed oil, karounidiol [20], had anticancer potential [19] and tumor inhibition effects [52]. This compound, likely a saponin, may not have been at a high enough concentration in the present extracts because the Gac seed kernels were defatted before they were extracted with the various solvents, which was consistent with a study by Le et al. [53], who found that Gac seed saponins were mainly associated with the fat component of the seeds.

5. Conclusions

Gac seeds, which are mostly considered as a waste product, could be a potentially useful source of anticancer candidates due to their cytotoxic activity against specific melanoma cells. The utilisation of Gac seeds to produce an anticancer product could reduce the waste burden on the environment and add value to the Gac fruit, which is cultivated in an increasing number of countries. This study found that water is suitable for the recovery of trypsin inhibitors and the preparation of an extract with significant anticancer potential. Butanol was found to be suitable to produce an extract enriched in saponins and phenolic compounds and with a high antioxidant activity. However, further studies are needed to fully understand what specific compounds are involved in the bioactivity of Gac seeds and their mechanism of action in order to better define their potential applications in the nutraceutical and pharmaceutical industries.

Author Contributions: Conceptualization, A.V.L., M.H.N., and P.D.R.; Methodology, A.V.L. and T.T.H.; Validation, A.V.L. and T.T.H.; Formal analysis, A.V.L., T.T.H.; Investigation, A.V.L.; Data curation, A.V.L., T.T.H., and P.D.R.; Writing—original draft preparation, A.V.L.; Writing—review & editing, A.V.L., T.T.H., P.D.R., M.H.N., and S.E.P.; Supervision, P.D.R. and M.H.N.

Acknowledgments: A.V.L. acknowledges the University of Newcastle and the Vietnamese Ministry of Education and Training (MOET) for their financial support.

References

1. Wimalasiri, D.; Piva, T.; Urban, S.; Huynh, T. Morphological and genetic diversity of *Momordica cochinchinenesis* (Cucurbitaceae) in Vietnam and Thailand. *Genet. Resour. Crop Evol.* **2016**, *63*, 19–33. [CrossRef]

2. Behera, T.; John, K.J.; Bharathi, L.; Karuppaiyan, R. Momordica. In *Wild Crop Relatives: Genomic and Breeding Resources*; Kole, C., Ed.; Springer: Heidelberg, Germany; New York, NY, USA, 2011; pp. 217–246.
3. Chuyen, H.V.; Nguyen, M.H.; Roach, P.D.; Golding, J.B.; Parks, S.E. Gac fruit (*Momordica cochinchinensis* Spreng): A rich source of bioactive compounds and its potential health benefits. *Int. J. Food Sci. Technol.* **2015**, *50*, 567–577. [CrossRef]
4. Huynh, T.; Nguyen, M.H.; Dao, N. Biomedical importance of *Momordica cochinchinensis* (GAC) fruit and future applications. *BJSTR* **2018**, *8*. in press.
5. Masayo, I.; Hikaru, O.; Tatsuo, Y.; Masako, T.; Yoshie, R.; Shuji, H.; Kunihide, M.; Ryuichi, H. Studies on the constituents of *Momordica cochinchinensis* Spreng. I. Isolation and characterization of the seed saponins, Momordica saponins I and II. *Chem. Pharm. Bull.* **1985**, *33*, 464–478. [CrossRef]
6. Chan, L.Y.; Wang, C.K.L.; Major, J.M.; Greenwood, K.P.; Lewis, R.J.; Craik, D.J.; Daly, N.L. Isolation and characterization of peptides from *Momordica cochinchinensis* seeds. *J. Nat. Prod.* **2009**, *72*, 1453–1458. [CrossRef] [PubMed]
7. Wong, R.C.; Fong, W.; Ng, T. Multiple trypsin inhibitors from *Momordica cochinchinensis* seeds, the Chinese drug mubiezhi. *Peptides* **2004**, *25*, 163–169. [CrossRef] [PubMed]
8. Chan, L.Y.; He, W.; Tan, N.; Zeng, G.; Craik, D.J.; Daly, N.L. A new family of cystine knot peptides from the seeds of *Momordica cochinchinensis*. *Peptides* **2013**, *39*, 29–35. [CrossRef] [PubMed]
9. Gao, X.M. (Ed.) Mu Bie Zi (*Semen momordicae*). In *Chinese Materia Medicia Beijing*; Traditional Chinese Materia Medica Press: Beijing, China, 2005; Volume 2, pp. 601–602.
10. Lin, Z.Y.; Liu, X.; Yang, F.; Yu, Y.Q. Structural characterization and identification of five triterpenoid saponins isolated from *Momordica cochinchinensis* extracts by liquid chromatography/tandem mass spectrometry. *Int. J. Mass Spectrom.* **2012**, *328*, 43–66. [CrossRef]
11. Kubola, J.; Siriamornpun, S. Phytochemicals and antioxidant activity of different fruit fractions (peel, pulp, aril and seed) of Thai gac (*Momordica cochinchinensis* Spreng). *Food Chem.* **2011**, *127*, 1138–1145. [CrossRef] [PubMed]
12. Kang, J.M.; Kim, N.; Kim, B.; Kim, J.-H.; Lee, B.-Y.; Park, J.H.; Lee, M.K.; Lee, H.S.; Jang, I.-J.; Kim, J.S.; et al. Gastroprotective action of cochinchina Momordica seed extract is mediated by activation of CGRP and inhibition of cPLA2/5-LOX pathway. *Dig. Dis. Sci.* **2009**, *54*, 2549–2560. [CrossRef] [PubMed]
13. Jung, K.; Chin, Y.-W.; Chung, Y.H.; Park, Y.H.; Yoo, H.; Min, D.S.; Lee, B.; Kim, J. Anti-gastritis and wound healing effects of Momordicae Semen extract and its active component. *Immunopharmacol. Immunotoxicol.* **2013**, *35*, 126–132. [CrossRef] [PubMed]
14. Kang, J.M.; Kim, N.; Kim, B.; Kim, J.-H.; Lee, B.-Y.; Park, J.H.; Lee, M.K.; Lee, H.S.; Kim, J.S.; Jung, H.C.; et al. Enhancement of gastric ulcer healing and angiogenesis by cochinchina Momordica seed extract in rats. *J. Korean Med. Sci.* **2010**, *25*, 875–881. [CrossRef] [PubMed]
15. Yu, J.S.; Kim, J.H.; Lee, S.; Jung, K.; Kim, K.H.; Cho, J.Y. Src/Syk-targeted anti-inflammatory actions of triterpenoidal saponins from Gac (*Momordica cochinchinensis*) Seeds. *Am. J. Chin. Med.* **2017**, 1–15. [CrossRef] [PubMed]
16. Jung, K.; Chin, Y.-W.; Yoon, K.D.; Chae, H.-S.; Kim, C.Y.; Yoo, H.; Kim, J. Anti-inflammatory properties of a triterpenoidal glycoside from Momordica cochinchinensis in LPS-stimulated macrophages. *Immunopharmacol. Immunotoxicol.* **2013**, *35*, 8–14. [CrossRef] [PubMed]
17. Tien, P.G.; Kayama, F.; Konishi, F.; Tamemoto, H.; Kasono, K.; Hung, N.T.; Kuroki, M.; Ishikawa, S.E.; Van Nguyen, C.; Kawakami, M. Inhibition of tumor growth and angiogenesis by water extract of Gac fruit (*Momordica cochinchinensis* Spreng). *Int. J. Oncol.* **2005**, *26*, 881–889. [CrossRef] [PubMed]
18. Zheng, L.; Zhang, Y.-M.; Zhan, Y.-Z.; Liu, C.-X. *Momordica cochinchinensis* seed extracts suppress migration and invasion of human breast cancer ZR-75-30 cells via down-regulating MMP-2 and MMP-9. *Asian Pac. J. Cancer Prev.* **2014**, *15*, 1105–1110. [CrossRef] [PubMed]
19. Akihisa, T.; Tokuda, H.; Ichiishi, E.; Mukainaka, T.; Toriumi, M.; Ukiya, M.; Yasukawa, K.; Nishino, H. Anti-tumor promoting effects of multiflorane-type triterpenoids and cytotoxic activity of karounidiol against human cancer cell lines. *Cancer Lett.* **2001**, *173*, 9–14. [CrossRef]
20. Kan, L.; Hu, Q.; Chao, Z.; Song, X.; Cao, X. Chemical constituents of unsaponifiable matter from seed oil of *Momordica cochinchinensis*. *China J. Chin. Mater. Med.* **2006**, *31*, 1441–1444.
21. Hernandez, J.F.; Gagnon, J.; Chiche, L.; Nguyen, T.M.; Andrieu, J.P.; Heitz, A.; Trinh Hong, T.; Pham, T.T.;

Le Nguyen, D. Squash trypsin inhibitors from *Momordica cochinchinensis* exhibit an atypical macrocyclic structure. *Biochemistry* **2000**, *39*, 5722–5730. [CrossRef] [PubMed]
22. Weidmann, J.; Craik, D.J. Discovery, structure, function, and applications of cyclotides: Circular proteins from plants. *J. Exp. Bot.* **2016**, *67*, 4801–4812. [CrossRef] [PubMed]
23. Sever, N.; Filipic, M.; Brzin, J.; Lah, T.T. Effect of cysteine proteinase inhibitors on murine B16 melanoma cell invasion in vitro. *Biol. Chem.* **2002**, *383*, 839–842. [CrossRef] [PubMed]
24. Heidtmann, H.-H.; Salge, U.; Abrahamson, M.; Bencina, M.; Kastelic, L.; Kopitar-Jerala, N.; Turk, V.; Lah, T.T. Cathepsin B and cysteine proteinase inhibitors in human lung cancer cell lines. *Clin. Exp. Metastasis* **1997**, *15*, 368–381. [CrossRef] [PubMed]
25. Clawson, G.A. Protease inhibitors and carcinogenesis: A review. *Cancer Investig.* **1996**, *14*, 597–608. [CrossRef]
26. Hocman, G. Chemoprevention of cancer: Protease inhibitors. *Int. J. Biochem.* **1992**, *24*, 1365–1375. [CrossRef]
27. Shamsi, T.N.; Parveen, R.; Afreen, S.; Azam, M.; Sen, P.; Sharma, Y.; Haque, Q.M.R.; Fatma, T.; Manzoor, N.; Fatima, S. Trypsin inhibitors from *Cajanus cajan* and *Phaseolus limensis* possess antioxidant, anti-Inflammatory, and antibacterial activity. *J. Diet. Suppl.* **2018**, 1–12. [CrossRef] [PubMed]
28. Samuelsson, G.; Kyerematen, G.; Farah, M.H. Preliminary chemical characterization of pharmacologically active compounds in aqueous plant extracts. *J. Ethnopharmacol.* **1985**, *14*, 193–201. [CrossRef]
29. Sasidharan, S.; Chen, Y.; Saravanan, D.; Sundram, K.; Latha, L.Y. Extraction, isolation and characterization of bioactive compounds from plants' extracts. *Afr. J. Tradit. Complement. Altern. Med.* **2011**, *8*, 1–10. [CrossRef] [PubMed]
30. Cheok, C.Y.; Salman, H.A.K.; Sulaiman, R. Extraction and quantification of saponins: A review. *Food Res. Int.* **2014**, *59*, 16–40. [CrossRef]
31. Mahatmanto, T.; Poth, A.G.; Mylne, J.S.; Craik, D.J. A comparative study of extraction methods reveals preferred solvents for cystine knot peptide isolation from *Momordica cochinchinensis* seeds. *Fitoterapia* **2014**, *95*, 22–33. [CrossRef] [PubMed]
32. Abascal, K.; Ganora, L.; Yarnell, E. The effect of freeze-drying and its implications for botanical medicine: A review. *Phytother. Res.* **2005**, *19*, 655–660. [CrossRef] [PubMed]
33. Klomklao, S.; Benjakul, S.; Kishimura, H.; Chaijan, M. Extraction, purification and properties of trypsin inhibitor from Thai mung bean (*Vigna radiata* (L.) R. Wilczek). *Food Chem.* **2011**, *129*, 1348–1354. [CrossRef]
34. Le, A.V.; Parks, S.E.; Nguyen, M.H.; Roach, P.D. Effect of solvents and extraction methods on recovery of bioactive compounds from defatted Gac (*Momordica cochinchinensis* Spreng.) seeds. *Separations* **2018**, *5*, 39. [CrossRef]
35. Makkar, H.P.; Siddhuraju, P.; Becker, K. Trypsin Inhibitor. In *Plant Secondary Metabolites*; Humana Press: New York, NY, USA, 2007; pp. 1–6.
36. Stauffer, C.E. Measuring trypsin inhibitor in soy meal: Suggested improvements in the standard method. *Cereal Chem.* **1990**, *67*, 296–302.
37. Tan, S.P.; Tuyen, K.C.; Parks, S.E.; Stathopoulos, C.E.; Roach, P.D. Effects of the spray-drying temperatures on the physiochemical properties of an encapsulated bitter melon aqueous extract powder. *Powder Technol.* **2015**, *281*, 65–75. [CrossRef]
38. Tan, S.P.; Vuong, Q.V.; Stathopoulos, C.E.; Parks, S.E.; Roach, P.D. Optimized aqueous extraction of saponins from bitter melon for production of a saponin-enriched bitter melon powder. *J. Food Sci.* **2014**, *79*, E1372–E1381. [CrossRef] [PubMed]
39. Thaipong, K.; Boonprakob, U.; Crosby, K.; Cisneros-Zevallos, L.; Byrne, D.H. Comparison of ABTS, DPPH, FRAP, and ORAC assays for estimating antioxidant activity from guava fruit extracts. *J. Food Compost. Anal.* **2006**, *19*, 669–675. [CrossRef]
40. Ishiyama, M.; Tominaga, H.; Shiga, M.; Sasamoto, K.; Ohkura, Y.; Ueno, K. A combined assay of cell vability and in vitro cytotoxicity with a highly water-soluble tetrazolium salt, neutral red and crystal violet. *Biol. Pharm Bull.* **1996**, *19*, 1518–1520. [CrossRef] [PubMed]
41. Wimalasiri, D. Genetic Diversity, Nutritional and Biological Activity of *Momordica cochinchinensis* (Cucurbitaceae). Ph.D. Thesis, RMIT University, Melbourne, Australia, 2015.
42. Arimatsu, P.; Sawangsook, O. Purification and characterization of Trypsin inhibitor from *Momordica cochinchinensis* Spreng. seed and its effects to Spodoptera litura. *Asian J. Plant Sci.* **2012**, *11*, 195–199. [CrossRef]
43. Cascales, L.; Henriques, S.T.; Kerr, M.C.; Huang, Y.-H.; Sweet, M.J.; Daly, N.L.; Craik, D.J. Identification and

characterization of a new family of cell-penetrating peptides cyclic cell-penetrating peptides. *J. Biol. Chem.* **2011**, *286*, 36932–36943. [CrossRef] [PubMed]

44. Anderson, R.L.; Wolf, W.J. Compositional changes in trypsin inhibitors, phytic acid, saponins and isoflavones related to soybean processing. *J. Nutr.* **1995**, *125*, 581S. [CrossRef] [PubMed]
45. Birk, Y. *Plant Protease Inhibitors as Cancer Chemopreventive Agents*; Springer: Berlin, Germany, 2003; ISBN 978-3-642-05514-0.
46. Troll, W.; Kennedy, A.R. *Protease Inhibitors as Cancer Chemopreventive Agents*; Plenum Pub Corp: New York, NY, USA, 1993; ISBN 0306443902.
47. Kennedy, A.R. Chemopreventive agents: Protease inhibitors. *Pharmacol. Ther.* **1998**, *78*, 167–209. [CrossRef]
48. Housman, G.; Byler, S.; Heerboth, S.; Lapinska, K.; Longacre, M.; Snyder, N.; Sarkar, S. Drug resistance in cancer: An overview. *Cancers* **2014**, *6*, 1769–1792. [CrossRef] [PubMed]
49. Chan, K.W.; Iqbal, S.; Khong, N.M.; Ooi, D.-J.; Ismail, M. Antioxidant activity of phenolics–saponins rich fraction prepared from defatted kenaf seed meal. *LWT-Food Sci. Technol.* **2014**, *56*, 181–186. [CrossRef]
50. Hostettmann, K.; Marston, A. *Chemistry and Pharmacology of Natural Products, Saponin*; Cambridge University Press: Cambridge, NY, USA, 1995; ISBN 0-521-32970-1.
51. US Food and Drug Administration (FDA). *Guidance for Industry*; USHaH Services, Ed.; US Food and Drug Administration (FDA): Silver Spring, MD, USA, 2012.
52. Yasukawa, K.; Akihisa, T.; Tamura, T.; Takido, M. Inhibitory effect of karounidiol on 12-O-tetradecanoylphorbol-13-acetate-induced tumor promotion. *Biol. Pharm Bull.* **1994**, *17*, 460–462. [CrossRef] [PubMed]
53. Le, A.V.; Parks, S.E.; Nguyen, M.H.; Roach, P.D. Optimisation of the microwave-assisted ethanol extraction of saponins from Gac (*Momordica cochinchinensis* Spreng) seeds. *Medicines* **2018**, *5*, 70. [CrossRef] [PubMed]

3

Resveratrol and Pterostilbene Exhibit Anticancer Properties Involving the Downregulation of HPV Oncoprotein E6 in Cervical Cancer Cells

Kaushiki Chatterjee [1,2], Dina AlSharif [2], Christina Mazza [2], Palwasha Syar [2], Mohamed Al Sharif [2] and Jimmie E. Fata [1,2,*]

1 Doctoral Program in Biology, CUNY Graduate Center, New York, NY 10016, USA; kaushiki.chatterjee@csi.cuny.edu

2 Department of Biology, College of Staten Island, New York, NY 10314, USA; dina95usa@aol.com (D.A.); Christinamazza19@gmail.com (C.M.); palwashasyar@yahoo.com (P.S.); Alsharif.mohamed@hotmail.com (M.A.S.)

* Correspondence: jimmie.fata@csi.cuny.edu;

Abstract: Cervical cancer is one of the most common cancers in women living in developing countries. Due to a lack of affordable effective therapy, research into alternative anticancer compounds with low toxicity such as dietary polyphenols has continued. Our aim is to determine whether two structurally similar plant polyphenols, resveratrol and pterostilbene, exhibit anticancer and anti-HPV (Human papillomavirus) activity against cervical cancer cells. To determine anticancer activity, extensive in vitro analyses were performed. Anti-HPV activity, through measuring E6 protein levels, subsequent downstream p53 effects, and caspase-3 activation, were studied to understand a possible mechanism of action. Both polyphenols are effective agents in targeting cervical cancer cells, having low IC50 values in the μM range. They decrease clonogenic survival, reduce cell migration, arrest cells at the S-phase, and reduce the number of mitotic cells. These findings were significant, with pterostilbene often being more effective than resveratrol. Resveratrol and to a greater extent pterostilbene downregulates the HPV oncoprotein E6, induces caspase-3 activation, and upregulates p53 protein levels. Results point to a mechanism that may involve the downregulation of the HPV E6 oncoprotein, activation of apoptotic pathways, and re-establishment of functional p53 protein, with pterostilbene showing greater efficacy than resveratrol.

Keywords: cervical cancer; resveratrol; pterostilbene; HPV E6; p53; cell cycle

---

1. Introduction

Cervical cancer is one of the most prevalent cancers affecting women worldwide. It is the second most common cancer in developing countries and 11th in developed countries—these regional differences are often attributed to the lack of Pap smears, a preventative procedure often absent in underdeveloped areas [1,2]. It is widely accepted that the etiological factor that causes cervical cancer is chronic infection of the human papilloma virus (HPV), which is considered the most common sexually transmitted infection [3]. Every year about 500,000 women acquire the disease and 75% are from the developing countries [4]. Moreover, recent evidence indicates that HPV infection is on the rise in men, leading to higher incidences of penile and oropharyngeal cancer [5]. HPVs can be clinically classified as "low-risk" (LR-HPV) or "high-risk" (HR-HPV) depending on the relative tendency of the HPV lesions to transform into malignancy. HPV 16 and HPV 18 are the two most important cancer-causing, high-risk HPV [6]. HPV progression to cancer is dependent on prolonged infection by these high risk HPV viruses. The progression of HPV lesions to a neoplastic stage is dependent on several co-factors. Although there are approved HPV vaccines and drugs available, a problem is the affordability of these drugs in low income areas [7]. Two such vaccines are Cervarix® and Gardasil® [8], which renders prophylactic actions against cervical lesions associated with the most common oncogenic HPV types, 16/18, but effective therapeutic measures for post-infection lesions are currently not available. The major concern for the common chemotherapeutic medicines like cisplatin and paclitaxel are their adverse side effects [9,10]. The development of natural chemoprotective drugs that effectively target HPV infection could drastically reduce the incidence and progression of cervical cancer worldwide if they are not cost inhibitive and have low side effects.

Of the varied groups of naturally occurring antioxidants, polyphenols have gained increased importance in cervical cancer since they have displayed potent antitumor properties in a number of cancers by targeting several pathways that are involved in cancer progression [11,12]. The current article uses cervical cancer cells to compare the tumor-inhibitory effects and mechanism of action of two such polyphenols, resveratrol and pterostilbene. Both resveratrol and pterostilbene are stilbenes, which is a class of natural polyphenolic compounds that have been studied for their anticarcinogenic activities. Resveratrol (3,4,5-trihydroxy-trans-stilbene) has been isolated from grapes, red wine, purple grape juice, peanuts, berries, and some medicinal plants [13]. Resveratrol is a widely studied stilbene compound having very low toxicity in the human system, and it is also known to modulate several pathways that are directly linked to cancer progression [14]. Both in vitro and in vivo cancer studies have shown resveratrol to inhibit cell proliferation and angiogenesis along with inducing pro-apoptotic properties [15]. The potential problem of using resveratrol as a chemoprotective agent is that it has low systemic bioavailability, which might lower its efficacy in the human system [16]. In order to overcome this, several efforts are being made to develop resveratrol derivatives with higher systemic bioavailability [17]. Pterostilbene (trans-3,5-dimethoxy-4-hydroxystilbene) is a naturally derived dimethylether analogue of resveratrol. Pterostilbene is believed to be produced in plants as a defense mechanism against some external microbial or fungal infection and is therefore considered a phytoalexin [18]. It has been isolated from grapevine leaves and blueberries [19]. Recently, pterostilbene has gained much attention as a possible anticancer agent, showing no toxicity in humans up to a dose of 250 mg/day [20].

Although the chemical structure of pterostilbene is closely related to resveratrol, the substitution of the hydroxyl group with a methoxy group in pterostilbene is believed to make the molecule more stable as well as increase its capacity to enter cells [21]. In addition, clinical studies have shown that the half-life and oral bioavailability of pterostilbene are significantly greater than those of resveratrol [20]. Studies on colon cancer cell lines have shown pterostilbene to be more potent than resveratrol in inhibiting DNA synthesis and in decreasing the expression of inflammatory genes responsible for cancer progression [22]. Although studies in other types of carcinomas show the potential efficacy of resveratrol and pterostilbene, there has been no study to the best of our knowledge that explores an anticancer mechanism that is specific for HPV-positive carcinoma. An in silico docking study has shown that resveratrol interacts with the p53 binding site of E6 residues [23]. E6 is a vital HPV oncoprotein essential for cervical cancer progression. E6 binds to tumor suppressor protein p53 and targets it for degradation by the ubiquitin proteasome pathway [24], thus causing uncontrolled cell proliferation. Here, we set out to compare the relative effectiveness of resveratrol against pterostilbene on cervical cancer cells, paying particular attention to their comparative IC_{50} values, changes in the levels of the HPV oncoprotein E6 and its target p53, as well as their comparative pro-apoptotic and anti-migratory capacities.

2. Materials and Methods

2.1. Cell Culture

Human cervical carcinoma HeLa cells were obtained from a commercial supplier (American Type Culture Collection, Manassas, VA, USA) and were cultured in Dulbecco's Modified Eagle

Medium: Nutrient Mixture F-12 (DMEM/F-12) (HyClone, GE Healthcare Life Sciences, Manassas, VA, USA), supplemented with 10% fetal calf serum (HyClone, GE Healthcare Life Sciences) and 0.1% Penicillin-Streptomycin Solution (HyClone). Cells were incubated in a 37 °C incubator with 5% CO_2.

2.2. *Determination of IC_{50} Using WST-1 Assay*

Seven thousand cells were plated on 96-well plates and allowed to grow for 24 h. Resveratrol (Acros, #430075000) or pterostilbene (TCI, #P1924) was serially diluted from 10–120 μM into DMEM/F-12 plus 1× insulin-transferrin-selenium (ITS) supplement (Invitrogen). Cells were treated with dilutions (in triplicate) for 24 h prior to performing a WST-1 (Water Soluble Tetrazolium salt-1) cell viability assay. The WST assay involved aspiration of the medium after treatment and rinsing three times with equal volumes of 1×Phosphate Buffered Saline (PBS), followed by the addition of 80 μL of 10% WST-1 (Clontech, Mountain View, CA, USA) in DMEM to each well. The plate was then incubated at 37 °C for 1 h and absorbance monitored at 440 nm using a plate reader. Results obtained were analyzed using GraphPad Prism 5 software to determine the IC_{50} using a standardized method [25,26].

2.3. *Live Imaging*

Images of untreated and treated (with resveratrol and pterostilbene) cells were taken every 10 min for 24 h to generate video files using a Zeiss Axio Observer Z1 microscope.

2.4. *Clonogenic Assay*

Two hundred thousand cells were plated on 6-well plates and allowed to grow for 24 h prior to treatment with pterostilbene (50 μM) and resveratrol (50 μM) for 24 h. After 24 h, cells were trypsinized to single cell suspensions. After cell counting, 150 viable cells from each treatment set were plated in one well from a 6-well plate and allowed to grow in complete DMEM/F-12 medium for 15 days. After said period of time, cells were washed once with 1× PBS then fixed and stained with 0.5% crystal violet in 6% glutaraldehyde for 30 min. The cells were briefly rinsed with tap water and allowed to air dry. Images of each well was taken and colonies were counted using ImageJ (NIH, Bethesda, Rockville, MD, USA). The plating efficiency and survival factor was calculated as determined previously [27].

2.5. *Scratch Assay*

Twelve thousand cells were grown on 96-well plates until a confluent monolayer was formed. A scratch was made with a sterile p200 tip in each well through the center of the culture. The debris was washed off with serum-free media and a marking was made on the bottom of the plate to take images at the same location. Cells were then treated with different concentrations (5 μM and 20 μM) of resveratrol or pterostilbene and brightfield images were taken after 48 h to allow closure of the control scratch. The images were analyzed using ImageJ and the area of closure was measured according to previous published methods [28].

2.6. *Flow Cytometry*

Two hundred and fifty thousand cells were cultured on 6-well plates and subsequently treated with resveratrol or pterostilbene (5 μM, 10 μM, and 15 μM) for 18 h. Cells were trypsinized, centrifuged, and washed with 0.1% Fetal Calf Serum (FCS) in 1× PBS solution and resuspended in 70% ethanol at −20 °C, which was added dropwise while shaking the samples vigorously. Fixed samples were kept at 4 °C for 1 h followed by washing twice in 1× PBS. Prior to flow cytometry, cells were incubated with RNase (500 μg/mL) for 30 min at 37 °C and then stained with propidium iodide (PI; 70 μM) for 30 mins. Cells were analyzed for DNA content by measuring PI fluorescence using an Accuri C6 flow cytometer (BD).

2.7. Western Blot Analysis

Two hundred and fifty thousand cells were cultured on 6-well plates and subsequently treated with resveratrol (10 μM, 50 μM) or pterostilbene (10 μM, 50 μM) for a period of 22 h. Extraction of proteins from cultured cells was performed using M-PER Mammalian protein extraction reagent (Thermo Fisher, Waltham, MA, USA) with protease and phosphatase inhibitors. The total amount of protein in each well was quantified using the Lowry method. To resolve the proteins, 25 μg of protein was subjected to sodium dodecyl sulfate-polyacrylamide gel electrophoresis using a 10% acrylamide separating gel and then transferred to nitrocellulose membrane for 1 h. The membrane was blocked at room temperature for 1 h with 5% nonfat dry milk in Tris Tween Buffered Saline (TTBS). The nitrocellulose membrane was then incubated overnight with a p53 antibody (sc-6243) followed by incubation at room temperature for 1 h with anti-rabbit IgG conjugated with horseradish peroxidase. SuperSignal West Pico chemiluminescence substrate (Pierce) was used for detection following the manufacturer's instructions. The membranes were scanned using APHA INNOTECH Fluorchem SP imaging system. Analysis of blots was done using ImageJ software.

2.8. Immunocytochemistry

Seven thousand HeLa cells were plated on 8-well chamber slides and allowed to grow for 48 h. Cells were then treated with different concentrations of resveratrol (5–50 μM) or pterostilbene (5–50 μM) for 22 h (for study of E6, p53 and cleaved caspase-3) and 18 h (for study of Phospho histone H3). All drug treatments were performed in serum-free DMEM/F-12 containing 1% supplement (ITS; insulin, transferrin, selenium; Gibco BRL, Grand Island, NY, USA). After treatment, cells were fixed in 4% paraformaldehyde at room temperature, rinsed with 1× PBS, and then permeabilized and blocked with 10% horse serum, 2% bovine serum albumin, and 0.5% Triton X-100 in PBS for 1 h. The cells were then incubated overnight with primary antibodies in blocking buffer. Subsequent to primary antibody treatment, the cells were washed and then incubated with the respective Fluorescein isothiocyanate (FITC) conjugated secondary antibodies for 3 h, followed by incubation with 4′,6-diamidino-2-phenylindole (DAPI) (10 μg/mL) and three washes with 1× PBS. The slides were then mounted with coverslips and cell images were acquired using a Zeiss Axio Observer Z1 microscope and an AxioVision 4.6.3-AP1. Images of different, randomly chosen fields were acquired with identical exposure times from each well for quantification. ImageJ was used to measure the fluorescence intensity and cell counting. The fluorescence intensities of E6 and P53 antibodies were normalized to DAPI intensity (blue).

Antibodies Used: E6 antibody (sc-460, Santa Cruz Biotechnology, Dallas, TX, USA), p53 antibody (sc-6243), cleaved caspase-3 antibody (D175, 9661, CST), Phospho Histone H3 (Ser 10) antibody (06–570, Millipore, Burlington, MA, USA).

2.9. Statistical Analysis

Statistical analyses were performed using Microsoft Excel® 2013 (Microsoft Corporation, Redmond, WA, USA) and GraphPad Prism® 5 (GraphPad Software, Inc., La Jolla, CA, USA). Means and standard deviations were calculated for each group. One-way ANOVA with Tukey test was used to compare three or more datasets and determine the significance between the groups. ANOVA is a test of variance and post hoc Tukey test used is for the determination of significance between groups [29,30]. $p < 0.05$ was considered as significant.

3. Results

3.1. Pterostilbene Is More Potent in Eliminating HPV+ HeLa Cells Compared to Resveratrol

In order to study the comparative cytotoxicity of pterostilbene and resveratrol on HeLa tumor cells, brightfield images (Figure 1A) and WST-1 cell viability assays (Figure 1B) were performed 24 h post-treatment. The brightfield images taken after 24 h of treatment (Figure 1A) showed that pterostilbene (40 µM) eliminates significantly more cells than resveratrol at the same concentration. Live imaging of cells treated with 60 µM of the two compounds show significantly more death and characteristic apoptotic blebbing in pterostilbene-treated cells when compared to untreated or resveratrol-treated cells (Supplementary Videos S1–S3). The WST-1 analysis revealed that although both pterostilbene and resveratrol eliminated HeLa cells significantly and in a dose-dependent manner, pterostilbene displayed a 1.97-fold lower IC_{50} when compared to resveratrol (42.3 µM vs. 83.5 µM; $p < 0.05$; Figure 1B). Additionally, both compounds, at 50 µM, significantly inhibited the clonogenicity of post-treated cells in a 15-day clonogenic assay (Figure 1C). Pterostilbene significantly reduced clonogenic survival by 87.5% compared to the control ($p < 0.05$), while resveratrol inhibited it by 63% ($p < 0.05$) (Figure 1C). Moreover, the difference between the survival percentages of the two treatment groups is significant ($p < 0.05$).

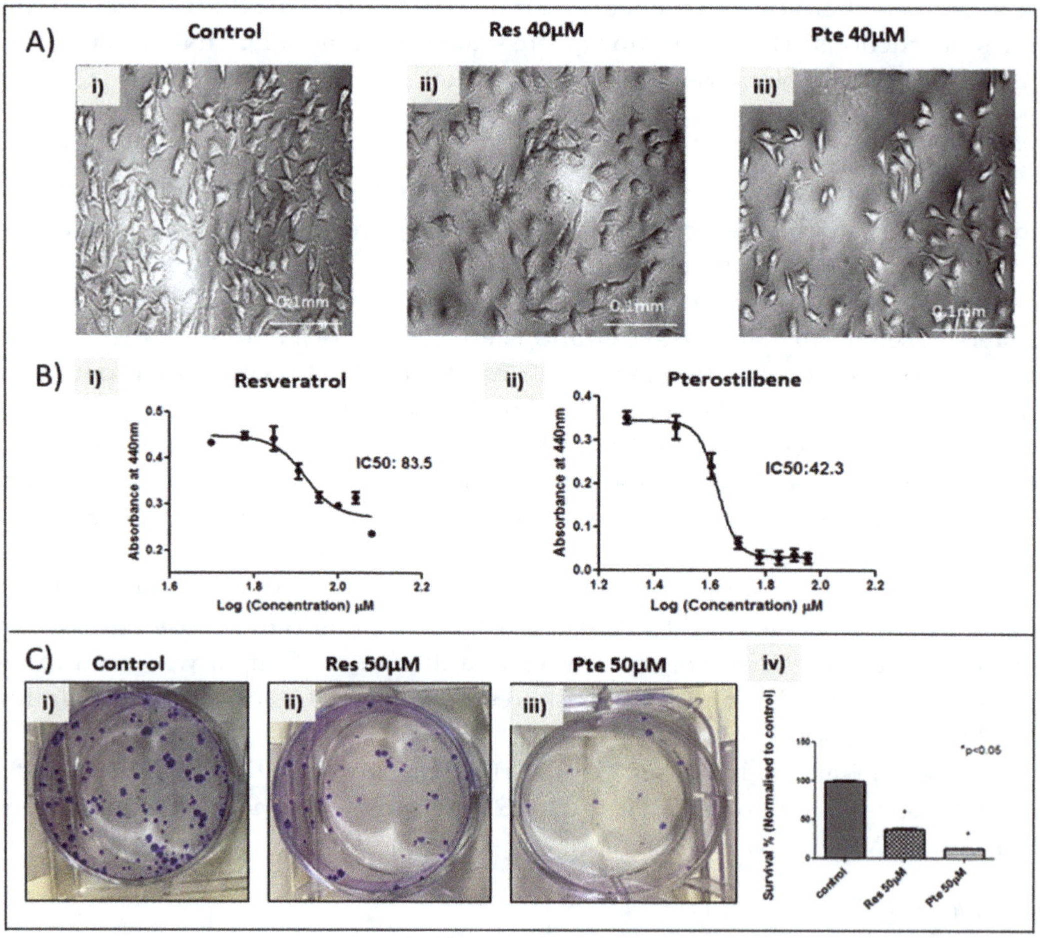

Figure 1. Pterostilbene is more potent in eliminating HeLa cervical cancer cells as compared to resveratrol: (**A**) Brightfield analysis of HeLa cells untreated (Ai) or treated for 24 h with 40 µM of resveratrol (Res; Aii) or 40 µM of pterostilbene (Pte; Aiii). Evidence of cell elimination was only seen robustly in cells treated with pterostilbene at 40 µM. (**B**) Analysis of IC_{50} values, generated by a Water Soluble Tetrazolium salt-1 (WST-1) assay after 24 h of exposure to resveratrol or pterostilbene indicates that pterostilbene (IC_{50} = 42.3 µM) is a more potent cytotoxic agent than resveratrol (IC_{50} = 83.5 µM; Bii). The graphs represent data from three independent experiments (mean ± S.E.M. (Standard error mean)). (**C**) Clonogenic assays performed to compare the relative effect of the two polyphenols on the clonogenicity of HeLa cells untreated (Ci) or treated with 50 µM of either resveratrol (Cii) or pterostilbene (Ciii). Results are from 15-days post-treatment and indicate that pterostilbene is more efficient in curbing the clonogenicity compared to resveratrol (Civ). Bar graph represents data from three independent experiments (mean ± S.E.M.; * $p < 0.05$; Civ).

3.2. *Inhibition of Cell Migration of HeLa Cells Treated with Pterostilbene and Resveratrol*

To determine the comparative efficacy of resveratrol and pterostilbene in inhibiting HeLa cell migration, two different sub-lethal concentrations of each compound were used in a 48-h scratch assay (Figure 2). Based on the WST-1 results and brightfield images (unpublished), we found that cells treated with a concentration below 25 µM showed no signs of cellular toxicity. To avoid any cytotoxicity, we used lower concentrations of 5 µM and 20 µM. At sub-lethal concentrations of 5 µM and 20 µM, both resveratrol and pterostilbene significantly inhibited HeLa cell migration relative to untreated cells ($p < 0.05$; Figure 2). Pterostilbene was more effective in inhibiting HeLa cell migration at 20 µM when compared to resveratrol; however, this result was not significant and no differences were seen between the two compounds at 5 µM (Figure 2). In an effort to analyze the effects of resveratrol and pterostilbene on cell migration, we normalized the amount of migration into the scratch (wound) by untreated cells, to 100%. Relative to this control, resveratrol-treated cells migrated only 71.2% (5 µM) and 63.7% (20 µM), while cells treated with pterostilbene migrated only 69.5% (5 µM) and 49.2% (20 µM) (Figure 2).

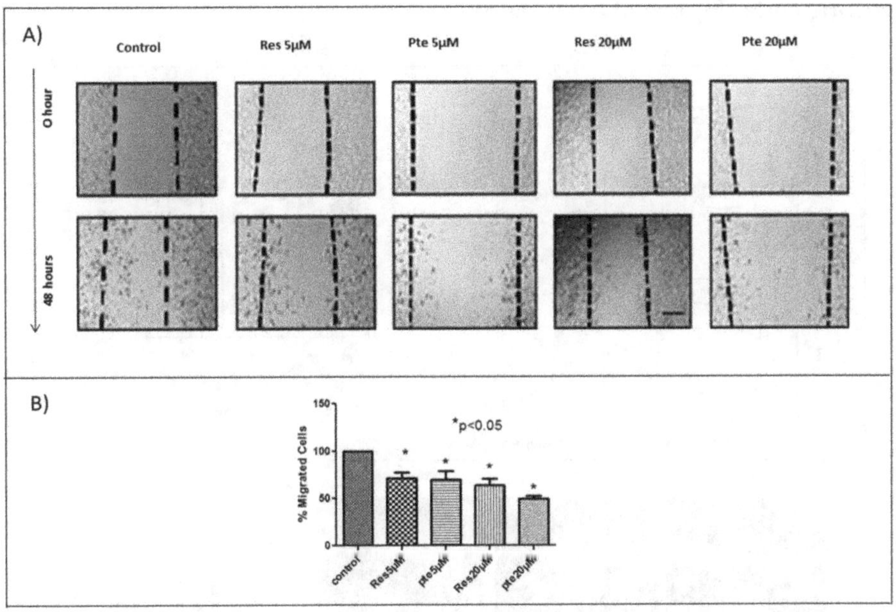

Figure 2. Resveratrol and pterostilbene inhibit cell migration: (**A**) HeLa cells were monitored for cell migration into a scratched "wound". Cells were either untreated or treated with sub-lethal concentrations (5 µM and 20 µM) of resveratrol (Res) or pterostilbene (Pte). The extent of migration into the scratched area was calculated after 48 h and revealed that both resveratrol and pterostilbene significantly inhibit cell migration, although pterostilbene had greater anti-migratory effect. (**B**) The graphs represents data from triplicate sample experiments normalized to the control (mean % migrated cells ± S.E.M.; * $p < 0.05$). Scale bar: 0.05 µm.

3.3. *Cell Cycle Arrest at S-Phase in HeLa Cells Treated with Low Concentrations of Resveratrol and Pterostilbene*

In order to compare the effect of sub-lethal doses of either resveratrol or pterostilbene on the cell cycle of HeLa cells, treatment was carried out with three different concentrations (5 µM, 10 µM, and 15 µM) of the two compounds for 18 h prior to flow cytometric analysis (Figure 3A). Flow cytometry analysis showed that the cells treated with either compound exhibited a significant decrease in the number of cells in the G2-M phase with respect to the control cells ($p < 0.05$) (Figure 3A,B, Table 1), indicating an S-phase cell cycle arrest. This effect corresponded with an increase in the number of cells arrested at the S-phase. Pterostilbene was significantly more potent than resveratrol in inhibiting cell cycle progression, showing effects at concentrations as low as

5 μM ($p < 0.05$) (Figure 3A,B, Table 1). At this concentration, pterostilbene had these percentages of cells in each phase: G1 = 53.4 ± 1.4, S = 34 ± 1.4, G2 =12.5 ± 0.2, while resveratrol had values of G1 = 64.8 ± 2.0, S = 16.3 ± 1.0, G2 = 18.3 ± 2.3. At a higher concentration (15 μM) both compounds significantly inhibited cells from entering into G2-M by arresting them in the S-phase, and difference between the extent of the arrest at this phase induced by the two compounds was significant ($p < 0.05$) (Figure 3A,B, Table 1).

To confirm the cell cycle data, which indicated that both compounds are potent inhibitors of cells entering into G2-M, we investigated the status of the M-phase mitotic marker phospho-histone-H3 by immunocytochemistry (Figure 3C,D). At concentrations of 10 μM, both compounds significantly suppressed the amount of cells positive for the mitotic marker phospho-histone-H3, when compared to the untreated cells control. Although resveratrol significantly suppressed the abundance of phospho-histone-H3 (mitotic cells) at 5 μM, when compared to the control cells, pterostilbene at this concentration was significantly more potent than resveratrol (Figure 3D). Relative to the control, which was set at 100%, cells treated with 5 μM pterostilbene exhibited only 13.8% mitotic cells positive for the marker, which was significantly lower than the resveratrol-treated sample at this concentration, which had 60% mitotic cells (Figure 3D; $p < 0.05$).

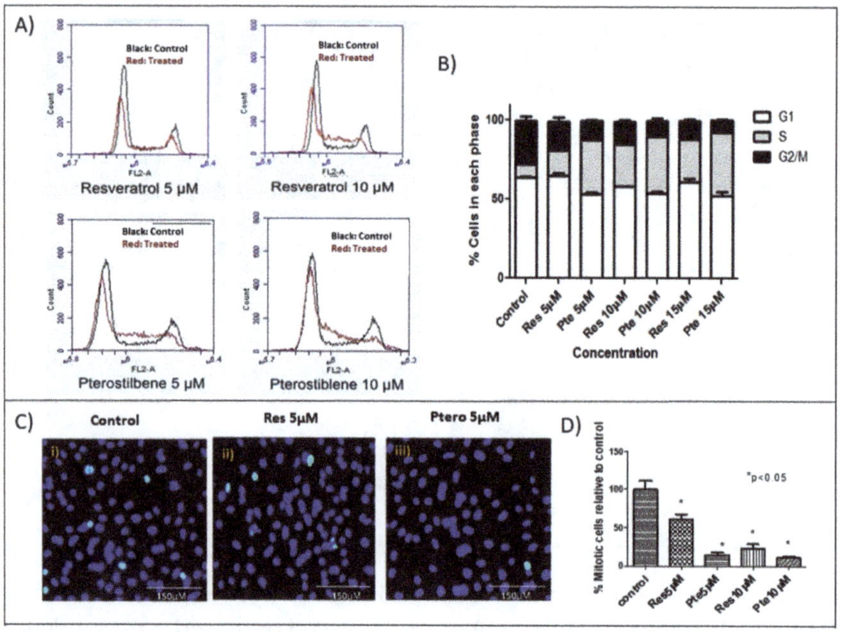

Figure 3. S-phase arrest in HeLa cells treated with low concentrations of resveratrol and pterostilbene: (**A**) Flow-cytometric evaluation of HeLa cells untreated or treated with sub-lethal doses of resveratrol (Res) and pterostilbene (Pte) for 18 h. Treated cells exhibited S-phase arrest and a subsequent decrease in the number of cells in G2/M. Pterostilbene was a more potent compound than resveratrol, showing a capacity to arrest cells at the S-phase at concentrations as low as 5 μM. (**B**) Graphical representation of the dose-dependent cell cycle effects induced by resveratrol and pterostilbene at three different concentrations (5 μM, 10 μM, and 15 μM). (**B**) The graph represents data from triplicate sample experiments normalized to the control (mean % cells in each phase ± S.E.M.) (**C**) Immunofluorescent images of HeLa cells probed for the M-phase marker phospho-histone-H3 (serine10). HeLa cells were untreated or treated with 5 μM and 10 μM of resveratrol or pterostilbene. Immunofluorescent images display a decrease of histone-H3 in cells treated with both the compounds, the effects at 5 μM of pterostilbene is much greater than those of resveratrol (at 5 μM). (**D**) Graphical representation of the percent of mitotic cells calculated from immunofluorescent images reveal that resveratrol and to a greater extent pterostilbene are effective in decreasing the number of mitotic HeLa cells. The graph represents data from experiments obtained from triplicate samples normalized to the control (mean % mitotic cells ± S.E.M.;* $p < 0.05$).

Table 1. Table showing the percentage of cells in each phase of the cell cycle (% ± S.E.M.) after treatment with different concentrations of resveratrol (Res) and pterostilbene (Pte).

	G1 ± S.E.M.	S ± S.E.M.	G2 ± S.E.M.
Control	64.1 ± 0.4	8.00 ± 2.5	27.7 ± 2.4
Res 5 μM	64.8 ± 2.0	16.3 ± 1.0	18.3 ± 2.3 ^
Pte 5 μM	53.4 ± 1.4 +	34.0 ± 1.4 *	12.5 ± 0.2 ^
Res 10 μM	58.5 ± 0.2	26.5 ± 0.2 *	14.4 ± 1.0 ^
Pte 10 μM	54.3 ± 0.8 +	35.6 ± 2.4 *	10.1 ± 1.5 ^
Res 15 μM	61.3 ± 1.9	27.1 ± 0.8 *,#	11.5 ± 1.2 ^
Pte 15 μM	52.3 ± 2.0 +	40.1 ± 3.4 *,#	7.7 ± 0.5 ^

+ $p < 0.05$ relative to G1 control, * $p < 0.05$ relative to S control, ^ $p < 0.05$ relative to G2 control, # $p < 0.05$ relative to each other.

3.4. Downregulation of Viral Oncoprotein E6 and Upregulation of Active-Caspase-3 in HeLa Cells Treated with Pterostilbene and Resveratrol

In order to investigate how resveratrol and pterostilbene were affecting HeLa cell survival and cell cycle progression, we treated cells with either of the two compounds at sub-lethal (10 μM) and higher (50 μM) concentrations prior to analysis by immunostaining for E6, active caspase-3, and p53 (Figure 4A–C). At 10 μM, both resveratrol and pterostilbene failed to significantly affect levels of E6 and active caspase-3 levels relative to the control (Figure 4A,B). However, at 50 μM both compounds significantly suppressed E6 levels and elevated cleaved caspase-3 levels in treated cells relative to the untreated cells (Figure 3A–C). At this concentration (50 μM), pterostilbene was significantly more potent than resveratrol at suppressing E6 levels (resveratrol = 0.77 ± 0.11: 23% decrease vs. pterostilbene = 0.57 ± 0.06: 43% decrease; $p < 0.05$) and simultaneously elevating active caspase-3. It should be noted that we were unable to detect any noticeable differences in the sub-cellular localization of E6 in treated cells (Figure 4A).

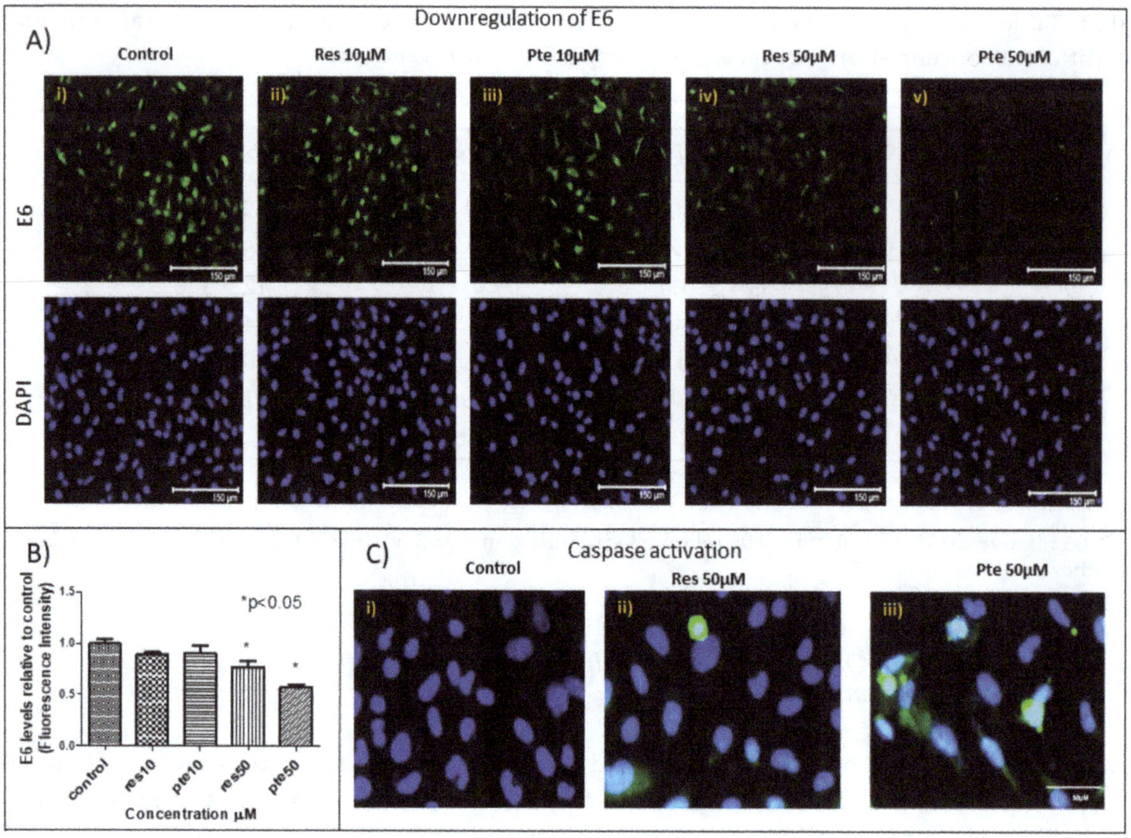

Figure 4. Downregulation of viral oncoprotein E6 and upregulation of active-caspase-3 in HeLa cells treated with resveratrol or pterostilbene: (**A**) HeLa cells immunostained for E6 levels (green) and counterstained with the nuclear dye 4′,6-diamidino-2-phenylindole (DAPI) (blue) after treatment with resveratrol (Res) and pterostilbene (Pte; 10 µM and 50 µM). Loss of E6 proteins are visually evident in cells treated with 50 µM of either resveratrol or pterostilbene. (**B**) Cell image analysis of the E6 fluorescent data revealed a significant 43% decrease of E6 protein levels in HeLa cells treated with pterostilbene at 50 µM and a 23% decrease of E6 levels in cells treated with resveratrol, both relative to the control. The graph represents data from experiments obtained from three independent experiments normalized to the control (mean % normalized to DAPI ± S.E.M.; * $p < 0.05$). (**C**) Immunofluorescent images probing for active-caspase-3 (green) shows a corresponding enhanced activation of this mediator of apoptosis by both resveratrol and pterostilbene.

3.5. Upregulation of Tumor Suppressor Protein p53 in HeLa Cells Treated with Pterostilbene and Resveratrol

Concomitant with E6 suppression, 50 µM pterostilbene treatment for 22 h caused an upregulation of p53 in HeLa cells (Figure 5A,B). When compared to the control, pterostilbene treatment elicited a 2-fold increase in p53 levels (staining normalized to DAPI; Figure 5B; $p < 0.05$). In comparison to the control, HeLa cells treated with 50 µM of resveratrol also caused an upregulation of p53 (1.75-fold increase; Figure 5A,B; $p < 0.05$) at 22 h.

Total protein levels of p53 were also analyzed by Western blot in cells treated with either resveratrol (10 µM and 50 µM) or pterostilbene (10 µM and 50 µM) for 22 h (Figure 5C,D). Both compounds elevated p53 levels at 50 µM; however, significance was only noted in cells treated with pterostilbene at this concentration (Figure 5C,D). Although cells treated with pterostilbene at 10 µM tended to have elevated p53 protein levels relative to both the control cells and cells treated with 10 µM of resveratrol, these differences were not significant based on an ANOVA test (Figure 5C,D).

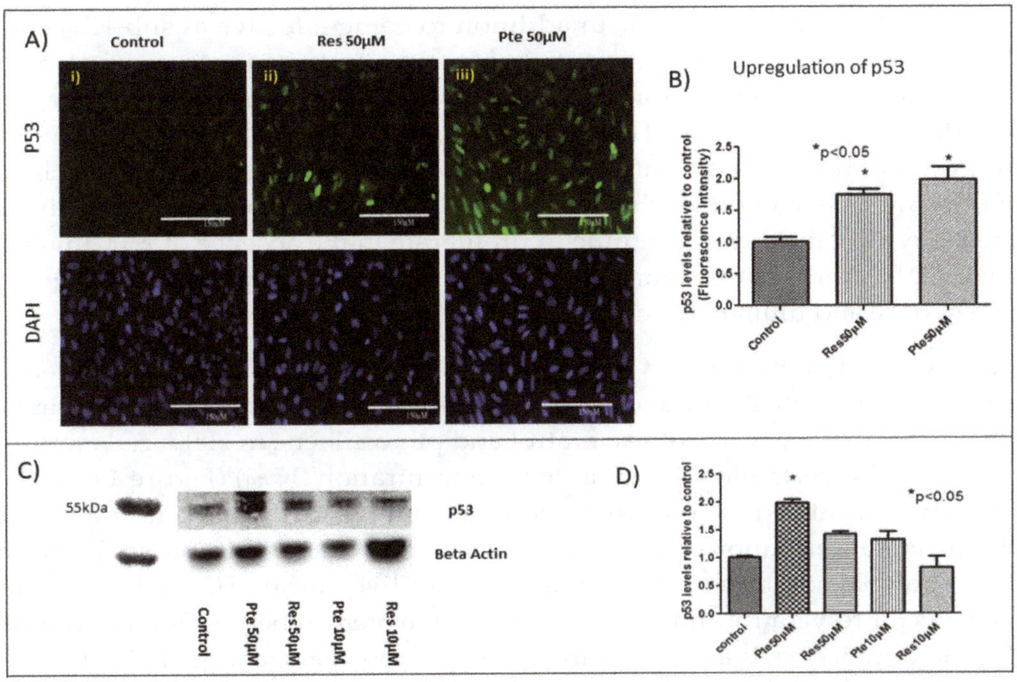

Figure 5. Upregulation of the tumor suppressor protein p53 in HeLa cells treated with resveratrol and pterostilbene: (**A**) Immunoflourescent images of p53 protein (green) untreated or after treatment with 50 μM of either resveratrol (Res) or pterostilbene (Pte) for 22 h. Levels of p53 are elevated in cells treated with either polyphenol. (**B**) Image analysis of p53 immunofluorescence indicates that pterostilbene treatment at 50 μM elicited a significant 2-fold increase in p53, while resveratrol exposure at similar concentrations induced a significant 1.75 increase in p53. The graph represents data from experiments obtained from three independent experiments normalized to the control (mean % normalized to DAPI ± S.E.M. * $p < 0.05$). (**C**) Western blot analysis also revealed that the elevation of p53 protein levels is evident in HeLa cells treated with 50 μM of resveratrol and pterostilbene; however, significant differences relative to the control were only reached with HeLa cells treated pterostilbene at 50 μM. (**D**) The graph represents data from experiments obtained from three independent experiments normalized to the control (mean % normalized to beta-actin ± S.E.M.; * $p < 0.05$).

4. Discussion and Conclusions

In the current study, for the first time to our knowledge, we have compared the antitumor potency of resveratrol and pterostilbene on E6+ cervical cancer cells in vitro. We demonstrated that pterostilbene was significantly more potent than resveratrol in eliminating and in abrogating the clonogenicity of these cervical cancer cells (Figure 1). To assess and study the effects of the two compounds, we used a wide range of concentrations. Sub IC_{50} concentrations ranging from 5–20 μM were used to understand the action of these polyphenols at a low concentration. The results show that at these concentrations the polyphenols can inhibit cell division and migration. To further understand the cytotoxic mechanisms, it was imperative for us to look at supra IC_{50} concentrations. We used 50 μM to understand the mechanism of action. The clonogenic assay using this high concentration elucidates the long-term effect of these polyphenols on surviving cells even after the removal of treatment. While sub-IC_{50} values of both compounds inhibited the migration of E6+ cervical cancer cells, a higher sub-lethal concentration of resveratrol (20 μM) was needed to exert any significant inhibitory effect. Nonetheless, pterostilbene caused a more significant degree of inhibition to cell migration, attesting its superior antitumor potency (Figure 2). It is a notion held by cancer researchers that sub-IC_{50} concentrations of chemotherapeutic drugs are ineffective in curtailing tumor malignancy. However, surprisingly, our data shows that even at a low sub-lethal concentration (5 μM), pterostilbene is more effective than resveratrol as an antiproliferative agent against cervical cancer cells by triggering cell cycle arrest at the S-phase (Figure 3). In addition to being effective at sub-IC_{50} concentrations, the supra-IC_{50} concentration of pterostilbene (50 μM) was also superior to resveratrol (at 50 μM) in suppressing E6 while upregulating p53 and active-caspase-3 expression, thus causing a greater degree of apoptosis-mediated cell elimination. This observed suppression of E6 and upregulation of p53 is of paramount importance because HPV infection and cancer progression in cervical cells relies on the expression of the viral E6 oncoprotein which targets p53 for degradation by the ubiquitination [24,31]. Thus, untreated cervical cancer cells continue to proliferate in the absence of p53, unable to respond to cell stress and DNA damage. Our data indicates that resveratrol and pterostilbene may restore an adequate p53 response and ultimately act as anticancer plant compounds.

A comparative study between resveratrol and pterostilbene on colon cancer cells had shown pterostilbene to be a more potent anticancer agent compared to resveratrol [15]. Our first approach to understand the comparative efficacy of resveratrol and pterostilbene in HeLa cells was a cytotoxicity analysis, in addition to ascertaining the inhibitory concentration (IC_{50}) (Figure 1 and Videos S1–S3). The results clearly indicated that pterostilbene could eliminate HeLa cells much faster and at a significantly lower concentration compared to resveratrol. We also further analyzed the cytotoxic potential of these polyphenols on a second cell line, E6-positive murine TC1 cells, and found a similar trend in IC_{50} results for resveratrol and pterostilbene, where pterostilbene is 2-fold more cytotoxic than resveratrol [32]. Since cancer cells are known to have enhanced clonogenecity [27,33], our study aimed to see the survival capability of the cells treated with supra-IC_{50} concentrations of either resveratrol or pterostilbene. Clonogenic studies show the long term-term effects of these polyphenols on cervical cancer cells after treatment for 24 h and then allowing the surviving cells to grow in normal growth medium for 15 days. Both compounds at supra-IC_{50} concentrations showed a dramatic decrease in the clonogenic capacity of the surviving cells. These results suggest that resveratrol and pterostilbene may suppress new tumor growth often seen in high-grade metastatic cervical cancer.

The migration of cancer cells is a very important factor responsible for the metastasizing of cancers [34]. Inhibition of migration can play a major role in checking the progression of cancer metastasis. Our study found that sub-cytotoxic doses of both compounds exhibit anti-migratory roles. These findings are supported by previous studies, which have shown that resveratrol shows anti-migratory activity by suppressing phorbol 12-myristate 13-acetate (PMA)-induced migration in cervical cancer cells [35]. Studies in hepatocellular carcinoma indicate that pterostilbene suppresses migration by downregulating MMP-9 expression [36]. These mechanisms might possibly be responsible for inhibiting migration in HeLa cells and remain to be determined in later studies.

Previous cell cycle arrest studies of resveratrol on HeLa cells showed that all the cells were arrested at the S-phase and none remained in the G2/M-phase [37,38]. Pterostilbene shows cell cycle arrest in several cancer studies [39]; however, to the best of our knowledge, no such study on cervical cancer has been carried out. Our current study showed that pterostilbene shows markedly better efficacy than resveratrol in arresting the cell cycle at the S-phase. To further analyze the effects of the two compounds on cell cycle arrest, we looked at phospho-histone H3 as a marker for mitosis [40]. Our observations strengthen and confirm the results obtained from flow cytometric analysis indicating that although both compounds are able to arrest mitosis, pterostilbene has enhanced capacity to arrest cancer cell growth.

Although we initially used sub-lethal concentrations of the two compounds on HeLa cells to decipher their antitumor mechanisms in the context of cell cycle arrest, it was imperative for us to delineate the possible mechanism of elimination of HeLa cells by these compounds at higher concentrations. Pterostilbene is known to be effective on cervical cancer cells by Endoplasmic reticulum (ER)-mediated stress development as well as by targeting the Nrf-2 pathway [41]. In HPV+ cancer cells, the oncoprotein E6 degrades the tumor-suppressor protein p53 by targeting it for proteasomal ubiquitination, which has been shown to augment the tumorigenic characteristics of cancer cells [24,42]. In contrast, inhibition of E6 expression in the cancer cells would be expected to allow p53 protein to trigger apoptosis and cell cycle arrest. Our findings support this latter statement, with resveratrol and pterostilbene activating caspase-3 while simultaneously downregulating E6 and upregulating p53. Our findings are partly supported by previous studies indicating that resveratrol treatment on cervical cancer cell lines upregulates p53 [43]. Our findings are the first to show a direct upregulation of p53 in HeLa cells by another polyphenol, namely, pterostilbene. Importantly previous studies have shown that p53 and simultaneous caspase-3 activation might be the key for triggering apoptosis in HeLa cells [44]. Our experiments support this finding and ascertain that resveratrol and pterostilbene act as robust agents capable of regulating the p53-dependent apoptotic pathway. The p53 protein, which is usually very low in HeLa cells, was upregulated by resveratrol and pterostilbene, leading us to hypothesize that reactivation of p53 in treated HeLa cells is a possible mechanism of action of these compounds.

Cervical cancer is a major concern in developing countries due to lack of affordable prophylaxis and treatment. As present modes of treatment like surgery, chemotherapy, or radiation involve high systemic toxicity, there is an urgent need to find affordable alternative therapies. Diet-based polyphenols like resveratrol and pterostilbene are therefore potential candidates for the effective therapy of cervical cancer with significantly low toxicity. We found pterostilbene to be a more potent anticancer agent than resveratrol in HeLa cells. This difference may be a function of pterostilbene being capable of upregulating p53 and downregulating E6 significantly more than resveratrol. As pterostilbene is non-toxic to normal cells [20], it has the potential to be a robust, cost-effective anti-E6+ tumor drug. Others have found that that pterostilbene possess greater bioavailability and stability [45] than resveratrol in vivo (80% vs. 20%). Resveratrol has been shown to be non-toxic to several cells lines like glial cells and neurons, even after a treatment dose of 100 μM for 48 h [46]. Other studies on normal fibroblasts also state the non-toxicity of resveratrol at our observed potent anticancer concentrations [47]. Additionally, pterostilbene shows no toxicity at these concentrations in normal skin fibroblasts and myoblasts [48]. According to clinical studies, the safe dosage for resveratrol and pterostilbene is 5 g/day [49] and 250 mg/day [20], respectively. Our initial in vivo studies in the laboratory using a non-toxic dosage of both resveratrol and pterostilbene has shown promising results in inhibiting tumor growth in a model of cervical cancer [32]. Taken together, our findings support the further evaluation of pterostilbene as a possible therapy against cervical cancer.

Here, we show that pterostilbene potently suppresses HPV E6 expression (Figure 4) and efficiently eliminates HPV+ cells in culture by p53-mediated apoptosis (Figures 1 and 5) while suppressing cell proliferation (Figure 3) and migration (Figure 2). We find that pterostilbene is a more promising agent against cervical cancer when compared to resveratrol. Based on such properties, the use of pterostilbene presents a relatively economical but highly hopeful therapeutic approach to treat HPV infections and cervical cancers. Our future studies will include signaling studies using HPV+ murine tumor models to confirm these observations in vivo.

Supplementary Materials:
Video S1: Pterostilbene induces enhanced cell death compared to resveratrol: Time lapse video of cells untreated; Video S2: Pterostilbene induces enhanced cell death compared to resveratrol: Time lapse video of cells treated with 60 μM resveratrol; Video S3: Pterostilbene induces enhanced cell death compared to resveratrol: Time lapse video of cells treated with 60 μM pterostilbene obtained for 24 h showing elevated blebbing and cell death in pterostilbene treatment.

Acknowledgments: Kaushiki Chatterjee was supported by a teaching assistantship from the College of Staten Island (CUNY) and a doctoral scholarship from Northwell Health. We are grateful to Sumit Mukherjee for providing technical assistance and research input for this manuscript.

Author Contributions: Kaushiki Chatterjee and Jimmie E. Fata conceived and designed the experiments. Kaushiki Chatterjee, Dina AlSharif, Christina Mazza, Palwasha Syar, and Mohamed Al Sharif carried out the experiments and analyzed the data. All the authors contributed to the research and shaping of the article.

References

1. Safaeian, M.; Solomon, D.; Castle, P.E. Cervical cancer prevention—Cervical screening: Science in evolution. *Obstet. Gynecol. Clin. N. Am.* **2007**, *34*, 739–760. [CrossRef] [PubMed]
2. Ferlay, J.; Soerjomataram, I.; Dikshit, R.; Eser, S.; Mathers, C.; Rebelo, M.; Parkin, D.M.; Forman, D.; Bray, F. Cancer incidence and mortality worldwide: Sources, methods and major patterns in GLOBOCAN 2012. *Int. J. Cancer* **2015**, *136*, E359–E386. [CrossRef] [PubMed]
3. Burd, E.M. Human papillomavirus and cervical cancer. *Clin. Microbiol. Rev.* **2003**, *16*, 1–17. [CrossRef] [PubMed]
4. Parkin, D.M.; Bray, F. Chapter 2: The burden of HPV-related cancers. *Vaccine* **2006**, *24*. [CrossRef] [PubMed]
5. Palefsky, J.M. Human papillomavirus-related disease in men: Not just a women's issue. *J. Adolesc. Health* **2010**, *46*, S12–S19. [CrossRef] [PubMed]
6. Serrano, B.; Brotons, M.; Bosch, F.X.; Bruni, L. Epidemiology and burden of HPV-related disease. *Best Pract. Res. Clin. Obstet. Gynaecol.* **2017**. [CrossRef] [PubMed]
7. Wigle, J.; Coast, E.; Watson-Jones, D. Human papillomavirus (HPV) vaccine implementation in low and middle-income countries (LMICs): Health system experiences and prospects. *Vaccine* **2013**, *31*, 3811–3817. [CrossRef] [PubMed]
8. Stanley, M. Potential mechanisms for HPV vaccine-induced long-term protection. *Gynecol. Oncol.* **2017**, *118*, S2–S7. [CrossRef] [PubMed]
9. Kitagawa, R.; Katsumata, N.; Shibata, T.; Kamura, T.; Kasamatsu, T.; Nakanishi, T.; Nishimura, S.; Ushijima, K.; Takano, M.; Satoh, T.; et al. Paclitaxel Plus Carboplatin Versus Paclitaxel Plus Cisplatin in Metastatic or Recurrent Cervical Cancer: The Open-Label Randomized Phase III Trial JCOG0505. *J. Clin. Oncol.* **2015**, *33*, 2129–2135. [CrossRef] [PubMed]
10. Astolfi, L.; Ghiselli, S.; Guaran, V.; Chicca, M.; Simoni, E.; Olivetto, E.; Lelli, G.; Martini, A. Correlation of adverse effects of cisplatin administration in patients affected by solid tumours: A retrospective evaluation. *Oncol. Rep.* **2013**, *29*, 1285–1292. [CrossRef] [PubMed]
11. Stoner, G.D.; Mukhtar, H. Polyphenols as cancer chemopreventive agents. *J. Cell. Biochem.* **1995**, *59*, 169–180. [CrossRef]
12. Mukherjee, S.; Ranjan Debata, P.; Hussaini, R.; Chatterjee, K.; NE Baidoo, J.; Sampat, S.; Navarra, J.P.; Fata, J.; Severinova, E.; Banerjee, P.; et al. Unique synergistic formulation of curcumin, epicatechin gallate and resveratrol, tricurin, suppresses HPV E6, eliminates HPV+ cancer cells, and inhibits tumor progression. *Oncotarget* **2017**, *8*, 60904–60916. [CrossRef] [PubMed]
13. Wang, D.-G.; Liu, W.-Y.; Chen, G.-T. A simple method for the isolation and purification of resveratrol from Polygonum cuspidatum. *J. Pharm. Anal.* **2013**, *3*, 241–247. [CrossRef] [PubMed]
14. Mukherjee, S.; Dudley, J.I.; Das, D.K. Dose-dependency of resveratrol in providing health benefits. *Dose Response* **2010**, *8*, 478–500. [CrossRef] [PubMed]
15. Nutakul, W.; Sobers, H.S.; Qiu, P.; Dong, P.; Decker, E.A.; McClements, D.J.; Xiao, H. Inhibitory effects of resveratrol and pterostilbene on human colon cancer cells: A side-by-side comparison. *J. Agric. Food Chem.* **2011**, *59*, 10964–10970. [CrossRef] [PubMed]
16. Francioso, A.; Mastromarino, P.; Masci, A.; d'Erme, M.; Mosca, L. Chemistry, stability and bioavailability of resveratrol. *Med. Chem.* **2014**, *10*, 237–245. [CrossRef] [PubMed]
17. Fulda, S. Resveratrol and derivatives for the prevention and treatment of cancer. *Drug Discov. Today* **2010**, *15*, 757–765. [CrossRef] [PubMed]
18. Langcake, P.; Cornford, C.A.; Pryce, R.J. Identification of pterostilbene as a phytoalexin from Vitis vinifera leaves. *Phytochemistry* **1979**, *18*, 1025–1027. [CrossRef]
19. McCormack, D.; McFadden, D. Pterostilbene and cancer: Current review. *J. Surg. Res.* **2012**, *173*. [CrossRef] [PubMed]
20. Riche, D.M.; McEwen, C.L.; Riche, K.D.; Sherman, J.J.; Wofford, M.R.; Deschamp, D.; Griswold, M. Analysis of safety from a human clinical trial with pterostilbene. *J. Toxicol.* **2013**, *2013*, 463595. [CrossRef] [PubMed]
21. Estrela, J.M.; Ortega, A.; Mena, S.; Rodriguez, M.L.; Asensi, M. Pterostilbene: Biomedical applications. *Crit. Rev. Clin. Lab. Sci. 50* **2013**, *50*, 65–78. [CrossRef] [PubMed]

22. Paul, S.; Rimando, A.M.; Lee, H.J.; Ji, Y.; Reddy, B.S.; Suh, N. Anti-inflammatory Action of Pterostilbene Is Mediated through the p38 Mitogen-Activated Protein Kinase Pathway in Colon Cancer Cells. *Cancer Prev. Res.* **2009**, *2*, 650–657. [CrossRef] [PubMed]
23. Kumar, S.; Jena, L.; Sahoo, M.; Kakde, M.; Daf, S.; Varma, A.K.; Hoory, T.; Monie, A.; Gravitt, P.; Wu, T.; et al. *In Silico* Docking to Explicate Interface between Plant-Originated Inhibitors and E6 Oncogenic Protein of Highly Threatening Human Papillomavirus 18. *Genom. Inform.* **2015**, *13*, 60. [CrossRef] [PubMed]
24. Scheffner, M.; Huibregtse, J.M.; Vierstra, R.D.; Howley, P.M. The HPV-16 E6 and E6-AP complex functions as a ubiquitin-protein ligase in the ubiquitination of p53. *Cell* **2017**, *75*, 495–505. [CrossRef]
25. Chung, E.; Prelli, F.; Dealler, S.; Lee, W.S.; Chang, Y.-T.; Wisniewski, T. Styryl-based and tricyclic compounds as potential anti-prion agents. *PLoS ONE* **2011**, *6*, e24844. [CrossRef] [PubMed]
26. Kusaczuk, M.; Krętowski, R.; Stypułkowska, A.; Cechowska-Pasko, M. Molecular and cellular effects of a novel hydroxamate-based HDAC inhibitor—belinostat—in glioblastoma cell lines: A preliminary report. *Invest. New Drugs* **2016**, *34*, 552–564. [CrossRef] [PubMed]
27. Munshi, A.; Hobbs, M.; Meyn, R.E. Clonogenic Cell Survival Assay. In *Chemosensitivity*; Humana Press: Totowa, NJ, USA, 2005; Volume 110, pp. 021–028.
28. Liang, C.-C.; Park, A.Y.; Guan, J.-L. In vitro scratch assay: A convenient and inexpensive method for analysis of cell migration in vitro. *Nat. Protoc.* **2007**, *2*, 329–333. [CrossRef] [PubMed]
29. Aumailley, L.; Warren, A.; Garand, C.; Dubois, M.J.; Paquet, E.R.; Le Couteur, D.G.; Marette, A.; Cogger, V.C.; Lebel, M. Vitamin C modulates the metabolic and cytokine profiles, alleviates hepatic endoplasmic reticulum stress, and increases the life span of Gulo-/- mice. *Aging (Albany NY)* **2016**, *8*, 458–483. [CrossRef] [PubMed]
30. Correa-Costa, M.; Braga, T.T.; Semedo, P.; Hayashida, C.Y.; Bechara, L.R.G.; Elias, R.M.; Barreto, C.R.; Silva-Cunha, C.; Hyane, M.I.; Gonçalves, G.M.; et al. Pivotal role of Toll-like receptors 2 and 4, its adaptor molecule MyD88, and inflammasome complex in experimental tubule-interstitial nephritis. *PLoS ONE* **2011**, *6*, e29004. [CrossRef] [PubMed]
31. DeFilippis, R.A.; Goodwin, E.C.; Wu, L.; DiMaio, D. Endogenous human papillomavirus E6 and E7 proteins differentially regulate proliferation, senescence, and apoptosis in HeLa cervical carcinoma cells. *J. Virol.* **2003**, *77*, 1551–1563. [CrossRef] [PubMed]
32. Chatterjee, K.; Mukherjee, S.; Vanmanen, J.; Banerjee, P.; Fata, J.E. CUNY Graduate Center, College of Staten Island. Unpublished work. 2018.
33. Pajonk, F.; Pajonk, K.; McBride, W.H. Inhibition of NF-κB, Clonogenicity, and Radiosensitivity of Human Cancer Cells. *JNCI J. Natl. Cancer Inst.* **1999**, *91*, 1956–1960. [CrossRef] [PubMed]
34. Yamaguchi, H.; Wyckoff, J.; Condeelis, J. Cell migration in tumors. *Curr. Opin. Cell Biol.* **2005**, *17*, 559–564. [CrossRef] [PubMed]
35. Kim, Y.S.; Sull, J.W.; Sung, H.J. Suppressing effect of resveratrol on the migration and invasion of human metastatic lung and cervical cancer cells. *Mol. Biol. Rep.* **2012**, *39*, 8709–8716. [CrossRef] [PubMed]
36. Pan, M.-H.; Chiou, Y.-S.; Chen, W.-J.; Wang, J.-M.; Badmaev, V.; Ho, C.-T. Pterostilbene inhibited tumor invasion via suppressing multiple signal transduction pathways in human hepatocellular carcinoma cells. *Carcinogenesis* **2009**, *30*, 1234–1242. [CrossRef] [PubMed]
37. Kramer, M.P.; Wesierska-Gadek, J. Monitoring of long-term effects of resveratrol on cell cycle progression of human HeLa cells after administration of a single dose. *Ann. N. Y. Acad. Sci.* **2009**, *1171*, 257–263. [CrossRef] [PubMed]
38. Zoberi, I.; Bradbury, C.M.; Curry, H.A.; Bisht, K.S.; Goswami, P.C.; Roti Roti, J.L.; Gius, D. Radiosensitizing and anti-proliferative effects of resveratrol in two human cervical tumor cell lines. *Cancer Lett.* **2002**, *175*, 165–173. [CrossRef]
39. Pan, M.-H.; Chang, Y.-H.; Badmaev, V.; Nagabhushanam, K.; Ho, C.-T. Pterostilbene Induces Apoptosis and Cell Cycle Arrest in Human Gastric Carcinoma Cells. *J. Agric. Food Chem.* **2007**, *55*, 7777–7785. [CrossRef] [PubMed]
40. Veras, E.; Malpica, A.; Deavers, M.T.; Silva, E.G. Mitosis-specific Marker Phospho-histone H3 in the Assessment of Mitotic Index in Uterine Smooth Muscle Tumors: A Pilot Study. *Int. J. Gynecol. Pathol.* **2009**, *28*, 316–321. [CrossRef] [PubMed]
41. Zhang, B.; Wang, X.-Q.; Chen, H.-Y.; Liu, B.-H. Involvement of the Nrf2 Pathway in the Regulation of Pterostilbene-Induced Apoptosis in HeLa Cells via ER Stress. *J. Pharmacol. Sci.* **2014**, *126*, 216–229. [CrossRef] [PubMed]

42. Yim, E.-K.; Park, J.-S. The role of HPV E6 and E7 oncoproteins in HPV-associated cervical carcinogenesis. *Cancer Res. Treat.* **2005**, *37*, 319–324. [CrossRef] [PubMed]
43. Athar, M.; Back, J.H.; Kopelovich, L.; Bickers, D.R.; Kim, A.L. Multiple molecular targets of resveratrol: Anti-carcinogenic mechanisms. *Arch. Biochem. Biophys.* **2009**, *486*, 95–102. [CrossRef] [PubMed]
44. Liu, Y.; McKalip, A.; Herman, B. Human papillomavirus type 16 E6 and HPV-16 E6/E7 sensitize human keratinocytes to apoptosis induced by chemotherapeutic agents: Roles of p53 and caspase activation. *J. Cell. Biochem.* **2000**, *78*, 334–349. [CrossRef]
45. Kapetanovic, I.M.; Muzzio, M.; Huang, Z.; Thompson, T.N.; McCormick, D.L. Pharmacokinetics, oral bioavailability, and metabolic profile of resveratrol and its dimethylether analog, pterostilbene, in rats. *Cancer Chemother. Pharmacol.* **2011**, *68*, 593–601. [CrossRef] [PubMed]
46. Shu, X.-H.; Li, H.; Sun, X.-X.; Wang, Q.; Sun, Z.; Wu, M.-L.; Chen, X.-Y.; Li, C.; Kong, Q.-Y.; Liu, J. Metabolic patterns and biotransformation activities of resveratrol in human glioblastoma cells: Relevance with therapeutic efficacies. *PLoS ONE* **2011**, *6*, e27484. [CrossRef] [PubMed]
47. Gosslau, A.; Chen, M.; Ho, C.-T.; Chen, K.Y. A methoxy derivative of resveratrol analogue selectively induced activation of the mitochondrial apoptotic pathway in transformed fibroblasts. *Br. J. Cancer* **2005**, *92*, 513–521. [CrossRef] [PubMed]
48. Dewi, N.I.; Yagasaki, K.; Miura, Y. Anti-proliferative effect of pterostilbene on rat hepatoma cells in culture. *Cytotechnology* **2015**, *67*, 671–680. [CrossRef] [PubMed]
49. Patel, K.R.; Scott, E.; Brown, V.A.; Gescher, A.J.; Steward, W.P.; Brown, K. Clinical trials of resveratrol. *Ann. N. Y. Acad. Sci.* **2011**, *1215*, 161–169. [CrossRef] [PubMed]

4

Report on Second International Conference on Natural Products for Cancer Prevention and Therapy Held in Kayseri, Turkey, 8–11 November 2017

Mükerrem Betül Yerer [1,*] and Anupam Bishayee [2,*]

1 Department of Pharmacology, Faculty of Pharmacy, University of Erciyes, Kayseri 38039, Turkey
2 Department of Pharmaceutical Sciences, College of Pharmacy, Larkin University, Miami, FL 33169, USA
* Correspondence: eczbetul@yahoo.com (M.B.Y.); abishayee@ularkin.org or abishayee@gmail.com (A.B.);

---

1. Preface

Scientific experts from eight countries gathered to share their views and experience on the latest research on natural products for cancer prevention and therapy. The traditionally used herbal medicines, medicinal plants, plant extracts, fractions, and phytochemicals for cancer prevention and therapy were discussed throughout the meeting. The scientific program comprised of 12 plenary lectures, 23 oral presentations, and 72 posters, providing an opportunity for more than 130 natural product scientists to present their research in three days. Abstracts for plenary talks, oral presentations, and posters were published as proceedings of the meeting in the special issue of Proceedings, Volume 1 and Issue 10 (http://www.mdpi.com/2504-3900/1/10). The aim of this biannual meeting was to foster discussion and disseminate the results of the research on natural products that are used for cancer prevention and therapy. During the meeting, the scientific committee members of the meeting who attended the conference had been selected as judges to evaluate all of the oral and poster presentations and the three best oral and poster presentation awards have been granted to the young scientists. The participants were able to network and engage in discussion for potential collaboration to advance our knowledge on utility of natural products for prevention and treatment of cancer.

2. Summary of the Scientific Presentations

2.1. Plenary Lectures

The meeting was successfully focused on the natural products being investigated for their efficiency in several cancer types and for their potency in cancer prevention. Only the plenary lectures have been summarized here in this manuscript, and all of the other oral and poster presentations have been listed where the abstracts can be reached from http://www.mdpi.com/2504-3900/1/10.

2.1.1. Growth Factors Responsible from the Cancer Progress: Role of Natural Products

Mükerrem Betül Yerer

Growth factors are one of the main factors responsible from the uncontrolled cell progress in cancer. Up to date many scientists have focused on these factors either as the marker or as the targets in several cancer types. Yerer has presented a plenary lecture on the natural products targeting these factors (Nerve growth factor (NGF), epidermal growth factor (EGF), hepatocyte growth factors (HGF), fibroblast growth factors (FGF), vascular endothelial growth factors (VEGF), platelet derived growth factor (PDGF), and transforming growth factor (TGF-β) (http://www.mdpi.com/2504-3900/1/10/979) [1].

2.1.2. Natural Products for Cancer Prevention and Therapy: Progress, Pitfalls and Promise

Anupam Bishayee

The presentation of Bishayee highlighted studies on cancer preventive and therapeutic attributes of various naturally occurring agents and underlying mechanisms of action, with special emphasis on results reported from our laboratory. Current limitations, challenges, and future directions of research for successful cancer drug development based on natural products will also be discussed (http://www.mdpi.com/2504-3900/1/10/982) [2].

2.1.3. Novel Anticancer Capacities of Saffron

Amr Amin

Amr Amin has presented a plenary lecture on the anticancer effects of the saffron's main active ingredient "safranal" against HCC using in vitro, in silico, and network analyses. In their studies, in addition to the unique and differential cell cycle arrest, safranal showed pro-apoptotic effect through activation of both intrinsic and extrinsic initiator caspases implicating ER stress-mediated apoptosis (http://www.mdpi.com/2504-3900/1/10/834) [3].

2.1.4. Cardiac Glycosides as Novel Modulators of Cancer Cell Survival

Marc Diederich

This plenary lecture focused on Cardiac Glycosides (GCs) can be considered as pharmacological agents, allowing for cancer cells to switch from one cell death modality to another. All the findings encourage to further explore a potential for CGs in general as cancer cell death modulators alone or in combination with other targeted treatments (http://www.mdpi.com/2504-3900/1/10/972) [4].

2.1.5. Ins and Outs of Flavonoids in Cancer Prevention vs. Cancer Therapy: A Lesson from Quercetin in Leukemia

Gian Luigi Russo, Maria Russo, Carmela Spagnuolo, Idolo Tedesco, Stefania Moccia

Russo et al. has critically reviewed the clinical and pre-clinical studies on the concept that polyphenols, being antioxidant compounds, can fight cancer. They suggest that a clear distinction must be done between the use of polyphenols, such as flavonoids, in cancer treatment versus cancer prevention, starting from adequate and specifically selected cellular models. As an example, he has present data on the potential application of quercetin against chronic lymphocytic leukemia (CLL) (http://www.mdpi.com/2504-3900/1/10/977) [5].

2.1.6. Anticancer Potential of Flavones

Randolph RJ Arroo, Didem Şöhretoğlu, Demetrios A Spandidos, Vasilis P Androutsopoulos

Flavones are abundantly present in common fruits and vegetables, many of which have been associated with cancer prevention. Taking into account that no flavonoid based drugs are clinically used in cancer therapy, Randolph has focused on the flavones—which constitute a subgroup of the flavonoids—show some structural analogy with estrogen, and are known to interact with human estrogen receptors, either as agonist or as antagonist. Thus, whereas epidemiological and pre-clinical data seem to indicate a high potential for flavonoids, from the point of view of the pharmaceutical industry and drug developers, they are considered poor candidates (http://www.mdpi.com/2504-3900/1/10/975) [6].

2.1.7. Resveratrol in Cancer Prevention and Treatment: Focusing on Molecular Targets and Mechanism of Action

Adriano Borriello

The relevance of these mechanisms and their translation in clinical therapy has been discussed in Borelli's plenary lecture. Resveratrol and its mechanism of action has been emphasized by her in cancer cells and in experimental models of senescence, inflammation, obesity, and metabolic diseases. Its molecular targets act at different levels: (1) specific molecular pathways (like p53, NF-kappaB, PKC, PI3K, MDM2, LATS1, STK3 and several others); (2) epigenetic control of gene transcription through sirtuin activation; (3) cell division cycle and differentiation; (4) apoptosis and autophagy; and, (5) cellular redox homeostasis (http://www.mdpi.com/2504-3900/1/10/976) [7].

2.1.8. Cynaropicrin: A Promising Natural Agent with Antitumor and Antiviral Activities

Mahmoud F. Elsebai, Jukka Hakkola, Mohamed Mehiri, Juana Diez

Human infection with HCV is currently recognized as the leading cause of hepatocellular carcinoma (HCC), which demands liver transplantation, which was estimated to result in ~10,000 deaths in the US only in the year 2011. Elsebai has presented a plenary lecture on cynaropicrin as a potential agent for treatment and prevention of HCC by indirect way through inhibition of HCV and in a direct way evidenced by the many antitumor activities in literature (http://www.mdpi.com/2504-3900/1/10/974) [8].

2.1.9. Relationship between Structure of Phenolics and Anticancer Activity

Müberra Koşar

Many phenolic compounds have been investigated for their potential use as cancer chemopreventive agents. Phenolic compounds consist of one or more hydroxyl substitution on the aromatic ring system. Koşar has emphasized that Cinnamic acid esters, such as caffeic acid phenethyl and benzyl esters, display selective antiproliferative activity against some types of cancer cells. Flavonoids consist of a large group of polyphenolic compounds having a benzo-γ-pyrone structure, and are ubiquitously present in plants. This structure can be responsible from the anticancer acitvities of these compounds (http://www.mdpi.com/2504-3900/1/10/978) [9].

2.1.10. Pristimerin is a Promising Natural Product against Breast Cancer In Vitro and In Vivo through Apoptosis and the Blockage of Autophagic Flux

Buse Cevatemre, Konstantinos Dimas, Bruno Botta and Engin Ulukaya

Ulukaya has given a lecture on the pristimerin's cytotoxic potential on particularly cancer stem cells (CSCs) should be much more important due to the CSCs' recent role in recurrence of cancer. He has presented their studies on Pristimerin that has been shown to suppress the proliferation of various cancer cell lines at relatively lower concentrations, of which, the IC50 values are around 0.5–4 μM (http://www.mdpi.com/2504-3900/1/10/973) [10].

2.1.11. Can Curcumin Be Employed to Promote the Integration of Oncology and Natural Products?

Mutlu Demiray and Fatemeh Bahadori

Curcumin is multi-targeted molecule with pleotropic nature, which inhibits NF-κB and related proteins promoting effectiveness of tyrosine kinase inhibitors (TKIs). Demiray has presented their clinical studies with curcumin on adenoid cystic carcinoma where they have treated patients for 72 months by oral curcumin and eight months by i.v curcumin. Disease control rate was 89.3% (15/17), and no any grade III-IV toxicities was observed related to curcumin reflecting the clinical use of curcumin on adenoid cystic carcinoma patients (http://www.mdpi.com/2504-3900/1/10/980) [11].

2.1.12. Therapeutic Potential of Black Pepper Compound for BRaf Resistant Melanoma

Neel M. Fofaria, Sharavan Ramachandran, and Sanjay K. Srivastava

Srivastava's presentation mainly focused on the combination of BRAF inhibitors with Mcl-1 inhibitor such as piperlongumine may have therapeutic advantage to melanoma patients with acquired resistance to BRAF inhibitors alone or in combination with MEK1/2 inhibitors (http://www.mdpi.com/2504-3900/1/10/981) [12].

2.2. Oral and Poster Presentations

Oral Presentations		
Title	**Authors**	**Link**
Effect of Pomegranate Extract and Tangeretin on Specific Pathways in the Rat Breast Cancer Model Induced with DMBA [13].	H. Fatih Gul et al.	http://www.mdpi.com/2504-3900/1/10/983
Synergistic Cytotoxic Effects of Resveratrol in Combination with Ceramide Metabolizing Enzymes in Ph + Acute Lymphoblastic Leukemia [14].	Osman Oğuz et al.	http://www.mdpi.com/2504-3900/1/10/984
Characterization of cycloartane-type sapogenol derivatives for prostate cancer chemoprevention [15].	Bilge Debelec-Butuner et al.	http://www.mdpi.com/2504-3900/1/10/985
Epibrassinolide treatment caused autophagy or apoptosis decision in a time-dependent manner through ER stress in colon cancer cells [16].	Pınar Obakan-Yerlikaya et al.	http://www.mdpi.com/2504-3900/1/10/986
Determination of Silymarin molecule activity in colon cancer by AgNOR technique [17].	Merve Alpay et al.	http://www.mdpi.com/2504-3900/1/10/987
The cytotoxic effect of *Lysimachia savranii* on the neuroblastoma cells [18].	Gonca Dönmez et al.	http://www.mdpi.com/2504-3900/1/10/988
Autocrine Growth Hormone-triggered curcumin resistance abolished by NF-κB signaling pathway dependent on inflammatory cytokines and active polyamine catabolic machinery in MCF-7, MDA-MB-453 and MDA-MB-231 breast cancer cells [19].	Ajda Çoker Gürkan et al.	http://www.mdpi.com/2504-3900/1/10/989
The effect of *Lysimachia savranii* on the migration of the breast cancer cells [20].	Işıl Aydemir et al.	http://www.mdpi.com/2504-3900/1/10/990
Investigation of cytotoxic effect of *Origanum minutiflorum* on cancer cells [21].	Oktay Özkan et al.	http://www.mdpi.com/2504-3900/1/10/991
Celastrol modulates lipid synthesis via PI3K/Akt/mTOR signaling axis to finalize cell death response in prostate cancer cells [22].	Elif Damla Arisan et al.	http://www.mdpi.com/2504-3900/1/10/992

Oral Presentations		
Title	**Authors**	**Link**
Investigation of the Effect of Paclitaxel and Pycnogenol on Mitochondrial Dynamics in Breast Cancer Therapy [23].	Suna Sayğılı et al.	http://www.mdpi.com/2504-3900/1/10/993
Effects of curcumin on lipid peroxidation and antioxidant enzymes in kidney, liver, brain and testis of mice bearing Ehrlich Solid Tumor [24].	Mustafa Nisari et al.	http://www.mdpi.com/2504-3900/1/10/994
Curcumin enhances the efficacy of 5-FU in Colo205 cell lines [25].	Ebru Öztürk et al.	http://www.mdpi.com/2504-3900/1/10/995
Effect of a New Sapogenol Derivative (AG-07) on Cell Death via Necrosis [26].	Yalcin Erzurumlu et al.	http://www.mdpi.com/2504-3900/1/10/996
Cytotoxic and Antiinflammatory Activity Guided Studies on *Plantago holosteum* Scop [27].	Yasin Genc et al.	http://www.mdpi.com/2504-3900/1/10/997
Continuously monitoring the cytotoxicity of API-1, α-chaconine and α-solanine on human lung carcinoma A549 [28].	Ebru Öztürk et al.	http://www.mdpi.com/2504-3900/1/10/998
The effects of α-chaconine on ER-α positive endometrium cancer cells [29].	Ayşe Kübra Karaboğa Arslan et al.	http://www.mdpi.com/2504-3900/1/10/999
Investigation of apoptotic effect of sinapic acid in Hep3B and HepG2 human hepatocellular carcinoma cells [30].	Canan Eroğlu et al.	http://www.mdpi.com/2504-3900/1/10/1000
Cytotoxic and Antioxidant Activity of four *Cousinia* Species of Stenocephalae Bunge. Section [31].	Leyla Paşayeva et al.	http://www.mdpi.com/2504-3900/1/10/1001
Apoptotic effect of Ginnalin A on MDA-MB-231 and MCF7 human breast cancer cell lines [32].	Ebru Avcı et al.	http://www.mdpi.com/2504-3900/1/10/1002
Cytotoxic effects of coumarin compounds imperatorin and osthole, alone and in combination with 5-fluorouracil in colon carcinoma cells [33].	Ayşe Eken et al.	http://www.mdpi.com/2504-3900/1/10/1003
Screening of some Apiaceae and Asteraceae plants for their cytotoxic potential [34].	Perihan Gürbüz et al.	http://www.mdpi.com/2504-3900/1/10/1004
Cyclodextrine Based Nanogels and Phase Solubility Studies of Flurbiprofen as a Chemopreventive Agent [35].	Ayşe Nur Oktay et al.	http://www.mdpi.com/2504-3900/1/10/1005
Poster Presentations		
Effect of a synthesized compound against cancerous cell line and synthesis of copper ion incorporated 1-(3,4-diaminophenyl) ethanone-based hybrid nanoflowers [36].	Burcu Somtürk Yılmaz et al.	http://www.mdpi.com/2504-3900/1/10/1006
Development of effective anticancer drug candidates against breast and colon cancers [37].	Senem Akkoç et al.	http://www.mdpi.com/2504-3900/1/10/1007

Poster Presentations		
Title	**Authors**	**Link**
Synthesis of copper ion incorporated aminoguanidine derivatives-based hybrid nanoflowers [38].	Sevtap Çağlar Yavuz et al.	http://www.mdpi.com/2504-3900/1/10/1008
Evaluation of anti-proliferative and cytotoxic properties of chlorogenic acid against breast cancer cell lines by real time monitoring [39].	Onur Bender et al.	http://www.mdpi.com/2504-3900/1/10/1009
Investigation of Apoptotic Effects of Usnic Acid on Hepatocellular Carcinoma [40].	Beste Yurdacan et al.	http://www.mdpi.com/2504-3900/1/10/1010
In vitro Cytotoxic Effect Evaluation of *Dioscorea communis* (L.) Caddick & Wilkin Rhizome and Stem Extracts on Hepatocellular Carcinoma Cells [41].	Ünal Egeli et al.	http://www.mdpi.com/2504-3900/1/10/1011
The Effect of Herbal Medicine on Neuroblastoma Cell Line in Culture [42].	Büşra Şen et al.	http://www.mdpi.com/2504-3900/1/10/1012
The foods containing miR-193b may inhibit the growth of breast cancer cells [43].	Dilek Asci Celik et al.	http://www.mdpi.com/2504-3900/1/10/1013
Is the dietary miR-193b a novel cell cycle arresting source for breast carcinoma? [44].	Nilgun Gurbuz et al.	http://www.mdpi.com/2504-3900/1/10/1014
The effects of Wortmannin and EGCG and combined treatments on MDA-MB-231 breast cancer cell lines via inactivation of PI3K signaling pathway [45].	Elgin Turkoz Uluer et al.	http://www.mdpi.com/2504-3900/1/10/1015
The effects of Paclitaxel and Metformin and combined treatments on TLR signaling pathway on MDA-MB-231 breast cancer cell lines [46].	Melike Ozgul et al.	http://www.mdpi.com/2504-3900/1/10/1016
Inhibition of telomerase activity by cucurbitacin I in colon cancer cell line, LS174T [47].	Emir Tosun et al.	http://www.mdpi.com/2504-3900/1/10/1017
Effect of cucurbitacin I on proliferation and migration in colorectal cancer cell line, LS174T [48].	Emir Tosun et al.	http://www.mdpi.com/2504-3900/1/10/1018
In vitro anticancer and cytotoxic activities of some plant extracts on HeLa and Vero cell lines [49].	Fulya Tugba Artun et al.	http://www.mdpi.com/2504-3900/1/10/1019
Anticancer Effects of Oleocanthal and *Pinus Pinaster* on Breast Cancer Cell in Culture [50].	Mahmud Özkut et al.	http://www.mdpi.com/2504-3900/1/10/1020
Antiproliferative and Apoptotic Effects of the Medicinal Plants on Breast Cancer Cell Lines [51].	Pınar Kılıçaslan Sönmez et al.	http://www.mdpi.com/2504-3900/1/10/1021
The role of trophoblastic stem cells conditioned media on JAR cell culture [52].	Hilal Kabadayı et al.	http://www.mdpi.com/2504-3900/1/10/1022
The effect of pycnogenol and paclitaxel on DNA damage in human breast cancer cell line [53].	Hülya Birinci et al.	http://www.mdpi.com/2504-3900/1/10/1023

Poster Presentations		
Title	**Authors**	**Link**
Investigation of the effects of paclitaxel and pycnogenol on inflammatory response (PTX3, BDNF, IGF2R) in human breast cancer cell line [54].	Hülya Birinci et al.	http://www.mdpi.com/2504-3900/1/10/1024
Is There Any Protective Effect of Pomegranate and Tangeretin on the DMBA-Induced Rat Breast Cancer Model? [55].	H. Fatih Gul et al.	http://www.mdpi.com/2504-3900/1/10/1025
The neurotoxic effects of *Origanum minutiflorum* [56].	İsmail Sari et al.	http://www.mdpi.com/2504-3900/1/10/1026
The Cytotoxic and Apoptotic Effects of Usnic Acid on Prostate Cancer versus Normal Cells [57].	Işıl Ezgi Eryılmaz et al.	http://www.mdpi.com/2504-3900/1/10/1027
Antiproliferative Effect of Methanolic Extract of *Linum arboretum* on A549 Cells [58].	Ozgur Vatan et al.	http://www.mdpi.com/2504-3900/1/10/1028
Investigation of *in vitro* Cytotoxic Effects of *Montivipera xanthina* on Healthy and Cancer Human Lung Cell Lines [59].	Huzeyfe Huriyet et al.	http://www.mdpi.com/2504-3900/1/10/1029
Development and Characterization of Paclitaxel-loaded PLGA Nanoparticles and Evaluation of Cytotoxicity on MCF-7 cell line by MTT Assay [60].	Merve Çelik Tekeli et al.	http://www.mdpi.com/2504-3900/1/10/1030
Effects of Fulvic Acid on Different Cancer Cell Lines [61].	S. Kerem Aydin et al.	http://www.mdpi.com/2504-3900/1/10/1031
Antioxidant, antibacterial and antiproliferative activities of Turkish rhubarb (*Rheum palmatum* L.) leaf extracts [62].	Mehmet Berköz et al.	http://www.mdpi.com/2504-3900/1/10/1032
The Effect of Herbal Medicine on Colon Cancer Cells in Culture [63].	Pelin Toros et al.	http://www.mdpi.com/2504-3900/1/10/1033
The Effect of Herbal Medicine on Prostate Cancer Cells in Culture [64].	Pelin Toro et al.	http://www.mdpi.com/2504-3900/1/10/1034
Determination of Antioxidant Capacity, Phenolic Acid Composition and Antiproliferative Effect Associated with Phenylalanine Ammonia Lyase (PAL) Activity in Some Plants Naturally Growing under Salt Stress [65].	Seda Şirin et al.	http://www.mdpi.com/2504-3900/1/10/1035
Development and Characterization of Paclitaxel-loaded PLGA Nanoparticles and Cytotoxicity Assessment by MTT assay on A549 cell line [66].	Sedat Ünal et al.	http://www.mdpi.com/2504-3900/1/10/1036
Evaluation of in vitro anti-proliferative activity of St. John's wort (*Hypericum perforatum* Linn.) plant extract on cervix adenocarcinoma [67].	Rana Kavurmacı et al.	http://www.mdpi.com/2504-3900/1/10/1037
The cytotoxic effect of *Annona muricata* leaf extract on triple negative breast cancer cell line [68].	Rana Kavurmacı et al.	http://www.mdpi.com/2504-3900/1/10/1038

Poster Presentations		
Title	**Authors**	**Link**
Cytotoxic activity of *Achillea coarctata* Poir. Extract [69].	Sevil Albayrak et al.	http://www.mdpi.com/2504-3900/1/10/1039
Cytotoxic activity of Endemic *Astragalus argaeus* Boiss. from Turkey [70].	Sevil Albayrak et al.	http://www.mdpi.com/2504-3900/1/10/1040
Lactic Acid Bacteria Mediated Apoptosis Induction: Natural way of colon cancer cells' inhibition [71].	Şebnem Kurhan et al.	http://www.mdpi.com/2504-3900/1/10/1041
Synthesized a new organic compound's cytotoxic activity quantum mechanics calculations and docking studies [72].	Senem Akkoç et al.	http://www.mdpi.com/2504-3900/1/10/1042
Anticancer Activity of *Centaurea babylonica* L. [73].	Elif Dündar et al.	http://www.mdpi.com/2504-3900/1/10/1043
Cytotoxic Effects of Functional Foods *Momordica charantia* L. and *Lycium barbarum* L. Extracts on Prostate Cancer Cells [74].	Guzide Satir Basaran et al.	http://www.mdpi.com/2504-3900/1/10/1044
Cytotoxic Effects of Kynurenic acid and Quinaldic acid in Hepatocellular Carcinoma (HepG2) cell line [75].	Pınar Atalay Dündar et al.	http://www.mdpi.com/2504-3900/1/10/1045
The Effects of Benzoxasol Derivate Compounds in Breast Cancer Cells [76].	Funda Kosova et al.	http://www.mdpi.com/2504-3900/1/10/1046
Potential Cytotoxic Activity of *Psephellus pyrrhoblepharus* Extracts [77].	Pelin Taştan et al.	http://www.mdpi.com/2504-3900/1/10/1047
Screening of *Onosma* species for Cytotoxic Activity [78].	Özge Güzel et al.	http://www.mdpi.com/2504-3900/1/10/1048
Apoptotic Effects of *Mount Bulgar Viper (Montivipera bulgardaghica)* PLA2 and SVMPs Venom Peptide fractions on HeLa and A549 Cancer Cells [79].	Yalcin Erzurumlu et al.	http://www.mdpi.com/2504-3900/1/10/1049
Turkish Propolis Extract Increases Apoptosis via Induction of Mitochondrial Membrane Potential Loss in MCF-7 Cells [80].	Sema Misir et al.	http://www.mdpi.com/2504-3900/1/10/1050
The Effect of Gilaburu (*Viburnum opulus*) Juice on Ehrlich Ascites Tumor (EAT) Cell Culture [81].	Özge Al et al.	http://www.mdpi.com/2504-3900/1/10/1051
Synthesis and characterizations of folate-conjugated PLGA-PEG nanoparticles loaded with dual agents [82].	Yüksel Öğünç et al.	http://www.mdpi.com/2504-3900/1/10/1052
Selective cytotoxic activity of *Scutellaria* species [83].	Zeynep Dogan et al.	http://www.mdpi.com/2504-3900/1/10/1053
The Antiproliferative Effect of Alpha Tocopherol in F98 Cell Culture [84].	Remzi Soner Cengiz et al.	http://www.mdpi.com/2504-3900/1/10/1054
Analysis of the Cytotoxic Effects of *Eryngium billardieri* Delar. Extracts on MCF7 Cell Line [85].	Leyla Paşayeva et al.	http://www.mdpi.com/2504-3900/1/10/1055
Cytotoxic Effects of *Alchemilla mollis* (Buser) Rothm. Extracts on MCF 7 cell line [86].	Selen İlgün et al.	http://www.mdpi.com/2504-3900/1/10/1056

Poster Presentations		
Title	**Authors**	**Link**
Comparative Evaluation of the cytotoxic effects of stem and flower extracts of *Rhaponticoides iconiensis* (Hub.-Mor.) M.V.Agab. & Greuter [87].	Eren Demirpolat et al.	http://www.mdpi.com/2504-3900/1/10/1057
Goji berry fruit extract suppresses cell proliferation of breast cancer cells by inhibiting EGFR/ERK signaling [88].	Hatice Bekci et al.	http://www.mdpi.com/2504-3900/1/10/1058
Biologically transformed Propolis Exhibits Cytotoxic Effect on A375 Malignant Melanoma Cells in vitro [89].	Hikmet Memmedov et al.	http://www.mdpi.com/2504-3900/1/10/1059
Rheum ribes extract increase the expression level of miR-200 family in human colorectal cancer cells [90].	Ilknur Cinar et al.	http://www.mdpi.com/2504-3900/1/10/1060
Potential effects of *Liquidambar orientalis* Mill. against HT-29 and HCT-116 cell lines [91].	Sumeyra Cetinkaya et al.	http://www.mdpi.com/2504-3900/1/10/1061
The Effect of Tocopherol-α On the Cell Viability in Caco-2 Cell Line [92].	Ayşenur Gök et al.	http://www.mdpi.com/2504-3900/1/10/1062
In vitro Antioxidant and Anticancer Activities of Some Local Plants from Bolu Province of Turkey [93].	Kadriye Nur Kasapoğlu et al.	http://www.mdpi.com/2504-3900/1/10/1063
Survey of the apoptotic effect of Ginnalin A on Hep3B human hepatocellular carcinoma cell line [94].	Pınar Özden et al.	http://www.mdpi.com/2504-3900/1/10/1064
Ameliorative effects of Carvacrol on Cyclophosphamide-induced testis damage and oxidative stress [95].	Mustafa Cengiz et al.	http://www.mdpi.com/2504-3900/1/10/1066
Synthesis of Anthocyanin-rich Red Cabbage Nanoflowers and Their Antimicrobial and Cytotoxic Properties [96].	Suheyl Furkan Konca et al.	http://www.mdpi.com/2504-3900/1/10/1067
Cytotoxic potentials of some Asteraceae plants from Turkey on HeLa cell line [97].	Kübra Uzun et al.	http://www.mdpi.com/2504-3900/1/10/1068
The Role of Lidocaine in the Dunning Model Rat Prostate Cancer Cells: Cell Kinetics and Motility [98].	Esma Purut et al.	http://www.mdpi.com/2504-3900/1/10/1069
Pelargonium endlicherianum Fenzl. Root extract suppresses cell proliferation of prostate cancer cells [99].	Selda Eren et al.	http://www.mdpi.com/2504-3900/1/10/1070
Assessment of antioxidant and cytotoxic activity of known antioxidants compared to neopterin [100].	Gözde Girgin et al.	http://www.mdpi.com/2504-3900/1/10/1071
Comparison of radical scavenging and cytotoxic activities of well-known non-enzymatic antioxidants [101].	Suna Sabuncuoğlu et al.	http://www.mdpi.com/2504-3900/1/10/1072
A Study on the Synthesis and Anticancer Activities of Novel 6-Methoxy Flavonyl Piperazine Derivatives [102].	Meltem Ceylan-Ünlüsoy et al.	http://www.mdpi.com/2504-3900/1/10/1073

Poster Presentations		
Title	**Authors**	**Link**
Effect of Paclitaxel Loaded Chitosan Nanoparticles and Quantum Dots on Breast Cancer [103].	Gülen Melike Demir et al.	http://www.mdpi.com/2504-3900/1/10/1074
Turkish Medicinal Plants Used in Cancer Treatment and Evaluation of Plant Usage in the Oncology Clinic of the İstanbul University Faculty of Medicine [104].	Büşra Teke et al.	http://www.mdpi.com/2504-3900/1/10/1075
Is Acteosid Effects on Colon Cancer Stem Cells Via Inflamation and/or Apoptosis? [105].	Fatma Firat et al.	http://www.mdpi.com/2504-3900/1/10/1076
Analysis of the Cytotoxic Effects of *Achillea millefolium* L. Extracts on MCF7 Cell Line [106].	Esra Köngül et al.	http://www.mdpi.com/2504-3900/1/10/1077

3. Author Affiliations

- Abdurrahim Kocyigit, Department of Medical Biochemistry, Faculty of Medicine, Bezmialem Vakif University, Sarıyer, Turkey
- Ademi Fahri Pirhan, Department of Biology, Faculty of Science, Ege University, Izmir, Turkey
- Adnan Ayhanci, Biology Department, Art and Science Faculty, Eskişehir Osmangazi University, Eskişehir, Turkey
- Adriana Borriello, Department of Biochemistry, Biophysics and General Pathology, University of Campania "L. Vanvitelli", Naples, Italy
- Ahmet Baysar, Department of Chemical Engineering, Inonu University, Malatya, Turkey
- Ahmet Cumaoglu, Department of Biochemistry, Faculty of Pharmacy, Erciyes University, Kayseri, Turkey
- Ahmet Savran, Department of Arts and Sciences, Faculty of Medicine, Niğde Ömer Halisdemir University, Niğde, Turkey
- Ajda Çoker-Gürkan, Department of Molecular Biology and Genetics, Istanbul Kultur University, Atakoy Campus, Istanbul, Turkey
- Ali Karagoz, Department of Molecular Biology and Genetics, Faculty of Science, Istanbul University, Istanbul, Turkey
- Amr Amin, Biology Department, UAE University, Abu Dhabi, United Arab Emirates
- Anupam Bishayee, Department of Pharmaceutical Sciences, College of Pharmacy, Larkin University, Miami, FL, USA
- Arzu Atalay, Biotechnology Institute, Ankara University, Ankara, Turkey
- Asuman Bozkir, Department of Pharmaceutical Technology, Faculty of Pharmacy, Ankara University, Ankara, Turkey
- Ayhan Altıntaş, Department of Pharmacognosy, Faculty of Pharmacy, Anadolu University, Eskişehir, Turkey
- Aynur Işık, Department of Molecular Biology and Genetics, Faculty of Science, Gazi University, Ankara, Turkey
- Ayse Baldemir, Department of Pharmaceutical botany, Faculty of Pharmacy, Erciyes University, Kayseri, Turkey
- Ayse Nalbantsoy, Department of Bioengineering, Faculty of Engineering, Ege University, Izmir, Turkey
- Aysun Adan, Molecular Biology and Genetics, Faculty of Life and Natural Sciences, Abdullah Gul University, Kayseri, Turkey

- Aysun Ökçesiz, Department of Pharmaceutical Toxicology, Faculty of Pharmacy, Erciyes University, Kayseri, Turkey
- Ayşe Eken, Department of Pharmaceutical Toxicology, Faculty of Pharmacy, Erciyes University, Kayseri, Turkey
- Ayşe Kübra Karaboğa Arslan, Department of Pharmacology, Faculty of Pharmacy, Erciyes University, Kayseri, Turkey
- Ayşe Nur Oktay, Department of Pharmaceutical Technology, Faculty of Pharmacy, Gazi University, Ankara, Turkey
- Ayşe Zeynep Ünal, Toxicology Department, Faculty of Pharmacy, Hacettepe University, Ankara, Turkey
- Ayşenur Gök, Ankara Unıversıty, Faculty of Veterinary Medicine, Ankara, Turkey
- Basseem Radwan, Department of Pharmacology, Faculty of Pharmacy, Erciyes University, Kayseri, Turkey
- Bayram Goçmen, Zoology Section, Department of Biology, Faculty of Science, Ege University, Izmir, Turkey
- Belma Aslım, Gazi University, Faculty of Science, Department of Biology, Teknikokullar, Ankara, Turkey
- Benjamin-Florian Hempel, Institut für Chemie, Technische Universitat Berlin, Strasse des 17. Juni 124, Berlin, Germany
- Beraat Özçelik, Department of Food Engineering, Faculty of Chemical and Metallurgical Enginerring, Istanbul Technical University, Turkey
- Berrin Tunca, Medical Biology Department, Faculty of Medicine, Uludag University, Bursa, Turkey
- Beste Yurdacan, Medical Biology Department, Faculty of Medicine, Uludag University, Gorukle, Bursa, Turkey
- Bijen Kıvçak, Deparment of Pharmacognosy, Faculty of Pharmacy, Ege University, İzmir, Turkey
- Bilge Debelec-Butuner, Department of Pharmaceutical Biotechnology, Faculty of Pharmacy, Ege University, Izmir, Turkey
- Bruno Botta, Dipartimento di Chimica e Tecnologie del Farmaco, Sapienza University of Roma, piazzale Aldo Moro 5, Roma, Italy
- Burak Durmaz, Department of Medical Biochemistry, Ege University, Turkey
- Burcu Somtürk Yılmaz, Department of Chemistry, Faculty of Sciences, Erciyes University, Kayseri, Turkey
- Burçin Türkmenoğlu, Department of Chemistry, Faculty of Sciences, Erciyes University, Kayseri, Turkey
- Buse Cevatemre, Department of Biology, Faculty of Arts and Sciences, Uludag University, Bursa, Turkey
- Büşra Şen, Department of Histology and Embryology, Faculty of Medicine, Celal Bayar University, Manisa, Turkey
- Büşra Teke, Faculty of Pharmacy, İstanbul University, Istanbul, Turkey
- Canan Eroğlu, Department of Medical Biology, Meram Faculty of Medicine, Necmettin Erbakan University, Konya, Turkey
- Canan Türkoğlu, Department of Biology, Faculty of Art and Life Sciences, Manisa Celal Bayar University, Manisa, Turkey
- Carmela Spagnuolo, Institute of Food Sciences, National Research Council, Avellino, Italy
- Çiğdem Yücel, Erciyes University Faculty of Pharmacy Department of Pharmaceutical Technology
- Damla Akogullari, Faculty of Medicine, Department of Histology & Embryology, Manisa Celal Bayar University, Manisa, Turkey

- Daniel Petras, Institut für Chemie, Technische Universitat Berlin, Strasse des 17. Juni 124, Berlin, Germany
- Demetrios A. Spandidos, Department of Toxicology, Medical School, University of Crete, Crete GR, Greece
- Didar Tasdemir, Department of Analytical Chemistry, Faculty of Pharmacy, Erciyes University, Kayseri, Turkey
- Didem Şöhretoğlu, Faculty of Pharmacy, Hacettepe Unıversıty, Ankara, Turkey
- Dilek Asci Celik, Department of Medical Biology, School of Medicine, Suleyman Demirel University, Isparta, Turkey
- Dilek Ceylan, Genome and Stem Cell Center, University of Erciyes, Kayseri, Turkey
- Ebru Avcı, Department of Medical Biology, Meram Faculty of Medicine, Necmettin Erbakan University, Konya, Turkey
- Ebru Öztürk, Department of Pharmacology, Faculty of Pharmacy, Erciyes University, Kayseri, Turkey
- Efe Kurtdede, Ankara, Turkey
- Elgin Turkoz Uluer, Department of Histology & Embryology, Faculty of Medicine, Manisa Celal Bayar University, Manisa, Turkey
- Elif Damla Arısan, Department of Molecular Biology and Genetics, Istanbul Kultur University, Atakoy Campus, Istanbul, Turkey
- Elif Dündar, Department of Pharmaceutical Botany, Graduate School of Health Sciences, Anadolu University, Eskişehir, Turkey
- Emin Sarıpınar, Department of Chemistry, Faculty of Sciences, Erciyes University, Kayseri, Turkey
- Emine Akalın Uruşak, Faculty of Pharmacy, İstanbul University, Istanbul, Turkey
- Emir Tosun, Department of Chemical Engineering, Inonu University, Malatya, Turkey
- Engin Ulukaya, Department of Clinical Biochemistry, Faculty of Medicine, Istinye University, Istanbul, Turkey
- Ercan Kurar, Department of Medical Biology, Meram Faculty of Medicine, Necmettin Erbakan University, Konya, Turkey
- Ercüment Ölmez, Faculty of Medicine, Department of Pharmacology, Celal Bayar University, Manisa, Turkey
- Erdal Bedir, Department of Bioengineering, Faculty of Engineering, Izmir Institute of Technology, Izmir, Turkey
- Erem Bilensoy, Hacettepe University Faculty of Pharmacy Department of Pharmaceutical Technology
- Eren Demirpolat, Department of Pharmacology, Faculty of Pharmacy, Erciyes University, Kayseri, Turkey
- Erkan Yilmaz, Biotechnology Institute, Ankara University, Ankara, Turkey
- Eser Yıldırım Sözmen, Department of Medical Biochemistry, Ege University, Turkey
- Esma Purut, Department of Biology, Faculty of Science, University of Istanbul, Istanbul, Turkey
- Esra Köngül, Department of Pharmacognosy, Faculty of Pharmacy, Erciyes University, Kayseri, Turkey
- Esra Küpeli Akkol, Department of Pharmaceutical Technology, Faculty of Pharmacy, Gazi University, Ankara, Turkey
- Evren Demircan, Department of Food Engineering, Faculty of Chemical and Metallurgical Enginerring, Istanbul Technical University, Turkey
- Ezgi Balkan, Department of Medical Biochemistry, Faculty of Medicine, Bezmialem Vakif University, Turkey
- Fatemeh Bahadori, Department of Pharmaceutical Biotechnology, Faculty of Pharmacy, Bezmialem Vakif University, Istanbul, Turkey

- Fatih Çöllü, Biology, Faculty of Science and Literature, Manisa Celal Bayar University, Manisa, Turkey
- Fatma Esin Kırık, Department of Medicinal Microbiology, Faculty of Medicine, Niğde Ömer Halisdemir University, Niğde, Turkey
- Fatma Firat, Department of Histology and Embryology, Faculty of Medicine, Manisa Celal Bayar University, Manisa, Turkey
- Feyzan Özdal Kurt, Department of Biology, Faculty of Art and Life Sciences, Manisa Celal Bayar University, Manisa, Turkey
- Fulya Tugba Artun, Institute of Science, Istanbul University, Istanbul, Turkey
- Funda Karbancıoğlu-Güler, Department of Food Engineering, Faculty of Chemical and Metallurgical Enginerring, Istanbul Technical University, Sarıyer, Turkey
- Funda Kosova, Faculty of Health Science, Celal Bayar University, Manisa, Turkey
- Funda Nuray Yalçın, Pharmacognosy Dept., Faculty of Pharmacy, Hacettepe University, Ankara, Turkey
- Gamze Güney Eskiler, Medical Biology Department, Faculty of Medicine, Sakarya University, Sakarya, Turkey
- Gian Luigi Russo Russo, Institute of Food Sciences, National Research Council, Avellino, Italy
- Gonca Dönmez, Department of Medicinal Biology, Faculty of Medicine, Niğde Ömer Halisdemir University, Niğde, Turkey
- Gorkem Kısmalı, Ankara, Turkey
- Gökçe Şeker Karatoprak, Erciyes University Faculty of Pharmacy Department of Pharmacognosy
- Gözde Girgin, Toxicology Department, Faculty of Pharmacy, Hacettepe University, Ankara, Turkey
- Gul Ozcan, Department of Biology, Faculty of Science, Istanbul University, Istanbul, Turkey
- Gulay Melikoglu, Department of Pharmacognosy, Faculty of Pharmacy, Istanbul University, Istanbul, Turkey
- Guzide Satır Basaran, Department of Biochemistry, Faculty of Pharmacy, Erciyes University, Kayseri, Turkey
- Gülen Melike Demir, Department of Pharmaceutical Technology, Faculty of Pharmacy, Gazi University, Ankara, Turkey
- Güliz Armagan, Department of Biochemistry, Faculty of Pharmacy, Ege University, İzmir, Turkey
- Gülşah Albayrak, Department of Histology and Embryology, Faculty of Medicine, Celal Bayar University, Manisa, Turkey
- Gülşah Çeçener, Medical Biology Department, Faculty of Medicine, Uludag University, Gorukle, Bursa, Turkey
- Gülşen Akalın Çiftçi, Department of Biochemistry, Faculty of Pharmacy, Anadolu University, Eskişehir, Turkey
- H. Fatih Gul, Department of Medical Biochemistry, Faculty of Medicine, Firat University, Elazig, Turkey
- H. Gul Dursun, Medical Biology Department, Meram Medical Faculty, Necmettin Erbakan University, Konya, Turkey
- H. Seda Vatansever, Department of Histology and Embryology, Faculty of Medicine, Manisa Celal Bayar University, Manisa, Turkey
- Hakkı Taştan, Department of Biology, Faculty of Science, Gazi University, Ankara, Turkey
- Harun Ülger, School of Medicine, Department of Anatomy, Erciyes University, Kayseri, Turkey
- Hasibe Vural, Department of Medical Biology, Meram Faculty of Medicine, Necmettin Erbakan University, Konya, Turkey
- Hatice Bekci, Department of Food Engineering, Engineering Faculty, Erciyes University, Kayseri, Turkey

- Hatice Kalkan Yıldırım, Faculty of Engineering Department of Food Engineering, Ege University, Turkey
- Hatice Susar, Department of Anatomy, Faculty of Medicine, Erciyes University, Kayseri, Turkey
- Hatice Yildirim, Department of Molecular Biology and Genetic, Balikesir University, Balikesir, Turkey
- Hikmet Memmedov, Department of Medical Biochemistry, Ege University, Turkey
- Hilal Kabadayı, Department of Histology and Embryology, School of Medicine, Manisa Celal Bayar University, Manisa, Turkey
- Hulusi Malyer, Botany Department, Faculty of Science and Art, Uludag University, Bursa, Turkey
- Huzeyfe Huriyet, Medical Biology Department, Faculty of Medicine, Uludag University, Bursa, Turkey
- Hülya Birinci, Department of Histology and Embryology, Faculty of Medicine, Celal Bayar University, Manisa, Turkey
- Hanifi Ozercan, Department of Medical Pathology, Faculty of Medicine, Firat University, Elazıg, Turkey
- Ibrahim Turan, Department of Genetic and Bioengineering, Faculty of Engineering and Natural Sciences, GumushaneUniversity, Gumushane, Turkey
- Iclal Saracoglu, Department of Pharmacognosy, Faculty of Pharmacy, Hacettepe University, Turkey
- Ilknur Cinar, Medical Biology Department, Meram Medical Faculty, Necmettin Erbakan University, Konya, Turkey
- Ismail Hakki Akgun, Department of Bioengineering, Faculty of Engineering, Ege University, Izmir, Turkey
- Ismail Ocsoy, Department of Analytical Chemistry, Faculty of Pharmacy, Erciyes University, Kayseri, Turkey
- Işıl Aydemir, Faculty of Medicine, Niğde Ömer Halisdemir University, Niğde, Turkey
- Işıl Ezgi Eryılmaz, Medical Biology Department, Faculty of Medicine, Uludag University, Bursa, Turkey
- İbrahim Çakir, Department of Food Engineering, Faculty of Engineering and Architecture, Abant İzzet Baysal University, Bolu, Turkey
- İbrahim Tuğlu, Department of Histology and Embryology, Medical of Faculty, Celal Bayar University, Manisa, Turkey
- İlhan Özer İlhan, Department of Chemistry, Faculty of Sciences, Erciyes University, Kayseri, Turkey
- İsmail Sari, Department of Medicinal Biochemistry, Faculty of Medicine, Niğde Ömer Halisdemir University, Niğde, Turkey
- İsmail Tuncer Değim, Department of Pharmaceutical Technology, Faculty of Pharmacy, Biruni University, Topkapı, İstanbul, Turkey
- Juana Diez, Department of Experimental and Health Sciences, Universitat Pompeu Fabra, Barcelona, Spain
- Jukka Hakkola, Pharmacology and Toxicology Unit, Institute of Biomedicne, University of Oulu, Oulu, Finland
- Kaan Adacan, Department of Molecular Biology and Genetics, Istanbul Kultur University, Atakoy Campus, Istanbul, Turkey
- Kadriye Nur Kasapoğlu, Department of Food Engineering, Faculty of Chemical and Metallurgical Enginerring, Istanbul Technical University, Turkey
- Kamil Vural, Department of Medicinal Pharmacology, Faculty of Medicine, Manisa Celal Bayar University, Manisa, Turkey
- Kemal Özbilgin, Department of Histology and Embryology, Faculty of Medicine, Celal Bayar University, Manisa, Turkey

- Kemal Sami Korkmaz, Department of Bioengineering, Faculty of Engineering, Ege University, Izmir, Turkey
- Konstantinos Dimas, Department of Pharmacology, Faculty of Medicine, University of Thessaly, Larissa, Greece
- Kübra Uzun, Pharmacognosy Dept., Faculty of Pharmacy, Erciyes University, Kayseri, Turkey
- Latife Merve Oktay, Faculty of Medicine Department of Medical Biology, Ege University, Turkey
- Leyla Paşayeva, Department of Pharmacognosy, Faculty of Pharmacy, Erciyes University, Kayseri, Turkey
- Mahmoud F. Elsebai, Pharmacognosy Department, Faculty of Pharmacy, Mansoura University, Mansoura, Egypt
- Mahmud Özkut, Department of Histology & Embryology, Faculty of Medicine, Manisa Celal Bayar University, Manisa, Turkey
- Marc Diederich, College of Pharmacy, Seoul National University, Seoul, Korea
- Maria usso, Institute of Food Sciences, National Research Council, Avellino, Italy
- Mehmet Berköz, Department of Pharmaceutical Biotechnology, Faculty of Pharmacy, Yuzuncu Yıl University, Van, Turkey
- Mehmet İbrahim Tuğlu, Department of Histology and Embryology, Faculty of Medicine, Manisa Celal Bayar University, Manisa, Turkey
- Mehmet Zülfü Yildiz, Zoology Section, Department of Biology, Faculty of Arts and Science, Adıyaman University, Adıyaman, Turkey
- Mehtap Nisari, Department of Anatomy, Faculty of Medicine, Erciyes University, Kayseri, Turkey
- Melike Ozgul, Department of Histology & Embryology, Faculty of Medicine, Manisa Celal Bayar University, Manisa, Turkey
- Meltem Ceylan-Ünlüsoy, Department of Pharmaceutical Chemistry, Faculty of Pharmacy, Ankara University, Ankara, Turkey
- Mert Burak Ozturk, Department of Bioengineering, Faculty of Engineering, Ege University, Izmir, Turkey
- Mert Ilhan, Department of Pharmaceutical Technology, Faculty of Pharmacy, Biruni University, İstanbul, Turkey
- Merve Alpay, Department of Biochemistry, Faculty of Medicine, Duzce University, Düzce, Turkey
- Merve Çelik Tekeli, Erciyes University Faculty of Pharmacy Department of Pharmaceutical Technology
- Merve Çelik, Department of Molecular Biology and Genetics, Faculty of Science and Letters, Istanbul Kultur University, Istanbul, Turkey
- Merve Karaman, Department of Biology, Balikesir University, Balikesir, Turkey
- Merve Uğur, Department of Molecular Biology and Genetics, Faculty of Science and Letters, Istanbul Kultur University, Istanbul, Turkey
- Metin Yıldırım, Department of Biochemistry, Faculty of Pharmacy, Mersin University, Mersin, Turkey
- Mirosław Krośniak, Department of Food Chemistry and Nutrition, Medical College, Jagiellonian University, Krakow, Poland
- Mohamed Mehiri, Nice, France
- Mustafa Cengiz, Department of Mathematics and Science Education, Education Faculty, Siirt University, Siirt, Turkey
- Mustafa Nisari, Department of Nutrition and Dietetics, Faculty of Health Sciences, University of Nuh Naci Yazgan, Kayseri, Turkey
- Mustafa Öztatlıcı, Department of Histology and Embryology, Faculty of Medicine, Manisa Celal Bayar University, Manisa, Turkey

- Mutlu Demiray, Department of Medical Oncology, KTO Karatay University, Konya, Turkey
- Müberra Koşar, Faculty of Pharmacy, Department of Pharmacognosy, Eastern Mediterranean University, Gazimağusa, North Cyprus via Mersin 10, Turkey
- Mükerrem Betül Yerer, Department of Pharmacology, Faculty of Pharmacy, Erciyes University, Kayseri, Turkey
- Müzeyyen Demirel, Department of Pharmaceutical Technology, Faculty of Pharmacy, Anadolu University, Tepebaşı, Turkey
- N. Nalan İmamoğlu, Department of Basic Sciences, Faculty of Pharmacy, Erciyes University, Kayseri, Turkey
- Nalan Özdemir, Department of Chemistry, Faculty of Sciences, Erciyes University, Talas Street, Kayseri, Turkey
- Narçın Palavan-Ünsal, Department of Molecular Biology and Genetics, Istanbul Kultur University, Atakoy Campus, Istanbul, Turkey
- Nazım Bozan, Department of Otorhinolaryngology, Faculty of Medicine, Yuzuncu Yil University, Van, Turkey
- Necip Ilhan, Department of Medical Biochemistry, Faculty of Medicine, Firat University, Elazig, Turkey
- Neel M. Fofaria, Department of Biomedical Sciences and Department of Immunotherapeutics and Biotechnology, Texas Tech University Health Sciences Center, Lubbock, USA
- Neriman İnanç, Department of Nutrition and Dietetics, Faculty of Health Sciences, University of Nuh Naci Yazgan, Kayseri, Turkey
- Nevin Çelebi, Department of Pharmaceutical Technology, Faculty of Pharmacy, Gazi University, Ankara, Turkey
- Nevin Ilhan, Department of Medical Biochemistry, Faculty of Medicine, Firat University, Elazıg, Turkey
- Nilgun Gurbuz, Department of Medical Biology, School of Medicine, Suleyman Demirel University, Isparta, Turkey
- Nilufer Cinkilic, Department of Biology, Science and Art Faculty, Uludag University, Bursa, Turkey
- Nur Selvi, Faculty of Medicine Department of Medical Biology, Ege University, Turkey
- Nurcan Silahtarlıoğlu, Graduate School Natural Applied Science, Erciyes University, Kayseri, Turkey
- Nurhayat Sutlupinar, Department of Pharmacognosy, Faculty of Pharmacy, Istanbul University, Istanbul, Turkey
- O. Faruk Kirlangic, Department of Molecular Biology and Genetic, Balikesir University, Balikesir, Turkey
- Oguzhan Tatar, Department of Medical Biochemistry, Faculty of Medicine, Firat University, Elazig, Turkey
- Oktay Özkan, Department of Medicinal Pharmacology, Faculty of Medicine, Niğde Ömer Halisdemir University, Niğde, Turkey
- Onur Bender, Biotechnology Institute, Ankara University, Ankara, Turkey
- Onur Kaya, Graduate School Natural Applied Science, Erciyes University, Kayseri, Turkey
- Oruc Allahverdiyev, Department of Pharmacology, Faculty of Pharmacy, Yuzuncu Yıl University, Van, Turkey
- Osman Oğuz, Molecular Biology and Genetics, Faculty of Life and Natural Sciences, Abdullah Gul University, Kayseri, Turkey
- Osman Tugay, Department of Biology Program of Botany, Faculty of Sciences, Selcuk University, Konya, Turkey

- Osman Üstün, Department of Pharmacognosy, Faculty of Pharmacy, Gazi University, Ankara, Turkey
- Oya Bozdağ-Dündar, Department of Pharmaceutical Chemistry, Faculty of Pharmacy, Ankara University, Ankara, Turkey
- Ozer Yılmaz, Department of Biology, Science and Art Faculty, Uludag University, Bursa, Turkey
- Ozgun Teksoy, Biology Department, Art and Science Faculty, Eskişehir Osmangazi University, Eskişehir, Turkey
- Ozgur Tag, Cancer Biology Laboratory, Department of Chemistry, Graduate School of Natural and Applied Sciences, Ege University, Izmir, Turkey
- Ozgur Vatan, Department of Biology, Science and Art Faculty, Uludag University, Bursa, Turkey
- Ömer Taş, Department of Pharmacognosy, Faculty of Pharmacy, Erciyes University, Kayseri, Turkey
- Özge Al, School of Medicine, Department of Anatomy, Erciyes University, Kayseri, Turkey
- Özge Güzel, Department of Bioengineering, Faculty of Engineering, Izmir Institute of Technology, Izmir, Turkey
- Özge Rencüzoğulları, Atakoy Campus, Department of Molecular Biology and Genetics, Istanbul Kultur University, Istanbul, Turkey
- Özlem Temiz-Arpacı, Department of Pharmaceutical Chemistry, Faculty of Pharmacy, Ankara University, Ankara, Turkey
- Pelin Taştan, Deparment of Pharmacognosy, Faculty of Pharmacy, Ege University, İzmir, Turkey
- Pelin Toros, Department of Histology & Embryology, Faculty of Medicine, Manisa Celal Bayar University, Manisa, Turkey
- Perihan Gürbüz, Pharmacognosy Dept., Faculty of Pharmacy, Erciyes University, Kayseri, Turkey
- Petek Ballar, Faculty of Pharmacy, Department of Biochemistry, Ege University, Izmir, Turkey
- Pınar Atalay Dündar, Department of Basic Sciences, Faculty of Pharmacy, Erciyes University, Kayseri, Turkey
- Pınar İkiz, Pharmacognosy Dept., Faculty of Pharmacy, Hacettepe University, Ankara, Turkey
- Pınar K. Sönmez, Department of Histology & Embryology, Faculty of Medicine, Manisa Celal Bayar University, Manisa, Turkey
- Pınar Kılıçaslan Sönmez, Department of Histology and Embryology, Faculty of Medicine, Celal Bayar University, Manisa, Turkey
- Pınar Obakan-Yerlikaya, Department of Molecular Biology and Genetics, Istanbul Kultur University, Atakoy Campus, Istanbul, Turkey
- Pınar Özden, Department of Medical Biology, Meram Faculty of Medicine, Necmettin Erbakan University, Konya, Turkey
- Pinar K. Sönmez, Department of Histology & Embryology, Faculty of Medicine, Manisa Celal Bayar University, Manisa, Turkey
- Rana Kavurmacı, Department of Advanced Technology, Ahi Evran University, Kırşehir, Turkey
- Randolph R. J. Arroo, Leicester School of Pharmacy, De Montfort University, The Gateway, Leicester LE1 9BH, UK
- Recep Eröz, Department of Genetics, Faculty of Medicine, Duzce University, Düzce, Turkey
- Remzi Soner Cengiz, Faculty of Veterinary Medicine, Turkey
- Remziye Kendirci, Department of Histology and Embryology, School of Medicine, Manisa Celal Bayar University, Manisa, Turkey
- Renata Francik, Department of Bioorganic Chemistry, Medical College, Jagiellonian University, Krakow, Poland
- Roderich D. Süssmuth, Institut für Chemie, Technische Universitat Berlin, Strasse des 17. Juni 124, Berlin, Germany

- Rojen Geylan, Department of Pharmacognosy, Faculty of Pharmacy, Erciyes University, Turkey
- Ruziye Daşkın, Botany Dept., Faculty of Science and Letters, Uludağ University, Bursa, Turkey
- S. Kerem Aydin, Sirri Yircali Anatolian High School, Balikesir, Turkey
- Sanjay K. Srivastava, Department of Biomedical Sciences and Department of Immunotherapeutics and Biotechnology, Texas Tech University Health Sciences Center, Lubbock, USA
- Seda Duman, Department of Bioengineering, Faculty of Engineering, Izmir Institute of Technology, Izmir, Turkey
- Seda Şirin, Gazi University, Faculty of Science, Department of Biology, Teknikokullar, Ankara, Turkey
- Sedat Ünal, Erciyes University Faculty of Pharmacy Department of Pharmaceutical Technology
- Seher Dalgic, Sirri Yircali Anatolian High School, Balikesir, Turkey
- Seher Yılmaz, School of Medicine, Department of Anatomy, Bozok University, Yozgat, Turkey
- Selda Eren, Faculty of Pharmacy, Erciyes University, Kayseri, Turkey
- Selen İlgün, Faculty of Pharmacy, Department of Pharmaceutical Botany, Erciyes University, Kayseri, Turkey
- Selim Demir, Department of Nutrition and Dietetics, Faculty of Health Sciences, Karadeniz Technical University, Trabzon, Turkey
- Sema Misir, Department of Biochemistry, Faculty of Pharmacy, Cumhuriyet University, Sivas, Turkey
- Senem Akkoç, Department of Chemistry, Faculty of Sciences, Erciyes University, Kayseri, Turkey
- Serap Yalcin, Department of Molecular Biology and Genetics, Ahi Evran University, Kırşehir, Turkey
- Serap Yalın, Department of Biochemistry, Faculty of Pharmacy, Mersin University, Mersin, Turkey
- Sevil Albayrak, Biology Department, Science Faculty, Erciyes University, Kayseri, Turkey
- Sevinç İnan, Department of Histology and Embryology, Faculty of Medicine, Celal Bayar University, Manisa, Turkey
- Sevtap Çağlar Yavuz, Department of Chemistry, Faculty of Sciences, Erciyes University, Kayseri, Turkey
- Seyhan Altun, Department of Biology, Faculty of Science, University of Istanbul, Istanbul, Turkey
- Sezin Anil, Department of Pharmacognosy, Faculty of Pharmacy, Istanbul University, Istanbul, Turkey
- Sharavan Ramachandran, Department of Biomedical Sciences and Department of Immunotherapeutics and Biotechnology, Texas Tech University Health Sciences Center, Lubbock, USA
- Sibel Gunes, Biology Department, Art and Science Faculty, Eskişehir Osmangazi University, Eskişehir, Turkey
- Sibel İlbasmiş Tamer, Department of Pharmaceutical Technology, Faculty of Pharmacy, Gazi University, Ankara, Turkey
- Sinem Yılmaz, Faculty of Pharmacy, Department of Biochemistry, Ege University, Izmir, Turkey
- Solmaz Susam, Department of Medical Biochemistry, Faculty of Medicine, Firat University, Elazig, Turkey
- Stefania Moccia, Institute of Food Sciences, National Research Council, Avellino, Italy
- Suheyl Furkan Konca, Department of Pharmaceutical Biotechnology, Faculty of Pharmacy, Erciyes University, Kayseri, Turkey
- Sukran Kultur, Department of Pharmaceutical Botany, Faculty of Pharmacy, Istanbul University, Istanbul, Turkey
- Sumeyra Cetinkaya, Medical Biology Department, Meram Medical Faculty, Necmettin Erbakan University, Konya, Turkey

- Suna Sabuncuoğlu, Toxicology Department, Faculty of Pharmacy, Hacettepe University, Ankara, Turkey
- Suna Sayğılı, Department of Histology and Embryology, Faculty of Medicine, Celal Bayar University, Manisa, Turkey
- Şamil Öztürk, Department of Histology & Embryology, Faculty of Medicine, Manisa Celal Bayar University, Manisa, Turkey
- Şebnem Kurhan, Novel Food Technologies Development, Application and Research Center, Abant İzzet Baysal University, Bolu, Turkey
- Taner Dağcı, Department of Physiology, Faculty of Medicine, Ege University, İzmir, Turkey
- Terken Baydar, Toxicology Department, Faculty of Pharmacy, Hacettepe University, Ankara, Turkey
- Tevhide Sel, Ankara University, Faculty of Veterinary Medicine, Turkey
- Tolga Cavas, Medical Biology Department, Faculty of Medicine, Uludag University, Bursa, Turkey
- Tolga Ertekin, School of Medicine, Department of Anatomy, Kocatepe University, Afyon, Turkey
- Tuna Onal, Department of Histology & Embryology, Faculty of Medicine, Manisa Celal Bayar University, Manisa, Turkey
- U. Sebnem Harput, Department of Pharmacognosy, Faculty of Pharmacy, Hacettepe University, Ankara, Turkey
- Ünal Egeli, Medical Biology Department, Faculty of Medicine, Uludag University, Bursa, Turkey
- Varol Sahinturk, Vocational School of Health Services, Eskişehir Osmangazi University, Eskişehir, Turkey
- Vasilis P. Androutsopoulos, Department of Toxicology, Medical School, University of Crete, Crete GR, Greece
- Veysel Kayser, Faculty of Pharmacy, The University of Sydney, Sydney, Australia
- Vildan Betül Yenigun, Department of Medical Biochemistry, Faculty of Medicine, Bezmialem Vakif University, Turkey
- Yalcin Erzurumlu, Faculty of Pharmacy, Department of Biochemistry, Ege University, Izmir, Turkey
- Yasemin Tekin, Biology Department, Art and Science Faculty, Eskişehir Osmangazi University, Eskişehir, Turkey
- Yasin Genc, Department of Pharmacognosy, Faculty of Pharmacy, Hacettepe University, Ankara, Turkey
- Yeşim Aktaş, Erciyes University Faculty of Pharmacy Department of Pharmaceutical Technology
- Yuksel Aliyazicioglu, Medicinal Plants, Traditional Medicine Practice and Research Center, Gumushane University, Gumushane, Turkey
- Yüksel Öğünç, Department of Biochemistry, Faculty of Pharmacy, Anadolu University, Eskişehir, Turkey
- Zerrin Seller, Department of Biochemistry, Faculty of Pharmacy, Anadolu University, Eskişehir, Turkey
- Zeynep Dogan, Department of Pharmacognosy, Faculty of Pharmacy, Hacettepe University, Ankara, Turkey

Acknowledgments: The authors are indebted to Erciyes University Rectorate and Erciyes University Faculty of Pharmacy and Larkin University, College of Pharmacy for their valuable contributions to the organization and to the Research Foundation of Erciyes University (Project Number: TSS-2017-7720) for their financial support of this symposium. Also to the local organizing committee members (Perihan Gürbüz, Eren Demirpolat, Ahmet Cumaoğlu, Gökçe Şeker Karatoprak, Ayşe Kübra Karaboğa Aslan, Ebru Öztürk and Görkem Kısmalı) for their accomplished work.

Author Contributions: M.B.Y. wrote the manuscript and A.B. reviewed and edited the document.

References

1. Yerer, M.B. Growth Factors Responsible from the Cancer Progress: Role of Natural Products. *Proceedings* **2017**, *1*, 979. [CrossRef]
2. Bishayee, A. Natural Products for Cancer Prevention and Therapy: Progress, Pitfalls and Promise. *Proceedings* **2017**, *1*, 982. [CrossRef]
3. Amin, A. Novel Anticancer Capacities of Saffron. *Proceedings* **2017**, *1*, 834. [CrossRef]
4. Diederich, M. Cardiac Glycosides as Novel Modulators of Cancer Cell Survival. *Proceedings* **2017**, *1*, 972. [CrossRef]
5. Russo, G.L.; Russo, M.; Spagnuolo, C.; Moccia, S. Ins and Outs of Flavonoids in Cancer Prevention vs. Cancer Therapy: A Lesson from Quercetin in Leukemia. *Proceedings* **2017**, *1*, 977. [CrossRef]
6. Arroo, R.R.J.; Şöhretoğlu, D.; Spandidos, D.A.; Androutsopoulos, V.P. Anticancer Potential of Flavones. *Proceedings* **2017**, *1*, 975. [CrossRef]
7. Borriello, A. Resveratrol in Cancer Prevention and Treatment: Focusing on Molecular Targets and Mechanism of Action. *Proceedings* **2017**, *1*, 976. [CrossRef]
8. Elsebai, M.F.; Hakkola, J.; Mehiri, M.; Diez, J. Cynaropicrin: A Promising Natural Agent with Antitumor and Antiviral Activities. *Proceedings* **2017**, *1*, 974. [CrossRef]
9. Koşar, M. Relationship between Structure of Phenolics and Anticancer Activity. *Proceedings* **2017**, *1*, 978. [CrossRef]
10. Cevatemre, B.; Dimas, K.; Botta, B.; Ulukaya, E. Pristimerin is a Promising Natural Product against Breast Cancer *in vitro* and *in vivo* through Apoptosis and the Blockage of Autophagic Flux. *Proceedings* **2017**, *1*, 973. [CrossRef]
11. Demiray, M.; Bahadori, F. Can Curcumin be Employed to Promote the Integration of Oncology and Natural Products? *Proceedings* **2017**, *1*, 980. [CrossRef]
12. Fofaria, N.M.; Ramachandran, S.; Srivastava, S.K. Therapeutic Potential of Black Pepper Compound for BRaf Resistant Melanoma. *Proceedings* **2017**, *1*, 981. [CrossRef]
13. Gul, H.F.; Ilhan, N.; Ilhan, N.; Ozercan, I.H. Effect of Pomegranate Extract and Tangeretin on Specific Pathways in the Rat Breast Cancer Model Induced with DMBA. *Proceedings* **2017**, *1*, 983. [CrossRef]
14. Oğuz, O.; Adan, A. Synergistic Cytotoxic Effects of Resveratrol in Combination with Ceramide Metabolizing Enzymes in Ph + Acute Lymphoblastic Leukemia. *Proceedings* **2017**, *1*, 984. [CrossRef]
15. Debelec-Butuner, B.; Ozturk, M.B.; Tag, O.; Akgun, I.H.; Bedir, E.; Korkmaz, K.S. Characterization of Cycloartane-Type Sapogenol Derivatives for Prostate Cancer Chemoprevention. *Proceedings* **2017**, *1*, 985. [CrossRef]
16. Obakan-Yerlikaya, P.; Adacan, K.; Arısan, E.D.; Çoker-Gürkan, A.; Palavan-Ünsal, N. Epibrassinolide Treatment Caused Autophagy or Apoptosis Decision in a Time-Dependent Manner through ER Stress in Colon Cancer Cells. *Proceedings* **2017**, *1*, 986. [CrossRef]
17. Alpay, M.; Eröz, R.; Kısmalı, G.; Kurtdede, E. Determination of Silymarin Molecule Activity in Colon Cancer by AgNOR Technique. *Proceedings* **2017**, *1*, 987. [CrossRef]
18. Dönmez, G.; Kırık, F.E.; Aydemir, I.; Sarı, İ.; Özkan, O.; Savran, A.; Tuğlu, M.İ. The Cytotoxic Effect of *Lysimachia savranii* on the Neuroblastoma Cells. *Proceedings* **2017**, *1*, 988. [CrossRef]
19. Gürkan, A.J.; Çelik, M.; Uğur, M.; Arisan, A.D.; Obakan Yerlikaya, P.; Palavan Ünsal, N. Autocrine Growth Hormone-Triggered Curcumin Resistance Abolished by NF-κB Signaling Pathway Dependent on Inflammatory Cytokines and Active Polyamine Catabolic Machinery in MCF-7, MDA-MB-453 and MDA-MB-231 Breast Cancer Cells. *Proceedings* **2017**, *1*, 989. [CrossRef]
20. Aydemir, I.; Sari, İ.; Dönmez, G.; Kırık, F.E.; Özkan, O.; Savran, A.; Tuğlu, M.İ. The Effect of *Lysimachia Savranii* on the Migration of the Breast Cancer Cells. *Proceedings* **2017**, *1*, 990. [CrossRef]
21. Özkan, O.; Aydemir, I.; Sarı, İ.; Dönmez, G.; Kırık, F.E.; Savran, A.; Tuğlu, M.İ. Investigation of Cytotoxic Effect of *Origanum Minutiflorum* on Cancer Cells. *Proceedings* **2017**, *1*, 991. [CrossRef]
22. Arisan, E.D.; Rencüzoğulları, Ö.; Çoker-Gürkan, A.; Obakan-Yerlikaya, P.; Palavan-Ünsal, N. Celastrol Modulates Lipid Synthesis via PI3K/Akt/mTOR Signaling Axis to finalize Cell Death Response in Prostate Cancer Cells. *Proceedings* **2017**, *1*, 992. [CrossRef]
23. Sayğılı, S.; Birinci, H.; Şen, B.; Öztatlıcı, M.; İnan, S.; Özbilgin, K. Investigation of the Effect of Paclitaxel and Pycnogenol on Mitochondrial Dynamics in Breast Cancer Therapy. *Proceedings* **2017**, *1*, 993. [CrossRef]

24. Nisari, M.; Yılmaz, S.; Ertekin, T.; Ceylan, D.; İnanç, N.; Al, Ö.; Ülger, H. Effects of Curcumin on Lipid Peroxidation and Antioxidant Enzymes in Kidney, Liver, Brain and Testis of Mice Bearing Ehrlich Solid Tumor. *Proceedings* **2017**, *1*, 994. [CrossRef]
25. Öztürk, E.; Karaboğa Arslan, A.K.; Radwan, B.; Yerer, M.B. Curcumin Enhances the Efficacy of 5-FU in Colo205 Cell Lines. *Proceedings* **2017**, *1*, 995. [CrossRef]
26. Erzurumlu, Y.; Tag, O.; Yılmaz, S.; Ballar, P.; Bedir, E. Effect of a New Sapogenol Derivative (AG-07) on Cell Death via Necrosis. *Proceedings* **2017**, *1*, 996. [CrossRef]
27. Genc, Y.; Harput, U.S.; Saracoglu, I. Cytotoxic and Antiinflammatory Activity Guided Studies on *Plantago holosteum* Scop. *Proceedings* **2017**, *1*, 997. [CrossRef]
28. Öztürk, E.; Karaboğa Arslan, A.K.; Yerer, M.B. Continuously Monitoring the Cytotoxicity of API-1, α-Chaconine and α-Solanine on Human Lung Carcinoma A549. *Proceedings* **2017**, *1*, 998. [CrossRef]
29. Karaboğa Arslan, A.K.; Yerer, M.B. The Effects of α-Chaconine on ER-α Positive Endometrium Cancer Cells. *Proceedings* **2017**, *1*, 999. [CrossRef]
30. Eroğlu, C.; Kurar, E.; Avcı, E.; Vural, H. Investigation of Apoptotic Effect of Sinapic Acid in Hep3B and HepG2 Human Hepatocellular Carcinoma Cells. *Proceedings* **2017**, *1*, 1000. [CrossRef]
31. Paşayeva, L.; Üstün, O.; Demirpolat, E.; Karatoprak, G.Ş.; Tugay, O.; Koşar, M. Cytotoxic and Antioxidant Activity of Four *Cousinia* Species of Stenocephalae Bunge Section. *Proceedings* **2017**, *1*, 1001. [CrossRef]
32. Avcı, E.; Eroğlu, C.; Özden, P.; Vural, H.; Kurar, E. Apoptotic Effect of Ginnalin A on MDA-MB-231 and MCF7 Human Breast Cancer Cell Lines. *Proceedings* **2017**, *1*, 1002. [CrossRef]
33. Eken, A.; Karaboğa Arslan, A.K.; Öztürk, E.; Ökçesiz, A.; Yerer, M.B. Cytotoxic Effects of Coumarin Compounds Imperatorin and Osthole, Alone and in Combination with 5-Fluorouracil in Colon Carcinoma Cells. *Proceedings* **2017**, *1*, 1003. [CrossRef]
34. Gürbüz, P.; Uzun, K.; Öztürk, E.; Yerer, M.B. Screening of Some Apiaceae and Asteraceae Plants for Their Cytotoxic Potential. *Proceedings* **2017**, *1*, 1004. [CrossRef]
35. Oktay, A.N.; İlbasmiş Tamer, S.; Çelebi, N. Cyclodextrine Based Nanogels and Phase Solubility Studies of Flurbiprofen as a Chemopreventive Agent. *Proceedings* **2017**, *1*, 1005. [CrossRef]
36. Somtürk Yılmaz, B.; Akkoç, S.; Özdemir, N. Effect of a Synthesized Compound against Cancerous Cell Line and Synthesis of Copper Ion Incorporated 1-(3,4-Diaminophenyl) Ethanone-Based Hybrid Nanoflowers. *Proceedings* **2017**, *1*, 1006. [CrossRef]
37. Akkoç, S.; Özer, İ.; Kayser, V. Development of Effective Anticancer Drug Candidates against Breast and Colon Cancers. *Proceedings* **2017**, *1*, 1007. [CrossRef]
38. Çağlar Yavuz, S.; Somtürk Yılmaz, B.; Özdemir, N.; Sarıpınar, E. Synthesis of Copper Ion Incorporated Aminoguanidine Derivatives-Based Hybrid Nanoflowers. *Proceedings* **2017**, *1*, 1008. [CrossRef]
39. Bender, O.; Atalay, A. Evaluation of Anti-Proliferative and Cytotoxic Properties of Chlorogenic Acid against Breast Cancer Cell Lines by Real Time Monitoring. *Proceedings* **2017**, *1*, 1009. [CrossRef]
40. Yurdacan, B.; Egeli, Ü.; Güney Eskiler, G.; Eryılmaz, I.E.; Çeçener, G.; Tunca, B. Investigation of Apoptotic Effects of Usnic Acid on Hepatocellular Carcinoma. *Proceedings* **2017**, *1*, 1010. [CrossRef]
41. Egeli, Ü.; Yurdacan, B.; Huriyet, H.; Güney Eskiler, G.; Eryılmaz, I.E.; Cavas, T.; Çeçener, G.; Malyer, H.; Tunca, B. In Vitro Cytotoxic Effect Evaluation of *Dioscorea communis* (L.) Caddick & Wilkin Rhizome and Stem Extracts on Hepatocellular Carcinoma Cells. *Proceedings* **2017**, *1*, 1011. [CrossRef]
42. Şen, B.; Toros, P.; Sönmez, P.K.; Özkut, M.; Öztürk, Ş.; Çöllü, F.; Inan, S.; Tuğlu, İ. The Effect of Herbal Medicine on Neuroblastoma Cell Line in Culture. *Proceedings* **2017**, *1*, 1012. [CrossRef]
43. Celik, D.A.; Gurbuz, N. The Foods Containing miR-193b May Inhibit the Growth of Breast Cancer Cells. *Proceedings* **2017**, *1*, 1013. [CrossRef]
44. Gurbuz, N.; Celik, D.A. Is the Dietary miR-193b a Novel Cell Cycle Arresting Source for Breast Carcinoma? *Proceedings* **2017**, *1*, 1014. [CrossRef]
45. Turkoz Uluer, E.; Ozgul, M.; Onal, T.; Ozbilgin, K.; Inan, S. The Effects of Wortmannin and EGCG and Combined Treatments on MDA-MB-231 Breast Cancer Cell Lines via Inactivation of PI3K Signaling Pathway. *Proceedings* **2017**, *1*, 1015. [CrossRef]
46. Ozgul, M.; Turkoz Uluer, E.; Onal, H.; Akogullari, D.; Ozbilgin, K.; Inan, S. The Effects of Paclitaxel and Metformin and Combined Treatments on TLR Signaling Pathway on MDA-MB-231 Breast Cancer Cell Lines. *Proceedings* **2017**, *1*, 1016. [CrossRef]

47. Tosun, E.; Baysar, A. Inhibition of Telomerase Activity by Cucurbitacin I in Colon Cancer Cell Line, LS174T. *Proceedings* **2017**, *1*, 1017. [CrossRef]
48. Tosun, E.; Baysar, A. Effect of Cucurbitacin I on Proliferation and Migration in Colorectal Cancer Cell Line, LS174T. *Proceedings* **2017**, *1*, 1018. [CrossRef]
49. Artun, F.T.; Karagoz, A.; Ozcan, G.; Melikoglu, G.; Anil, S.; Kultur, S.; Sutlupinar, N. In Vitro Anticancer and Cytotoxic Activities of Some Plant Extracts on HeLa and Vero Cell Lines. *Proceedings* **2017**, *1*, 1019. [CrossRef]
50. Özkut, M.; Albayrak, G.; Kılıçaslan Sönmez, P.; Şen, B.; Toros, P.; Öztürk, Ş.; Çöllü, F.; İnan, S.; Tuğlu, M.İ. Anticancer Effects of Oleocanthal and Pinus Pinaster on Breast Cancer Cell in Culture. *Proceedings* **2017**, *1*, 1020. [CrossRef]
51. Kılıçaslan Sönmez, P.; Albayrak, G.; Özkut, M.; Şen, B.; Toros, P.; Öztürk, Ş.; Çöllü, F.; İnan, S.; Tuğlu, M.İ. Antiproliferative and Apoptotic Effects of the Medicinal Plants on Breast Cancer Cell Lines. *Proceedings* **2017**, *1*, 1021. [CrossRef]
52. Kabadayı, H.; Kendirci, R.; Vatansever, H.S. The Role of Trophoblastic Stem Cells Conditioned Media on JAR Cell Culture. *Proceedings* **2017**, *1*, 1022. [CrossRef]
53. Birinci, H.; Şen, B.; Sayğılı, S.; Ölmez, E.; Türköz Uluer, E.; Özbilgin, K. The Effect of Pycnogenol and Paclitaxel on DNA Damage in Human Breast Cancer Cell Line. *Proceedings* **2017**, *1*, 1023. [CrossRef]
54. Birinci, H.; Şen, B.; Sayğılı, S.; Ölmez, E.; İnan, S.; Özbilgin, K. Investigation of the Effects of Paclitaxel and Pycnogenol on Inflammatory Response (PTX3, BDNF, IGF2R) in Human Breast Cancer Cell Line. *Proceedings* **2017**, *1*, 1024. [CrossRef]
55. Gul, H.F.; Ilhan, N.; Susam, S.; Tatar, O.; Ilhan, N. Is There Any Protective Effect of Pomegranate and Tangeretin on the DMBA-Induced Rat Breast Cancer Model? *Proceedings* **2017**, *1*, 1025. [CrossRef]
56. Sari, İ.; Dönmez, G.; Kırık, F.E.; Aydemir, I.; Özkan, O.; Savran, A.; Vural, K.; Tuğlu, M.İ. The Neurotoxic Effects of *Origanum minutiflorum*. *Proceedings* **2017**, *1*, 1026. [CrossRef]
57. Eryılmaz, I.E.; Güney Eskiler, G.; Yurdacan, B.; Egeli, Ü.; Çeçener, G.; Tunca, B. The Cytotoxic and Apoptotic Effects of Usnic Acid on Prostate Cancer versus Normal Cells. *Proceedings* **2017**, *1*, 1027. [CrossRef]
58. Vatan, O.; Yılmaz, O.; Huriyet, H.; Cavas, T.; Cinkılıç, N. Antiproliferative Effect of Methanolic Extract of Linum arboreum on A549 Cells. *Proceedings* **2017**, *1*, 1028. [CrossRef]
59. Huriyet, H.; Cavas, T.; Vatan, O.; Cinkilic, N. Investigation of In Vitro Cytotoxic Effects of Montivipera xanthina on Healthy and Cancer Human Lung Cell Lines. *Proceedings* **2017**, *1*, 1029. [CrossRef]
60. Tekeli, M.Ç.; Yücel, Ç.; Ünal, S.; Şeker Karatoprak, G.; Aktaş, Y.; Bilensoy, E. Development and Characterization of Paclitaxel-loaded PLGA Nanoparticles and Evaluation of Cytotoxicity on MCF-7 cell line by MTT Assay. *Proceedings* **2017**, *1*, 1030. [CrossRef]
61. Aydin, S.K.; Dalgic, S.; Karaman, M.; Kirlangic, O.F.; Yildirim, H. Effects of Fulvic Acid on Different Cancer Cell Lines. *Proceedings* **2017**, *1*, 1031. [CrossRef]
62. Berköz, M.; Yıldırım, M.; Allahverdiyev, O.; Krośniak, M.; Francik, R.; Bozan, N.; Yalın, S. Antioxidant, Antibacterial and Antiproliferative Activities of Turkish Rhubarb (*Rheum palmatum* L.) leaf Extracts. *Proceedings* **2017**, *1*, 1032. [CrossRef]
63. Toros, P.; Şen, B.; Sönmez, P.K.; Özkut, M.; Öztürk, Ş.; Çöllü, F.; İnan, S.; Tuğlu, İ. The Effect of Herbal Medicine on Colon Cancer Cells in Culture. *Proceedings* **2017**, *1*, 1033. [CrossRef]
64. Toros, P.; Şen, B.; Sönmez, P.K.; Özkut, M.; Öztürk, Ş.; Çöllü, F.; İnan, S.; Tuğlu, S. The Effect of Herbal Medicine on Prostate Cancer Cells in Culture. *Proceedings* **2017**, *1*, 1034. [CrossRef]
65. Şirin, S.; Aslım, B. Determination of Antioxidant Capacity, Phenolic Acid Composition and Antiproliferative Effect Associated with Phenylalanine Ammonia Lyase (PAL) Activity in Some Plants Naturally Growing under Salt Stress. *Proceedings* **2017**, *1*, 1035. [CrossRef]
66. Ünal, S.; Yücel, Ç.; Çelik Tekeli, M.; Şeker Karatoprak, G.; Aktaş, Y.; Bilensoy, E. Development and Characterization of Paclitaxel-Loaded PLGA Nanoparticles and Cytotoxicity Assessment By MTT Assay on A549 Cell Line. *Proceedings* **2017**, *1*, 1036. [CrossRef]
67. Kavurmacı, R.; Yalcin, S. Evaluation of In Vitro Anti-Proliferative Activity of St. John's Wort (*Hypericum perforatum* Linn.) Plant Extract on Cervix Adenocarcinoma. *Proceedings* **2017**, *1*, 1037. [CrossRef]
68. Kavurmacı, R.; Yalcin, S. The Cytotoxic Effect of Annona muricata Leaf Extract on Triple Negative Breast Cancer Cell Line. *Proceedings* **2017**, *1*, 1038. [CrossRef]
69. Albayrak, S.; Silahtarlıoğlu, N. Cytotoxic Activity of *Achillea coarctata* Poir. Extract. *Proceedings* **2017**, *1*, 1039. [CrossRef]

70. Albayrak, S.; Kaya, O. Cytotoxic Activity of Endemic *Astragalus argaeus* Boiss. from Turkey. *Proceedings* **2017**, *1*, 1040. [CrossRef]
71. Kurhan, Ş.; Çakir, İ. Lactic Acid Bacteria Mediated Apoptosis Induction: Natural Way of Colon Cancer Cells' Inhibition. *Proceedings* **2017**, *1*, 1041. [CrossRef]
72. Akkoç, S.; Türkmenoğlu, B.; Çağlar Yavuz, S. Synthesized a New Organic Compound's Cytotoxic Activity Quantum Mechanics Calculations and Docking Studies. *Proceedings* **2017**, *1*, 1042. [CrossRef]
73. Dündar, E.; Akalın Çiftçi, G.; Altıntaş, A. Anticancer Activity of Centaurea babylonica L. *Proceedings* **2017**, *1*, 1043. [CrossRef]
74. Satir Basaran, G.; Bekci, H.; Baldemir, A.; İlgün, S.; Cumaoğlu, A. Cytotoxic Effects of Functional Foods *Momordica charantia* L. and *Lycium barbarum* L. Extracts on Prostate Cancer Cells. *Proceedings* **2017**, *1*, 1044. [CrossRef]
75. Atalay Dündar, P.; İmamoğlu, N.N. Cytotoxic Effects of Kynurenic Acid and Quinaldic Acid in Hepatocellular Carcinoma (HepG2) Cell Line. *Proceedings* **2017**, *1*, 1045. [CrossRef]
76. Kosova, F.; Temiz-Arpacı, Ö.; Ölmez, E.; Tuğlu, İ. The Effects of Benzoxasol Derivate Compounds in Breast Cancer Cells. *Proceedings* **2017**, *1*, 1046. [CrossRef]
77. Taştan, P.; Armagan, G.; Dağcı, T.; Kıvçak, B. Potential Cytotoxic Activity of Psephellus pyrrhoblepharus Extracts. *Proceedings* **2017**, *1*, 1047. [CrossRef]
78. Güzel, Ö.; Duman, S.; Yılmaz, S.; Pirhan, A.F.; Bedir, E. Screening of Onosma Species for Cytotoxic Activity. *Proceedings* **2017**, *1*, 1048. [CrossRef]
79. Erzurumlu, Y.; Petras, D.; Goçmen, B.; Hempel, B.F.; Heiss, P.; Yildiz, M.Z.; Süssmuth, R.D.; Nalbantsoy, A. Apoptotic Effects of Mount Bulgar Viper (*Montivipera bulgardaghica*) PLA2 and SVMPs Venom Peptide fractions on HeLa and A549 Cancer Cells. *Proceedings* **2017**, *1*, 1049. [CrossRef]
80. Misir, S.; Demir, S.; Turan, I.; Aliyazicioglu, Y. Turkish Propolis Extract Increases Apoptosis via Induction of Mitochondrial Membrane Potential Loss in MCF-7 Cells. *Proceedings* **2017**, *1*, 1050. [CrossRef]
81. Al, Ö.; Ülger, H.; Eetekin, T.; Nisari, M.; Susar, H.; Ceylan, D.; Şeker Karatoprak, G. The Effect of Gilaburu (*Viburnum opulus*) Juice on Ehrlich Ascites Tumor (EAT) Cell Culture. *Proceedings* **2017**, *1*, 1051. [CrossRef]
82. Öğünç, Y.; Demirel, M.; Seller, Z. Synthesis and Characterizations of Folate-Conjugated PLGA-PEG Nanoparticles Loaded with Dual Agents. *Proceedings* **2017**, *1*, 1052. [CrossRef]
83. Dogan, Z.; Saracoglu, I. Selective Cytotoxic Activity of Scutellaria Species. *Proceedings* **2017**, *1*, 1053. [CrossRef]
84. Cengiz, R.S.; Gök, A.; Kurtdede, E.; Kısmalı, G.; Sel, T. The Antiproliferative Effect of Alpha Tocopherol in F98 Cell Culture. *Proceedings* **2017**, *1*, 1054. [CrossRef]
85. Paşayeva, L.; Köngül, E.; Geylan, R.; Şeker Karatoprak, G.; Tugay, O. Analysis of the Cytotoxic Effects of Eryngium billardieri Delar. Extracts on MCF7 Cell Line. *Proceedings* **2017**, *1*, 1055. [CrossRef]
86. İlgün, S.; Şeker Karatoprak, G.; Koşar, M. Cytotoxic Effects of Alchemilla mollis (Buser) Rothm. Extracts on MCF 7 Cell Line. *Proceedings* **2017**, *1*, 1056. [CrossRef]
87. Demirpolat, E.; Paşayeva, L.; Tugay, O. Comparative Evaluation of the Cytotoxic Effects of Stem and Flower Extracts of *Rhaponticoides iconiensis* (Hub.-Mor.) M.V.Agab. & Greuter. *Proceedings* **2017**, *1*, 1057. [CrossRef]
88. Bekci, H.; Satır Basaran, G.; Baldemir, A.; Cumaoglu, A. Goji Berry Fruit Extract Suppresses Cell Proliferation of Breast Cancer Cells by Inhibiting EGFR/ERK Signalling. *Proceedings* **2017**, *1*, 1058. [CrossRef]
89. Memmedov, H.; Durmaz, B.; Merve Oktay, L.; Selvi, N.; Kalkan Yıldırım, H.; Yıldırım Sözmen, E. Biologically Transformed Propolis Exhibits Cytotoxic Effect on A375 Malignant Melanoma Cells In Vitro. *Proceedings* **2017**, *1*, 1059. [CrossRef]
90. Cinar, I.; Cetinkaya, S.; Dursun, H.G. Rheum ribes Extract Increase the Expression Level of miR-200 Family in Human Colorectal Cancer Cells. *Proceedings* **2017**, *1*, 1060. [CrossRef]
91. Cetinkaya, S.; Cinar, I.; Dursun, H.G. Potential Effects of *Liquidambar orientalis* Mill. Against HT-29 and HCT-116 Cell Lines. *Proceedings* **2017**, *1*, 1061. [CrossRef]
92. Gök, A.; Kurtdede, E.; Cengiz, R.S.; Kısmalı, G.; Sel, T. The Effect of Tocopherol-α on the Cell Viability in Caco-2 Cell Line. *Proceedings* **2017**, *1*, 1062. [CrossRef]
93. Kasapoğlu, K.N.; Kocyigit, A.; Yenigun, V.B.; Balkan, E.; Demircan, E.; Karbancıoğlu-Güler, F.; Özçelik, B. In Vitro Antioxidant and Anticancer Activities of Some Local Plants from Bolu Province of Turkey. *Proceedings* **2017**, *1*, 1063. [CrossRef]

94. Özden, P.; Avcı, E.; Vural, H. Survey of the Apoptotic Effect of Ginnalin A on Hep3b Human Hepatocellular Carcinoma Cell Line. *Proceedings* **2017**, *1*, 1064. [CrossRef]
95. Cengiz, M.; Teksoy, O.; Sahinturk, V.; Tekin, Y.; Gunes, S.; Ayhanci, A. Ameliorative Effects of Carvacrol on Cyclophosphamide-Induced Testis Damage and Oxidative Stress. *Proceedings* **2017**, *1*, 1066. [CrossRef]
96. Konca, S.F.; Tasdemir, D.; Aydogdu, G.; Yilmaz, E.; Bozkir, A.; Ocsoy, I. Synthesis of Anthocyanin-Rich Red cabbage Nanoflowers and Their Antimicrobial and Cytotoxic Properties. *Proceedings* **2017**, *1*, 1067. [CrossRef]
97. Uzun, K.; İkiz, P.; Daşkın, R.; Gürbüz, P.; Yalçın, F.N. Cytotoxic Potentials of Some Asteraceae Plants from Turkey on HeLa Cell Line. *Proceedings* **2017**, *1*, 1068. [CrossRef]
98. Purut, E.; Altun, S. The Role of Lidocaine in the Dunning Model Rat Prostate Cancer Cells: Cell Kinetics and Motility. *Proceedings* **2017**, *1*, 1069. [CrossRef]
99. Eren, S.; Bekci, H.; Satır Basaran, G.; Seker Karatoprak, G.; Cumaoglu, A. *Pelargonium endlicherianum* Fenzl. Root Extract Suppresses Cell Proliferation of Prostate Cancer Cells. *Proceedings* **2017**, *1*, 1070. [CrossRef]
100. Girgin, G.; Sabuncuoğlu, S.; Ünal, A.Z.; Baydar, T. Assessment of Antioxidant and Cytotoxic Activity of Known Antioxidants Compared to Neopterin. *Proceedings* **2017**, *1*, 1071. [CrossRef]
101. Sabuncuoğlu, S.; Ünal, A.Z.; Girgin, G. Comparison of Radical Scavenging and Cytotoxic Activities of Well-Known Non-Enzymatic Antioxidants. *Proceedings* **2017**, *1*, 1072. [CrossRef]
102. Ceylan-Ünlüsoy, M.; Bozdağ-Dündar, O. A Study on the Synthesis and Anticancer Activities of Novel 6-Methoxy Flavonyl Piperazine Derivatives. *Proceedings* **2017**, *1*, 1073. [CrossRef]
103. Demir, G.M.; Ilhan, M.; Küpeli Akkol, E.; Taştan, H.; Işık, A.; Tuncer Değim, İ. Effect of Paclitaxel Loaded Chitosan Nanoparticles and Quantum Dots on Breast Cancer. *Proceedings* **2017**, *1*, 1074. [CrossRef]
104. Teke, B.; Akalın Uruşak, E. Turkish Medicinal Plants Used in Cancer Treatment and Evaluation of Plant Usage in the Oncology Clinic of the İstanbul University Faculty of Medicine. *Proceedings* **2017**, *1*, 1075. [CrossRef]
105. Firat, F.; Türkoğlu, C.; Özdal Kurt, F.; Vatansever, H.S. Is Acteosid Effects On Colon Cancer Stem Cells via Inflamation and/or Apoptosis? *Proceedings* **2017**, *1*, 1076. [CrossRef]
106. Köngül, E.; Taş, Ö.; Paşayeva, L.; Şeker Karatoprak, G. Analysis of the Cytotoxic Effects of *Achillea millefolium* L. Extracts on MCF7 Cell Line. *Proceedings* **2017**, *1*, 1077. [CrossRef]

5

The Dual Antioxidant/Prooxidant Effect of Eugenol and its Action in Cancer Development and Treatment

Daniel Pereira Bezerra [1], Gardenia Carmen Gadelha Militão [2], Mayara Castro de Morais [3] and Damião Pergentino de Sousa [3,*]

1 Instituto Gonçalo Moniz, Fundação Oswaldo Cruz (IGM-FIOCRUZ/BA), Salvador 40296-710, Bahia, Brazil; danielpbezerra@gmail.com
2 Departamento de Fisiologia, Universidade Federal de Pernambuco, Recife 50670-901, Pernambuco, Brazil; gcgadelha@yahoo.com.br
3 Departamento de Ciências Farmacêuticas, Universidade Federal da Paraíba, João Pessoa 58051-970, Paraíba, Brazil; mayaracastrodemorais@gmail.com
* Correspondence: damiao_desousa@yahoo.com.br;

Abstract: The formation of reactive oxygen species (ROS) during metabolism is a normal process usually compensated for by the antioxidant defense system of an organism. However, ROS can cause oxidative damage and have been proposed to be the main cause of age-related clinical complications and diseases such as cancer. In recent decades, the relationship between diet and cancer has been more studied, especially with foods containing antioxidant compounds. Eugenol is a natural compound widely found in many aromatic plant species, spices and foods and is used in cosmetics and pharmaceutical products. Eugenol has a dual effect on oxidative stress, which can action as an antioxidant or prooxidant agent. In addition, it has anti-carcinogenic, cytotoxic and antitumor properties. Considering the importance of eugenol in the area of food and human health, in this review, we discuss the role of eugenol on redox status and its potential use in the treatment and prevention of cancer.

Keywords: reactive oxygen species; metabolism; antitumor activity; antioxidant activity; phenylpropanoid; natural products; essential oils; clove; *Syzygium aromaticum*

---

1. Introduction

Reactive oxygen species (ROS) are a heterogeneous group of molecules that are, along with endogenous antioxidants, ubiquitously present in all organisms. They are implicated in various diseases including malignant transformations [1]. The term "oxidative stress" refers to an imbalance in which pro-oxidants overwhelm the capacity of antioxidant defense systems [2]; it has been shown to contribute to the development of some types of cancer [3].

The report of anticancer potential of aromatic compounds found in foods and plants have increased in the recent decades [4–8] and there are advanced studies of mechanisms of action and clinical approaches in progress. This chemical class of natural products show interesting potential as health promoting agents and, consequently, with application to improving the quality of life. These include the polyphenols that are important components of human diet. Interestingly, some of these compounds may act as either antioxidants or pro-oxidants to exert protective effects against cancer [9–11]. Eugenol (4-allyl-2-methoxyphenol) (Figure 1) is an aromatic phenylpropanoid phenol contained in clove (*Syzygium aromaticum*, Myrtaceae), which is well-known for its culinary uses. Eugenol also occurs in soybeans, mung beans [12], coffee [13], bananas [14] and in herbs such as nutmeg (*Myristica fragrans*, Myristicaceae), cinnamon (*Cinnamomum verum*, Lauraceae) and basil (*Ocimum basilicum*, Lamiaceae); however, *Syzygium aromaticum* can be considered the principal natural source of this compound (45% or 90% of the total oil) [15]. Clove has been used for a long time by civilizations because of its flavor and its properties make it important for culinary and medicinal uses. Eugenol has been included as a spicy flavoring in whisky, ice cream, baked goods and candy in restricted concentrations [16–18]. Eugenol has dual effect on the oxidative stress, which can action as an antioxidant or prooxidant agent. In addition, it has anti-carcinogenic, cytotoxic and antitumor properties. Considering the importance of eugenol in the area of food and human health, in this review, we discuss the role of eugenol on redox status and its potential use in the treatment and prevention of cancer. Searches were performed in the scientific literature database PubMed comprising all papers in English published until September 2017 using the following key words: eugenol with oxidant; antioxidant; cancer; cytotoxic; or antitumor. No exclusion criteria were performed.

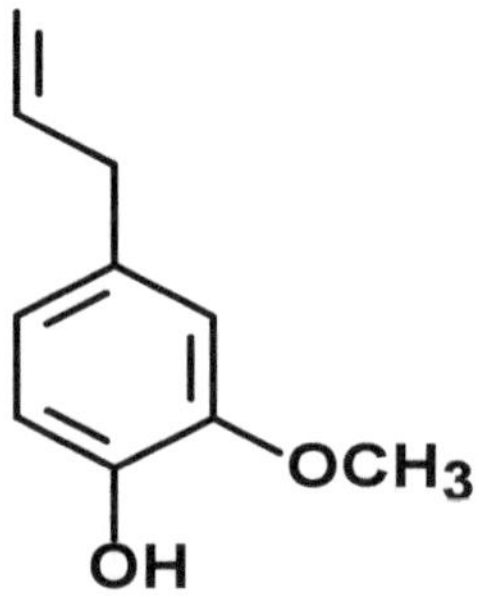

Figure 1. Chemical structure of eugenol.

2. Anti-Carcinogenic/Chemopreventive Effect of Eugenol and Its Relation to the Inhibition of Oxidative Stress

The ability to inhibit oxidative stress has been described as a protective effect against cancer formation (carcinogenesis or tumorigenesis); on the other hand, once a cancer has already formed, the antioxidant effect can contribute to the cancer's development, while the pro-oxidant effect can induce cancer cell death by several signaling pathways [19]. Interestingly, eugenol has been described as an agent with a double effect, antioxidant and pro-oxidant, presenting beneficial effects in the prevention of cancer formation and in cancer treatment (Figure 2). Despite some contradictory studies, there are many articles evaluating these biochemical and pharmacologic aspects.

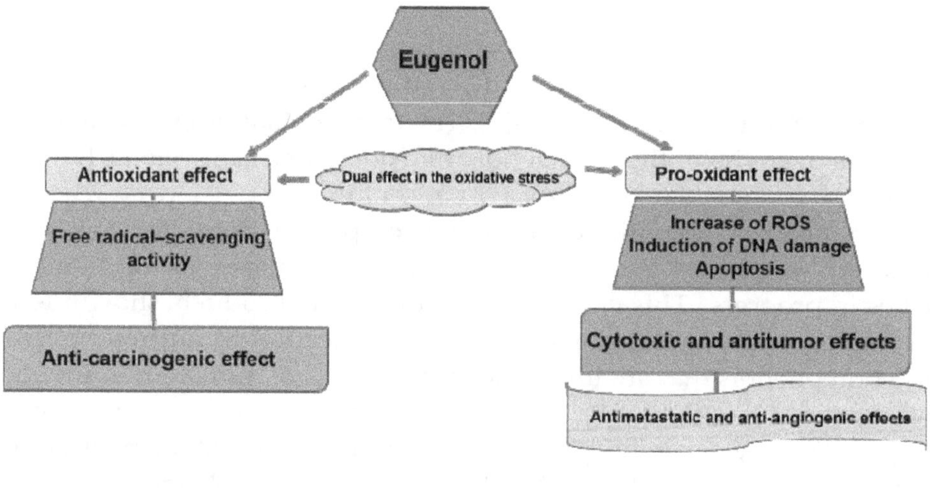

Figure 2. The dual effect of eugenol in the oxidative stress and its action in cancer development and treatment.

The anti-carcinogenic effect of eugenol had been investigated in several models [20–28]. The anti-carcinogenic effect of eugenol against skin carcinogenesis was investigated by Kaur et al. [20]. Skin cancer was initiated by applying 160 nmol 7,12-dimethylbenz[a]anthracene (DMBA) and promoted by twice weekly applications of 8.5 nmol 12-otetradecanoylphorbol-13-acetate (TPA) for 28 weeks and was followed by eugenol treatment. DMBA is a polycyclic aromatic hydrocarbon pro-carcinogen that requires metabolic conversion to its ultimate carcinogenic diol epoxide metabolites by oxidation, which is carried out through cytochrome P450 family 1 subfamily A member 1 (CYP1A1) and cytochrome P450 family 1 subfamily B member 1 (CYP1B1). Therefore, the carcinogenic effect of DMBA depends on the level of the oxidative metabolism of cytochrome P450 family 1. Two protocols were established: an anti-initiation protocol (topical application of 200 μL eugenol at 15% v/v in acetone one week before, one hour prior and two times after DMBA application); and an anti-promotion protocol (topical application of 30 μL eugenol at 15% v/v in acetone, 30 min prior to every TPA application). The treatment with eugenol did not prevent tumor formation but led to a reduction in tumor size. The control group presented tumor size of 9.7 g, and eugenol treatment showed tumor size of 5.6 g in the anti-initiation protocol and 2.8 g in the anti-promotion protocol. In addition, topical application of eugenol prior to TPA exposure led to the development of papillomatous keratoacanthoma with minimal cell proliferation but without squamous cell carcinoma. The anti-carcinogenic effect of eugenol was attributed to its anti-inflammatory activity, because some markers of inflammation, including inducible nitric oxide synthase (iNOS) and cyclooxygenase-2 (COX-2) expression and the levels of pro-inflammatory cytokines interleukin-6 (IL-6), tumor necrosis factor alpha (TNF-α) and prostaglandin E2 (PGE2), were reduced in DMBA/TPA-exposed animals after treatment with eugenol. Furthermore, eugenol was found to suppress the activation of nuclear factor kappa B (NF-κB) in mouse skin with TPA-induced inflammation [20].

Additionally, eugenol treatment (~100 mg/kg) inhibited the tumor formation in mouse skin model induced by application of DMBA as initiator and croton oil as promotor via radical scavenging activity of eugenol, downregulation of Myc (proto-oncogene), H-ras (harvey rat sarcoma virus oncogene) and Bcl-2 (B-cell lymphoma 2, apoptosis regulator) expression along with upregulation of p53, Bax (BCL2 associated X, apoptosis regulator) and active caspase-3 expression in the skin lesions [21,22]. Topical administration of eugenol also partially inhibited the benzo[a]pyrene-induced skin carcinogenesis in Swiss mice [23]. However, topical application of eugenol had minimal protection in reducing DMBA-induced skin carcinogenesis in Swiss mice [24].

The chemopreventive effect of eugenol on *N*-methyl-*N*′-nitro-*N*-nitrosoguanidine (MNNG)-induced gastric carcinogenesis in Wistar rats was also performed [25,26]. MNNG (150 mg/kg) was administered by intragastric intubation three times with a gap of two weeks in between the treatments and eugenol (100 mg/kg) was administered by intragastric route, three times per week starting on the day following the first exposure to MNNG and continued until the end of the experimental period. The incidence of gastric tumors in MNNG-treated rats was 100% with a mean tumor burden of 274.38 mm^3 and eugenol treatment decreased the tumor incidence to 16.66% with a tumor burden of 14.78 mm^3. Administration of eugenol induced apoptosis via the mitochondrial pathway by modulating the Bcl-2 family proteins, apoptotic protease activating factor 1 (Apaf-1), cytochrome c and caspases and inhibiting of invasion and angiogenesis as evidenced by changes in the activities of matrix metalloproteinases (MMP) and the expression of MMP-2 and -9, vascular endothelial growth factor (VEGF), vascular endothelial growth factor receptor 1 (VEGFR1), tissue inhibitor of metalloproteinase-2 (TIMP-2) and reversion-inducing-cysteine-rich protein with kazal motifs (RECK). Moreover, reduction in the NF-κB activation along with increasing of its inhibitor family members, IκB kinase α (IκBα) and inhibitor of kappa B (IKKβ), reduction of cyclin D1, cyclin B and proliferating cell nuclear antigen (PCNA) and increasing of p53, $p21^{waf1}$ and growth arrest and DNA damage-inducible 45 (Gadd45) were observed in eugenol-treated animals [25,26].

Using MCF 10A breast epithelial cells and H-ras transfected MCF 10A (MCF 10A-ras) as a model of cancer progression, eugenol exhibited cytotoxicity in μM range to MCF 10A-ras cells but not in MCF 10A cells [27]. In addition, eugenol reduced the ATP generation and inhibited oxidative phosphorylation and fatty acid oxidation via downregulating of c-Myc/PGC-1β/ERRα signaling pathway and inhibiting ROS production in H-ras transfected MCF 10A breast epithelial cells, indicating that eugenol can prevent breast cancer progression by regulation of cellular energy metabolism [27]. On the other hand, eugenol treatment does not exert modifying effects on lung carcinogenesis induced by urethane [28]. No significant differences in the incidences and multiplicities of lung lesions were observed between eugenol and control groups. In this model of lung carcinogenesis, transgenic mice with the human prototype c-Ha-ras gene received a single intraperitoneal injection of 250 mg/kg urethane, followed by a diet containing 6000 ppm eugenol or basal diet for 26 weeks [28]. The Table 1 summarize the anti-carcinogenic effect of eugenol.

Table 1. Summary of anti-carcinogenic effect of eugenol.

Carcinogenesis Model	Carcinogen	Eugenol Administration	Effect	References
Skin carcinogenesis	DMBA + TPA	Topical	Reduction in tumor incidence and size; and/or development of papillomatous keratoacanthoma with minimal cell proliferation but without squamous cell carcinoma	[20]
Skin carcinogenesis	DMBA + croton oil	Topical	Inhibition of tumor formation ~60%	[21,22]
Skin carcinogenesis	benzo[a]pyrene	Topical	Inhibition of tumor formation ~50%	[23]
Skin Carcinogenesis	DMBA	Topical	Minimal protection	[24]
Gastric carcinogenesis	MNNG	Intragastric	Inhibition of tumor formation ~75%	[25,26]
Lung carcinogenesis	Urethane	Oral	No protection	[28]

DMBA: 7,12-dimethylbenz[a]anthracene; TPA: 12-otetradecanoylphorbol-13-acetate; MNNG: *N*-methyl-*N*′-nitro-*N*-nitrosoguanidine.

The anti-carcinogenic effect of eugenol can also be attributed to its antioxidant property. Eugenol has been reported to have antioxidant activity, as assessed by diverse models [12,29–35]. Eugenol reacts with 2,2-diphenyl-1-picrylhydrazyl (DPPH) and shows high DPPH free radical-scavenging activity [29–33]. The concentration of eugenol required for 50% DPPH scavenging (IC_{50}: half maximal inhibitory concentration) activity ranged from 98 to 138 μM [31,35]. Eugenol also exhibits effective antioxidant activity in the linoleic acid emulsion system by inhibiting lipid peroxidation at 91 μM. In addition, eugenol has ferric ion (Fe^{3+}) reducing ability and electron donor properties for neutralizing free radicals by forming stable products [31]. Eugenol inhibits malonaldehyde (MA) formation from cod liver oil by 91% at ~1 mM [12]. Furthermore, eugenol inhibits microsomal lipid peroxidation (IC_{50} about 80 μM) as well as iron and OH radical-initiated lipid peroxidation in rat liver mitochondria, with IC_{50} values of 10 and 14 μM, respectively. The antioxidant effect was determined by the inhibition of thiobarbituric acid-reactive substances (TBARS) formation [29,30].

The effect of eugenol on in vivo lipid peroxidation mediated by carbon tetrachloride (CCl_4) has also been evaluated [30]. The CCl_4 model has been used for many years to investigate the effect of antioxidants in the liver xenobiotic metabolism. When eugenol was given at 5 mg/kg orally at three different times—i.e., prior to (−1 h), along with (0 h), or after (+3 h)—in relation to the time of CCl_4 dosing (i.p. administration of 0.4 mg/kg), it prevented significantly the rise in serum glutamic-oxaloacetic transaminase (SGOT) activity, lipid peroxidation and liver necrosis. However, eugenol failed to prevent a decrease in glucose-6-phosphatase activity, suggesting that the damage to endoplasmic reticulum (ER) is not protected by eugenol. Thus, the protective action of eugenol can be explained by the interception of secondary radicals derived from ER lipids rather than interference with the primary radicals of CCl_4 ($\bullet CCl_3/CCl_3OO\bullet$) [30]. In addition, the in vivo antioxidant effect of eugenol on liver danger induced by thioacetamide (TA) was also performed [36]. TA is frequently used to produce liver danger in animals due to generation of ROS and instigation of oxidative stress, which causes liver damage. Adult male Wistar rats were treated with eugenol (10.7 mg/kg/day) orally for 15 days. TA was administered (300 mg/kg, i.p.) for the last two days at 24 h intervals and the rats were sacrificed on the 16th day. Pretreatment with eugenol controlled the levels of lipid peroxidation and protein oxidation products with consequent reduction of TBARS, lipid hydroperoxides and protein carbonyl formation in plasma and the liver. Increased expression of the COX-2 gene as well as increases in pro-inflammatory cytokine TNF-α and IL-6 plasma levels induced by TA was also partially reverted by eugenol pretreatment. The protective effect of eugenol can be attributed to the reduction of cytochrome P450 family 2 subfamily E member 1 (CYP2E1) activity, the main enzyme responsible for TA-induced hepatotoxicity and oxidative stress [36].

Genotoxicity and mutagenicity of xenobiotics are also involved in the carcinogenic process and may occur as a result of oxidative stress. Interestingly, the antimutagenic and anti-genotoxic effects of eugenol has been also reported. Eugenol suppressed the mutagenicity induced by furylfuramide, 4-nitroquinoline 1-oxide, aflatoxin B in *Salmonella typhimurium* [37]. Eugenol also inhibits detoxification enzymes and prevents DMBA-induced DNA damage in MCF-7 (human breast adenocarcinoma) cell line [38,39]. Eugenol at dose of 50–500 mg/kg administered by gavage prevents the genotoxicity-induced by cyclophosphamide, procarbazine, *N*-methyl-*N*′-nitro-*N*-nitrosoguanidine and urethane [40]. In addition, the mutagenicity of benzo[a]pyrene but not DMBA and aflatoxin B1, in the *S. typhimurium* mutagenicity assay was reduced in liver S-9 fractions prepared from rats treated orally with eugenol (1000 mg/kg) [41]. In contrast, eugenol causes intrachromosomal recombination in yeast *Saccharomyces cerevisiae* in logarithmic phase cultures [42] and although eugenol induces no mutagenesis in Ames test, it causes chromosomal aberrations and increased the incidence of sister chromatid exchanges in Chinese hamster ovary cells [43,44]. At μM range, eugenol is not able to prevent the DNA lesions induced by hydrogen peroxide (H_2O_2) [33]. However, eugenol protected the supercoiled pBR322 plasmid DNA oxidative damage induced by Fe^{2+} and H_2O_2 at mM range [35]. Moreover, eugenol, at concentrations above 50 μM, inhibited the DNA oxidative damage induced by hydroxyl radicals produced by Fenton reactions using Fe^{2+} and H_2O_2 [32].

3. Cytotoxic and Antitumor Effects of Eugenol and Its Relation to the Induction of Oxidative Stress

Controversial results have been found for the cytotoxic activity of eugenol. Some studies have shown that eugenol is capable of inducing cytotoxicity at concentrations in the μM range, whereas other studies show that eugenol is capable of inducing cytotoxic effects only at concentrations in the mM range. Nevertheless, eugenol is able to induce cytotoxicity to cancer cell lines with different histological types, including skin, breast, colon, prostate, cervical, hepatocellular, lung, oral squamous cells and leukemia. In addition, the ability to induce oxidative stress has been also ascribed to eugenol in cell-based assays.

Eugenol in the μM range inhibits the growth of melanoma cells—Sbcl2 (primary melanoma), WM3211 (primary radial growth phase), WM98-1 (primary vertical growth phase) and WM1205Lu (metastatic melanoma)—accompanied by cell cycle arrest at the S phase, followed by apoptosis [45]. Using cDNA array analysis, it was demonstrated that eugenol modulates expression of E2F family members. In addition, eugenol was able to inhibit the E2F1 transcriptional activity and, as overexpression of E2F1 restores melanoma cell proliferation, this indicates that eugenol targets E2F functions in melanoma cells [45]. In addition, eugenol in the μM range inhibits the growth of HL-60 (human promyelocytic leukemia), U-937 (human histiocytic lymphoma), HepG2 (human hepatocellular carcinoma), 3LL (Lewis mouse lung carcinoma) and SNU-C5 (human colon carcinoma) lines [46]. Eugenol-treated HL-60 cells display DNA fragmentation, ROS production, loss of mitochondrial transmembrane potential, bax translocation, Bcl-2 reduction, cytochrome c release and caspase-9 and -3 activation, suggesting that eugenol causes apoptotic cell death. Moreover, pretreatment of HL-60 cells with *N*-acetyl-L-cysteine (an antioxidant), Z-VAD-FMK (a pan caspase inhibitor) and Z-DEVD-FMK (a caspase-3 inhibitor) decreases the eugenol-induced apoptosis, indicating that eugenol activates the caspase- and ROS-mediated apoptosis pathways [46]. Moreover, treatment of HL-60 cells with eugenol, produced formation of three DNA adducts and incubation of HL-60 cells with the combination of 100 μM eugenol and 100 μM H_2O_2 potentiated the levels of DNA adduct in HL-60 cells. Oxidative base damage was also observed. The DNA adducts formed were inhibited by the addition of either ascorbic acid or glutathione [47]. Eugenol in the μM range is also cytotoxic to DU-145 (androgen-insensitive prostate cancer cells) and KB (oral squamous carcinoma cells) [48].

Using LNCaP (androgen responsive human prostate carcinoma) and PC-3 (androgen independent human prostate carcinoma) cell lines, eugenol induces cytotoxicity in the μM range and causes an increase in G_2/M phase [49]. Apoptotic cell death was not detected at the concentrations used; however, eugenol in combination with 2-methoxyestradiol causes apoptosis along with a reduction of the expression of anti-apoptotic protein Bcl-2 and enhancement of the expression of the pro-apoptotic protein Bax. The apoptosis induced by this combination is not affected in PC-3 cells with overexpression or lack of Bcl-2 but is associated with the loss of mitochondrial membrane potential [49]. Eugenol in μM concentrations causes cytotoxicity to MCF-7, T47-D (human breast carcinoma) and MDA-MB-231 (human breast adenocarcinoma) cells through down-regulation of E2F1 and its downstream anti-apoptosis target, surviving independently of the status of p53 and ERα [50]. Eugenol inhibits the breast cancer related oncogenes, NF-κB and cyclin D1 and up-regulates the cyclin-dependent kinase inhibitor $p21^{WAF1}$ protein; On the other hand, eugenol was also cytotoxic to non-cancer cell line MCF 10A (human breast epithelial) with IC_{50} value of 2.2 μM [50]. Júnior et al. [51] also assessed the cytotoxicity of eugenol in the μM range on MDA-MB-231, MCF-7, SIHA (human cervix carcinoma), SK-Mel-28 (human melanoma) and A2058 (human melanoma) cells; it was accompanied by ROS production, causing G2/M phase block and, consequently, clastogenesis. Eugenol also induced downregulation of PCNA (proliferation cell nuclear antigen), decreased the mitochondria transmembrane potential and upregulated Bax [51].

Controversially, some studies have indicated that eugenol has no cytotoxic activity or has cytotoxicity only when present in the mM range [52–73]. In studies with HSG (human submandibular gland adenocarcinoma) and HSC-2 (human oral squamous cell carcinoma) cells, eugenol caused cytotoxicity when in the mM range but no ROS induction was observed [58,59]. On the other hand, Atsumi et al. [60] stated that eugenol caused a biphasic ROS production that was enhanced at 5–10 μM and decreased at 500 μM in HSG, treated with H_2O_2 plus horseradish peroxidase or with visible light irradiation. In HL-60 cells, eugenol presents IC_{50} of 0.38 mM that is accompanied by internucleosomal DNA fragmentation. The expression of the mRNAs and the activity of manganese superoxide dismutase and copper- and zinc-containing superoxide dismutase are inhibited by eugenol, suggesting that eugenol targets the oxidative stress in cancer cells. In contrast, eugenol-induced cytotoxicity is enhanced by *N*-acetyl-L-cysteine or glutathione treatment [58,61]. On the other hand, eugenol induces cytotoxicity and ROS generation in HSG cells in which glutathione or cysteine are protecting from damage [62,63].

Pisano et al. [64] demonstrated that eugenol has no cytotoxic effect at 100 μM in malignant melanoma cell lines WM266-4, SK-Mel-28, LCP-Mel, LCM-Mel, PNP-Mel, CN-MelA, 13443 and GR-Mel. In human melanoma G361 cells, eugenol in the mM range inhibits the viability of G361 cells. Eugenol-treated G361 cells present caspase-3 and -6 cleavage and activation. The caspase-3 substrates poly(ADP-ribose)polymerase (PARP) and DNA fragmentation factor 45 (DFF45) are cleaved in eugenol-induced apoptosis, suggesting induction of caspase-dependent apoptosis [65]. Interestingly, similar results were found in human osteosarcoma HOS cells, suggesting that eugenol can also induce caspase-dependent apoptosis pathways in HOS cells [66].

In a study with human cervical carcinoma cell line (HeLa), eugenol presented cytotoxicity in the mM range and in a synergistic combination with sulforaphane, downregulated the expression of Bcl-2, COX-2 and IL-β. It also produced a synergistic effect when combined with gemcitabine, causing downregulation of the expression of Bcl-2, COX-2 and IL-β [67,68]. Also, in the mM range, eugenol was cytotoxic and induced apoptosis to colon carcinoma cell lines HCT-15 and HT-29. The loss of the membrane mitochondrial potential and generation of ROS were accompanied in the eugenol-induced apoptosis. Augmented ROS generation resulted in the DNA fragmentation and activation of PARP, p53 and caspase-3 [69]. Eugenol in the mM range also inhibits the growth of human breast carcinoma MCF-7 cells, accompanied by cell shrinkage and an increase in the percentage of apoptotic cells and DNA fragments. A depleted level of intracellular glutathione and increased level of lipid peroxidation are also observed [70]. In another study with MCF-7 cells, eugenol presented an IC_{50} value of 0.9 mM, increased the ROS production, decreased the ATP level and induced the loss of the mitochondrial membrane potential and release of the cytochrome c and lactate. Cell viability and ROS production were restored by pretreatment with the antioxidants. On the other hand, the eugenol effect was not affected in MCF-7 cells with overexpression of Bcl-2 [71]. Human oral squamous cell carcinoma cell line HSC-2 treated with a concentration of eugenol in the mM range presented metabolic changes including reduction of ATP utilization, oxidative stress and an increase in the polyamines and glycolytic metabolites [72]. In HepG2 and Caco-2 (human colon carcinoma) cells, the treatment with eugenol-loaded nanoemulsions and free eugenol caused increasing in the cell death by apoptosis and ROS generation [73]. The Table 2 summarize the in vitro cytotoxic effect of eugenol.

Table 2. Summary of in vitro cytotoxic effects of eugenol against cancer and non-cancer cell lines.

Cell Lines	Histological Type	Origin	IC_{50} (μM)	References
Cancer cells				
Sbcl2	Primary melanoma	Human	~0.5	[45]
WM3211	Primary melanoma	Human	~0.5	[45]
WM98-1	Primary melanoma	Human	~0.5	[45]
WM1205Lu	Metastatic melanoma	Human	~0.5	[45]
SK-Mel-28	Melanoma	Human	7.2	[51]
A2058	Melanoma	Human	12.2	[51]
WM266-4	Melanoma	Human	>100	[64]
SK-Mel-28	Melanoma	Human	>100	[64]
LCP-Mel	Melanoma	Human	>100	[64]
LCM-Mel	Melanoma	Human	>100	[64]
PNP-Mel	Melanoma	Human	>100	[64]
CN-MelA	Melanoma	Human	>100	[64]
13443	Melanoma	Human	>100	[64]
GR-Mel	Melanoma	Human	>100	[64]
HSG	Submandibular gland adenocarcinoma	Human	~100	[59]
			396	[60]
T47-D	Breast carcinoma	Human	0.9	[50]
MDA-MB-231	Breast adenocarcinoma	Human	1.7	[50]
			15.1	[51]
			~1600	[71]
MCF-7	Breast adenocarcinoma	Human	1.5	[50]
			22.8	[51]
			~400	[70]
			900	[71]

Table 2. *Cont.*

Cell Lines	Histological Type	Origin	IC_{50} (μM)	References
HCT-15	Colon adenocarcinoma	Human	300	[69]
HT-29	Colon adenocarcinoma	Human	500	[69]
Caco-2	Colon carcinoma	Human	~750	[73]
SNU-C5	Colon carcinoma	Human	129.4	[46]
LNCaP	Prostate adenocarcinoma	Human	~550	[49]
PC-3	Prostate carcinoma	Human	~180	[49]
DU-145	Prostate carcinoma	Human	30.4	[48]
SIHA	Cervical carcinoma	Human	18.3	[51]
HeLa	Cervical carcinoma	Human	500	[72]
HepG2	Hepatocellular carcinoma	Human	118.6	[46]
			~500	[73]
3LL	Lewis lung carcinoma	Mouse	89.6	[46]
KB	Oral squamous cell carcinoma	Human	28.5	[48]
HSC-2	Oral squamous cell carcinoma	Human	~700	[72]
HOS	Osteosarcoma	Human	1500	[66]
HL-60	Promyelocytic leukemia	Human	23.7	[46]
			380	[61]
U-937	Histocytic lymphoma	Human	39.4	[46]
Non-cancer cells				
MCF 10A	Breast epithelial	Human	2.2	[50]

IC_{50}: half maximal inhibitory concentration.

In vivo antitumor effects of eugenol have been also investigated [45,50,74]. Using B6D2F1 mice bearing B16 melanoma, eugenol treatment (125 mg/kg/i.p. of body weight twice a week) caused the in vivo antitumor effect [45]. On day 15, the size of tumors in the eugenol-treated group was 62% less than the control group, with an increase of 19% in the survival rate. At the end of the treatment, 50% of the animals in the control group presented metastases but no eugenol-treated animals showed any signs of invasion or metastasis [45]. Moreover, eugenol (100 mg/kg/i.p.) was able to inhibit the growth of the Ehrlich ascites model by 28.88% and inhibited 24.35% tumor growth in the Ehrlich solid tumor model [74].

In mice engrafted with human breast adenocarcinoma MDA-MB-231 cells subcutaneously, eugenol treatment with a dose of 100 mg/kg every two days for four weeks inhibited tumor growth [50]. Moreover, eugenol downregulated E2F1, survivin, NF-κB and cyclin D1 and increased the levels of $p21^{WAF1}$, Bax, cleaved PARP-1 and the active form of caspase-9 in tumor xenografts [50]. The Table 3 summarize the in vivo antitumor effect of eugenol. Regarding the antimetastatic potential of eugenol, it exerts inhibitory effects on matrix metallopeptidase 9 (MMP-9) via inhibition of extracellular signal-regulated kinase (ERK) phosphorylation in human fibrosarcoma HT1080 cells [32].

Table 3. Summary of in vivo antitumor effect of eugenol.

Tumor	Histological Type	Origin	Dose (mg/kg)	Treatment	Route	Inhibition Rate (%)	References
B16	Melanoma	Mouse	125	Twice a week	i.p.	62	[45]
Ehrlich (ascites model)	Carcinoma	Mouse	100	Every two days for four weeks	i.p.	28.9	[74]
Ehrlich (solid model)	Carcinoma	Mouse	100	Every two days for four weeks	i.p.	24.4	[74]
MDA-MB-231	Breast adenocarcinoma	Human	100	Every two days for four weeks	i.p.	~66	[50]

i.p.: intraperitoneal.

Although there are a large number of papers on the cytotoxic properties of eugenol, controversial results delay the completion of preclinical efficacy and safety studies as well as clinical trials. However, the ability of eugenol to induce oxidative stress, as observed in cell-based assays, appears to be related to its cytotoxic and antitumor effect. Other compounds with dual antioxidant and prooxidant effect have a dose/concentration-response relationship, for example, at low doses/concentrations present antioxidant effect and at high doses/concentrations show prooxidant effect [75–78]; however, we do not find this relationship with the data published with eugenol. Problems related to the degree of purity of the compound, its evaporation (for volatile compounds for example) during the experiments, the methods used to quantify these data (since different cellular and animal models may present divergent results and interpretations) and some laboratory and interpretation errors (including the use of cell lines contaminated with *Mycoplasma* sp., errors in cell line authentication, etc.) may contribute to explain these controversial results.

In relation to the structure-activity relationship of eugenol, the cytotoxicity of eugenol-related compounds has been associated with the activity of the production of phenoxyl radicals, their stability of the subsequent quinonemethide and the hydrophobicity [79]. In relation to the antioxidant activity, the number of hydroxyl groups in the phenol ring of eugenol enhanced it antioxidant action [31,80]. Moreover, the presence of bromine substituent in ortho-position to the OH-group increases its antioxidant activity [81].

4. Conclusions

The studies presented in this review reveal the therapeutic potential of eugenol in cancer prevention and treatment and the relationship with its antioxidant and pro-oxidant activities. The Figure 3 summarize the molecular mechanisms of eugenol. Therefore, the consumption of vegetables containing this compound in significant quantities might well be useful in inhibiting the free radicals responsible for tumor development. In addition, the data reported are in accordance with the scientific understanding that a better quality of life and increased longevity may be obtained via healthy food, with the health promoting effects of its bioactive constituents.

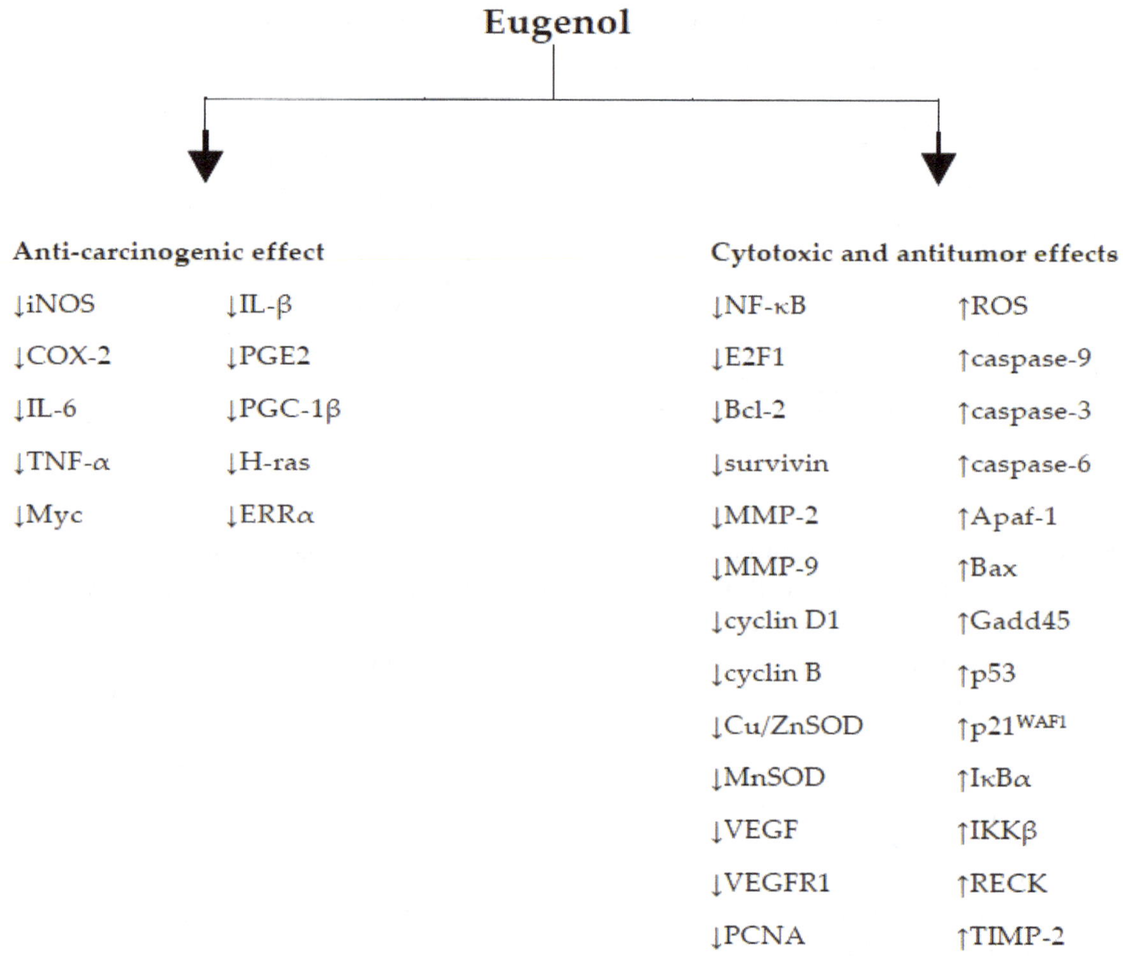

Figure 3. Molecular mechanisms of eugenol. ↑: upregulation; ↓: downregulation; Apaf-1: apoptotic protease activating factor 1; Bax: BCL2 associated X, apoptosis regulator; Bcl-2: B-cell lymphoma 2, apopstosis regulator; COX-2: cycloxygenase-2; Cu/ZnSOD: copper- and zinc-containing superoxide dismutase; ERRα: estrogen-related receptor alpha; Gadd45: growth arrest and DNA damage-inducible 45: IKKβ: IκB kinase α; IL-6: interleukin 6; iNOS: inducible nitric oxide synthase; IκBα: inhibitor of kappa B; MMP-2: matrix metalloproteinase-2; MMP-9: matrix metalloproteinase-9; MnSOD: manganese superoxide dismutase; NF-κB: nuclear factor-kappa B; PCNA: proliferating cell nuclear antigen; PGC-1β: peroxisome proliferator-activated receptor gamma coactivator 1-beta; PGE2: prostaglandin E2; RECK: reversion-inducing-cysteine-rich protein with kazal motifs; ROS: reactive oxygen species; TIMP-2: tissue inhibitor of metalloproteinase-2; TNF-α: tumor necrosis factor alpha; VEGF: vascular endothelial growth factor; VEGFR1: vascular endothelial growth factor receptor 1.

Acknowledgments: This work was supported by the Brazilian agencies: Conselho Nacional de Desenvolvimento Científico e Tecnológico (CNPq) and Coordenação de Aperfeiçoamento de Pessoal de Nível Superior (CAPES).

Author Contributions: Daniel Pereira Bezerra surveyed the data and wrote the pharmacological part of the review. Gardenia Carmen Gadelha Militão was responsible for the analysis of these data and wrote the pharmacological part. Damião Pergentino de Sousa wrote the chemical content, revised and planned the study. Mayara Castro de Morais was responsible for formatting the manuscript.

Abbreviations

Apaf-1	Apoptotic protease activating factor 1
Bax	BCL2 associated X, apoptosis regulator
Bcl-2	B-cell lymphoma 2, apopstosis regulator
COX-2	Cyclooxygenase-2

CYP 1A1	Cytochrome P450 family 1 subfamily A member 1
CYP1B1	Cytochrome P450 family 1 subfamily B member 1
DFF45	DNA fragmentation factor 45
DMBA	7,12-dimethylbenz[a]anthracene
DNA	Deoxyribonucleic acid
DPPH	2,2-diphenyl-1-picrylhydrazyl
ER	Endoplasmic reticulum
Gadd45	Growth arrest and DNA damage-inducible 45
IC_{50}	Half maximal inhibitory concentration
IKKβ	Inhibitor of kappa B
IL-6	Interleukin-6
iNOS	Inducible nitric oxide synthase
IκBα	IκB Kinase α
MA	Malonaldehyde
MCF 10A-ras	H-ras transfected MCF 10A
MMP	Matrix metalloproteinases
MNNG	*N*-Methyl-*N*′-nitro-*N*-nitrosoguanidine
NF-κB	Nuclear factor kappa B
PARP	Poly(ADP-ribose)polymerase
PCNA	Proliferating cell nuclear antigen
PGE2	Prostaglandin E2
RECK	Reversion-inducing-cysteine-rich protein with kazal motifs
ROS	Reactive Oxygen Species
SGOT	Serum glutamic-oxaloacetic transaminase
TA	Thioacetamide
TBARS	Thiobarbituric acid-reactive substances
TIMP-2	Tissue inhibitor of metalloproteinase-2
TNF-α	Tumor necrosis factor alpha
TPA	12-otetradecanoylphorbol-13-acetate
VEGF	Vascular endothelial growth factor
VEGFR1	Vascular endothelial growth factor receptor 1

References

1. Selim, K.A.; Abdelrasoul, H.; Aboelmagd, M.; Tawila, A.M. The role of the MAPK signaling, topoisomerase and dietary bioactives in controlling cancer incidence. *Diseases* **2017**, *5*, 13. [CrossRef] [PubMed]
2. Gào, X.; Schöttker, B. Reduction-oxidation pathways involved in cancer development: A systematic review of literature reviews. *Oncotarget* **2017**, *8*, 51888–51906. [CrossRef] [PubMed]
3. Fiaschi, T.; Chiarugi, P. Oxidative stress, tumor microenvironment, and metabolic reprogramming: A diabolic liaison. *Int. J. Cell Biol.* **2012**, 762825. [CrossRef] [PubMed]
4. Bezerra, D.P.; Soares, A.K.; de Sousa, D.P. Overview of the role of vanillin on redox status and cancer development. *Oxid. Med. Cell Longev.* **2016**, 9734816. [CrossRef] [PubMed]
5. Carvalho, A.A.; Andrade, L.N.; De Sousa, E.B.; De Sousa, D.P. Antitumor phenylpropanoids found in essential oils. *Biomed. Res. Int.* **2015**, 392674. [CrossRef] [PubMed]
6. Sobral, M.V.; Xavier, A.L.; Lima, T.C.; De Sousa, D.P. Antitumor activity of monoterpenes found in essential oils. *Sci. World J.* **2014**, 953451. [CrossRef] [PubMed]
7. De Sousa, D.P. *Bioactive Essential Oils and Cancer*; Springer: New York, NY, USA, 2015.
8. Ferraz, R.P.; Bomfim, D.S.; Carvalho, N.C.; Soares, M.B.; da Silva, T.B.; Machado, W.J.; Prata, A.P.; Costa, E.V.; Moraes, V.R.; Nogueira, P.C.; et al. Cytotoxic effect of leaf essential oil of *Lippia gracilis* Schauer (Verbenaceae). *Phytomedicine* **2013** *20*, 615–621. [CrossRef] [PubMed]

9. Khan, H.Y.; Zubair, H.; Ullah, M.F.; Ahmad, A.; Hadi, S.M. A prooxidant mechanism for the anticancer and chemopreventive properties of plant polyphenols. *Curr. Drug Targets* **2012**, *13*, 1738–1749. [CrossRef] [PubMed]
10. Forester, S.C.; Lambert, J.D. The role of antioxidant versus pro-oxidant effects of green tea polyphenols in cancer prevention. *Mol. Nutr. Food Res.* **2011**, *55*, 844–854. [CrossRef] [PubMed]
11. Assi, M. The differential role of reactive oxygen species in early and late stages of cancer. *Am. J. Physiol. Regul. Integr. Comp. Physiol.* **2017**, *313*, R646–R653. [CrossRef] [PubMed]
12. Lee, K.-G.; Shibamoto, T. Antioxidant properties of aroma compounds isolated from soybeans and mung beans. *J. Agric. Food Chem.* **2000**, *48*, 4290–4293. [CrossRef] [PubMed]
13. Charalambous, G. *The Quality of Foods and Beverages V2: Chemistry and Technology*, 1st ed.; Academic Press: New York, NY, USA, 1981; p. 408.
14. Jordán, M.J.; Tandon, K.; Shaw, P.E.; Goodner, K.L. Aromatic profile of aqueous banana essence and banana fruit by gas chromatography-mass spectrometry (GC-MS) and gas chromatography-olfactometry (GC-O). *J. Agric. Food Chem.* **2001**, *49*, 4813–4817. [CrossRef] [PubMed]
15. Kamatou, G.P.; Vermaak, I.; Viljoen, A.M. Eugenol-from the remote maluku islands to the international market place: A review of a remarkable and versatile molecule. *Molecules* **2012**, *17*, 6953–6981. [CrossRef] [PubMed]
16. Lee, K.-Y.M.; Patterson, A.; Piggot, J.R.; Richardson, G.D. Origins of flavour in whiskies and a revised flavour wheel: A review. *J. Inst. Brew.* **2001**, *107*, 287–313. [CrossRef]
17. Bohnert, H.J.; Nguyen, H.R.; Lewis, N.G. *Bioengineering and Molecular Biology of Plant Pathways*; Elsevier: San Diego, CA, USA, 2008.
18. Srinivasan, K. Antioxidant potential of spices and their active constituents. *Crit. Rev. Food Sci. Nutr.* **2014**, *54*, 352–372. [CrossRef] [PubMed]
19. Gorrini, C.; Harris, I.S.; Mak, T.W. Modulation of oxidative stress as an anticancer strategy. *Nat. Rev. Drug Discov.* **2013**, *12*, 931–947. [CrossRef] [PubMed]
20. Kaur, G.; Athar, M.; Alam, M.S. Eugenol precludes cutaneous chemical carcinogenesis in mouse by preventing oxidative stress and inflammation and by inducing apoptosis. *Mol. Carcinog.* **2010**, *49*, 290–301. [CrossRef] [PubMed]
21. Sukumaran, K.; Unnikrishnan, M.C.; Kuttan, R. Inhibition of tumour promotion in mice by eugenol. *Indian J. Physiol. Pharmacol.* **1994**, *38*, 306–308. [PubMed]
22. Pal, D.; Banerjee, S.; Mukherjee, S.; Roy, A.; Panda, C.K.; Das, S. Eugenol restricts DMBA croton oil induced skin carcinogenesis in mice: Downregulation of c-Myc and H-ras, and activation of p53 dependent apoptotic pathway. *J. Dermatol. Sci.* **2010**, *59*, 31–39. [CrossRef] [PubMed]
23. Van Duuren, B.L.; Goldschmidt, B.M. Cocarcinogenic and tumor-promoting agents in tobacco carcinogenesis. *J. Natl. Cancer Inst.* **1976**, *56*, 1237–1242. [CrossRef] [PubMed]
24. Azuine, M.A.; Amonkar, A.J.; Bhide, S.V. Chemopreventive efficacy of betel leaf extract and its constituents on 7,12-dimethylbenz(a)anthracene induced carcinogenesis and their effect on drug detoxification system in mouse skin. *Indian J. Exp. Biol.* **1991**, *29*, 346–351. [PubMed]
25. Manikandan, P.; Murugan, R.S.; Priyadarsini, R.V.; Vinothini, G.; Nagini, S. Eugenol induces apoptosis and inhibits invasion and angiogenesis in a rat model of gastric carcinogenesis induced by MNNG. *Life Sci.* **2010**, *86*, 936–941. [CrossRef] [PubMed]
26. Manikandan, P.; Vinothini, G.; Vidya Priyadarsini, R.; Prathiba, D.; Nagini, S. Eugenol inhibits cell proliferation via NF-κB suppression in a rat model of gastric carcinogenesis induced by MNNG. *Invest. New Drugs* **2011**, *29*, 110–117. [CrossRef] [PubMed]
27. Yan, X.; Zhang, G.; Bie, F.; Lv, Y.; Ma, Y.; Ma, M.; Wang, Y.; Hao, X.; Yuan, N.; Jiang, X. Eugenol inhibits oxidative phosphorylation and fatty acid oxidation via downregulation of c-Myc/PGC-1β/ERRα signaling pathway in MCF10A-ras cells. *Sci. Rep.* **2017**, *7*, 12920. [CrossRef] [PubMed]
28. Koujitani, T.; Yasuhara, K.; Tamura, T.; Onodera, H.; Takagi, H.; Takizawa, T.; Hirose, M.; Hayashi, Y.; Mitsumori, K. Lack of modifying effects of eugenol on development of lung proliferative lesions induced by urethane in transgenic mice carrying the human prototype c-Ha-ras gene. *J. Toxicol. Sci.* **2001**, *26*, 129–139. [CrossRef] [PubMed]

29. Ito, M.; Murakami, K.; Yoshino, M. Antioxidant action of eugenol compounds: Role of metal ion in the inhibition of lipid peroxidation. *Food Chem. Toxicol.* **2005**, *43*, 461–466. [CrossRef] [PubMed]
30. Nagababu, E.; Rifkind, J.M.; Boindala, S.; Nakka, L. Assessment of antioxidant activity of eugenol in vitro and in vivo. *Methods Mol. Biol.* **2010**, *610*, 165–180. [PubMed]
31. Gülçin, İ. Antioxidant activity of eugenol: A structure-activity relationship study. *J. Med. Food* **2011**, *14*, 975–985. [CrossRef] [PubMed]
32. Nam, H.; Kim, M.M. Eugenol with antioxidant activity inhibits MMP-9 related to metastasis in human fibrosarcoma cells. *Food Chem. Toxicol.* **2013**, *55*, 106–112. [CrossRef] [PubMed]
33. Horvathova, E.; Navarova, J.; Galova, E.; Sevcovicova, A.; Chodakova, L.; Snahnicanova, Z.; Melusova, M.; Kozics, K.; Slamenova, D. Assessment of antioxidative, chelating, and DNA-protective effects of selected essential oil components (eugenol, carvacrol, thymol, borneol, eucalyptol) of plants and intact *Rosmarinus officinalis* oil. *J. Agric. Food Chem.* **2014**, *62*, 6632–6639. [CrossRef] [PubMed]
34. Mahapatra, S.K.; Roy, S. Phytopharmacological approach of free radical scavenging and anti-oxidative potential of eugenol and *Ocimum gratissimum* Linn. *Asian Pac. J. Trop. Med.* **2014**, *7S1*, S391–S397. [CrossRef]
35. Zhang, L.L.; Zhang, L.F.; Xu, J.G.; Hu, Q.P. Comparison study on antioxidant, DNA damage protective and antibacterial activities of eugenol and isoeugenol against several foodborne pathogens. *Food Nutr. Res.* **2017**, *61*, 1353356. [CrossRef] [PubMed]
36. Yogalakshmi, B.; Viswanathan, P.; Anuradha, C.V. Investigation of antioxidant, anti-inflammatory and DNA-protective properties of eugenol in thioacetamide-induced liver injury in rats. *Toxicology* **2010**, *268*, 204–212. [CrossRef] [PubMed]
37. Miyazawa, M.; Hisama, M. Suppression of chemical mutagen-induced SOS response by alkylphenols from clove (*Syzygium aromaticum*) in the *Salmonella typhimurium* TA1535/pSK1002 umu test. *J. Agric. Food Chem.* **2001**, *49*, 4019–4025. [CrossRef] [PubMed]
38. Rompelberg, C.J.; Verhagen, H.; van Bladeren, P.J. Effects of the naturally occurring alkenylbenzenes eugenol and trans-anethole on drug-metabolizing enzymes in the rat liver. *Food Chem. Toxicol.* **1993**, *31*, 637–645. [CrossRef]
39. Han, E.H.; Hwang, Y.P.; Jeong, T.C.; Lee, S.S.; Shin, J.G.; Jeong, H.G. Eugenol inhibit 7,12-dimethylbenz[a]anthracene-induced genotoxicity in MCF-7 cells: Bifunctional effects on CYP1 and NAD(P)H: Quinone oxidoreductase. *FEBS Lett.* **2007**, *581*, 749–756. [CrossRef] [PubMed]
40. Abraham, S.K. Anti-genotoxicity of trans-anethole and eugenol in mice. *Food Chem. Toxicol.* **2001**, *39*, 493–498. [CrossRef]
41. Rompelberg, C.J.; Evertz, S.J.; Bruijntjes-Rozier, G.C.; van den Heuvel, P.D.; Verhagen, H. Effect of eugenol on the genotoxicity of established mutagens in the liver. *Food Chem. Toxicol.* **1996**, *34*, 33–42. [CrossRef]
42. Schiestl, R.H.; Chan, W.S.; Gietz, R.D.; Mehta, R.D.; Hastings, P.J. Safrole, eugenol and methyleugenol induce intrachromosomal recombination in yeast. *Mutat. Res.* **1989**, *224*, 427–436. [CrossRef]
43. Stich, H.F.; Stich, W.; Lam, P.P.S. Potentiation of genotoxicity by concurrent application of compounds found in betel quid: Arecoline, eugenol, quercetin, chlorogenic acid and Mn^{2+}. *Mutat. Res.* **1981**, *90*, 355–363. [CrossRef]
44. National Toxicology Program (NTP). Carcinogenesis Studies of Eugenol (CAS No. 97–53–0) in F344/N Rats and B6C3F1 Mice (Feed Studies). *Natl. Toxicol. Program Tech. Rep. Ser.* **1983**, *223*, 1–159.
45. Ghosh, R.; Nadiminty, N.; Fitzpatrick, J.E.; Alworth, W.L.; Slaga, T.J.; Kumar, A.P. Eugenol causes melanoma growth suppression through inhibition of E2F1 transcriptional activity. *J. Biol. Chem.* **2005**, *280*, 5812–5819. [CrossRef] [PubMed]
46. Yoo, C.B.; Han, K.T.; Cho, K.S.; Ha, J.; Park, H.J.; Nam, J.H.; Kil, U.H.; Lee, K.T. Eugenol isolated from the essential oil of Eugenia caryophyllata induces a reactive oxygen species-mediated apoptosis in HL-60 human promyelocytic leukemia cells. *Cancer Lett.* **2005**, *225*, 41–52. [CrossRef] [PubMed]
47. Bodell, W.J.; Ye, Q.; Pathak, D.N.; Pongracz, K. Oxidation of eugenol to form DNA adducts and 8-hydroxy-2′-deoxyguanosine: Role of quinone methide derivative in DNA adduct formation. *Carcinogenesis* **1998**, *19*, 437–443. [CrossRef] [PubMed]
48. Carrasco, A.; Espinoza, C.; Cardile, V.; Gallardo, C.; Cardona, W.; Lombardo, L.; Catalán, M.; Cuellar, F.; Russo, A. Eugenol and its synthetic analogues inhibit cell growth of human cancer cells. *J. Braz. Chem. Soc.* **2008**, *19*, 543–548. [CrossRef]

49. Ghosh, R.; Ganapathy, M.; Alworth, W.L.; Chan, D.C.; Kumar, A.P. Combination of 2-methoxyestradiol (2-ME2) and eugenol for apoptosis induction synergistically in androgen independent prostate cancer cells. *J. Steroid Biochem. Mol. Biol.* **2009**, *113*, 25–35. [CrossRef] [PubMed]
50. Al-Sharif, I.; Remmal, A.; Aboussekhra, A. Eugenol triggers apoptosis in breast cancer cells through E2F1/survivin down-regulation. *BMC Cancer* **2013**, *13*, 600. [CrossRef] [PubMed]
51. Júnior, P.L.; Câmara, D.A.; Costa, A.S.; Ruiz, J.L.; Levy, D.; Azevedo, R.A.; Pasqualoto, K.F.; de Oliveira, C.F.; de Melo, T.C.; Pessoa, N.D.; et al. Apoptotic effect of eugenol envolves G2/M phase abrogation accompanied by mitochondrial damage and clastogenic effect on cancer cell in vitro. *Phytomedicine* **2016**, *23*, 725–735. [CrossRef] [PubMed]
52. Young, S.C.; Wang, C.J.; Hsu, J.D.; Hsu, J.L.; Chou, F.P. Increased sensitivity of Hep G2 cells toward the cytotoxicity of cisplatin by the treatment of piper betel leaf extract. *Arch Toxicol.* **2006**, *80*, 319–327. [CrossRef] [PubMed]
53. Fujimoto, A.; Sakanashi, Y.; Matsui, H.; Oyama, T.; Nishimura, Y.; Masuda, T.; Oyama, Y. Cytometric analysis of cytotoxicity of polyphenols and related phenolics to rat thymocytes: Potent cytotoxicity of resveratrol to normal cells. *Basic Clin. Pharmacol. Toxicol.* **2009**, *104*, 455–462. [CrossRef] [PubMed]
54. Slamenová, D.; Horváthová, E.; Wsólová, L.; Sramková, M.; Navarová, J. Investigation of anti-oxidative, cytotoxic, DNA-damaging and DNA-protective effects of plant volatiles eugenol and borneol in human-derived HepG2, Caco-2 and VH10 cell lines. *Mutat. Res.* **2009**, *677*, 46–52. [CrossRef] [PubMed]
55. Jaganathan, S.K.; Supriyanto, E. Antiproliferative and molecular mechanism of eugenol-induced apoptosis in cancer cells. *Molecules* **2012**, *17*, 6290–6304. [CrossRef] [PubMed]
56. Koh, T.; Machino, M.; Murakami, Y.; Umemura, N.; Sakagami, H. Cytotoxicity of dental compounds towards human oral squamous cell carcinoma and normal oral cells. *In Vivo* **2013**, *27*, 85–95. [PubMed]
57. Sharma, U.K.; Sharma, A.K.; Gupta, A.; Kumar, R.; Pandey, A.; Pandey, A.K. Pharmacological activities of cinnamaldehyde and eugenol: Antioxidant, cytotoxic and anti-leishmanial studies. *Mol. Cell. Biol.* **2017**, *63*, 73–78. [CrossRef] [PubMed]
58. Fujisawa, S.; Atsumi, T.; Satoh, K.; Kadoma, Y.; Ishihara, M.; Okada, N.; Nagasaki, M.; Yokoe, I.; Sakagami, H. Radical generation, radical-scavenging activity, and cytotoxicity of eugenol-related compounds. *In Vitro Mol. Toxicol.* **2000**, *13*, 269–280.
59. Fujisawa, S.; Atsumi, T.; Ishihara, M.; Kadoma, Y. Cytotoxicity, ROS-generation activity and radical-scavenging activity of curcumin and related compounds. *Anticancer Res.* **2004**, *24*, 563–569. [PubMed]
60. Atsumi, T.; Fujisawa, S.; Tonosaki, K. A comparative study of the antioxidant/prooxidant activities of eugenol and isoeugenol with various concentrations and oxidation conditions. *Toxicol. In Vitro* **2005**, *19*, 1025–1033. [CrossRef] [PubMed]
61. Okada, N.; Hirata, A.; Murakami, Y.; Shoji, M.; Sakagami, H.; Fujisawa, S. Induction of cytotoxicity and apoptosis and inhibition of cyclooxygenase-2 gene expression by eugenol-related compounds. *Anticancer Res.* **2005**, *25*, 3263–3269. [PubMed]
62. Atsumi, T.; Iwakura, I.; Fujisawa, S.; Ueha, T. Reactive oxygen species generation and photo-cytotoxicity of eugenol in solutions of various pH. *Biomaterials* **2001**, *22*, 1459–1466. [CrossRef]
63. Fujisawa, S.; Atsumi, T.; Satoh, K.; Sakagami, H. Interaction between 2-ethoxybenzoic acid (EBA) and eugenol, and related changes in cytotoxicity. *J. Dent. Res.* **2003**, *82*, 43–47. [CrossRef] [PubMed]
64. Pisano, M.; Pagnan, G.; Loi, M.; Mura, M.E.; Tilocca, M.G.; Palmieri, G.; Fabbri, D.; Dettori, M.A.; Delogu, G.; Ponzoni, M.; et al. Antiproliferative and pro-apoptotic ctivity of eugenol-related biphenyls on malignant melanoma cells. *Mol. Cancer* **2007**, *6*, 8–20. [CrossRef] [PubMed]
65. Kim, G.C.; Choi, D.S.; Lim, J.S.; Jeong, H.C.; Kim, I.R.; Lee, M.H.; Park, B.S. Caspases-dependent apoptosis in human melanoma cell by eugenol. *Korean J. Anat.* **2006**, *39*, 245–253.
66. Shin, S.H.; Park, J.H.; Kim, G.C. The mechanism of apoptosis induced by eugenol in human osteosarcoma cells. *J. Korean Assoc. Oral Maxillofac. Surg.* **2007**, *33*, 20–27.
67. Hussain, A.; Brahmbhatt, K.; Priyani, A.; Ahmed, M.; Rizvi, T.A.; Sharma, C. Eugenol enhances the chemotherapeutic potential of gemcitabine and induces anticarcinogenic and anti-inflammatory activity in human cervical cancer cells. *Cancer Biother. Radiopharm.* **2011**, *26*, 519–527. [CrossRef] [PubMed]
68. Hussain, A.; Priyani, A.; Sadrieh, L.; Brahmbhatt, K.; Ahmed, M.; Sharma, C. Concurrent sulforaphane and eugenol induces differential effects on human cervical cancer cells. *Integr. Cancer Ther.* **2012**, *11*, 154–165. [CrossRef] [PubMed]

69. Jaganathan, S.K.; Mazumdar, A.; Mondhe, D.; Mandal, M. Apoptotic effect of eugenol in human colon cancer cell lines. *Cell Biol. Int.* **2011**, *35*, 607–615. [CrossRef] [PubMed]
70. Vidhya, N.; Devaraj, S.N. Induction of apoptosis by eugenol in human breast cancer cells. *Indian J. Exp. Biol.* **2011**, *49*, 871–878. [PubMed]
71. Al Wafai, R.; El-Rabih, W.; Katerji, M.; Safi, R.; El Sabban, M.; El-Rifai, O.; Usta, J. Chemosensitivity of MCF-7 cells to eugenol: Release of cytochrome-c and lactate dehydrogenase. *Sci. Rep.* **2017**, *7*, 43730. [CrossRef] [PubMed]
72. Koh, T.; Murakami, Y.; Tanaka, S.; Machino, M.; Onuma, H.; Kaneko, M.; Sugimoto, M.; Soga, T.; Tomita, M.; Sakagami, H. Changes of metabolic profiles in an oral squamous cell carcinoma cell line induced by eugenol. *In Vivo* **2013**, *27*, 233–243. [PubMed]
73. Majeed, H.; Antoniou, J.; Fang, Z. Apoptotic effects of eugenol-loaded nanoemulsions in human colon and liver cancer cell lines. *Asian Pac. J. Cancer Prev.* **2014**, *15*, 9159–9164. [CrossRef] [PubMed]
74. Jaganathan, S.K.; Mondhe, D.; Wani, Z.A.; Pal, H.C.; Mandal, M. Effect of honey and eugenol on ehrlich ascites and solid carcinoma. *J. Biomed. Biotechnol* **2010**, 989163:1–989163:5. [CrossRef] [PubMed]
75. Osseni, R.A.; Rat, P.; Bogdan, A.; Warnet, J.M.; Touitou, Y. Evidence of prooxidant and antioxidant action of melatonin on human liver cell line HepG2. *Life Sci.* **2000**, *68*, 387–399. [CrossRef]
76. Schwartz, J.L. The dual roles of nutrients as antioxidants and prooxidants: Their effects on tumor cell growth. *J. Nutr.* **1996**, *126*, 1221S–1227S. [PubMed]
77. Shi, M.; Xu, B.; Azakami, K.; Morikawa, T.; Watanabe, K.; Morimoto, K.; Komatsu, M.; Aoyama, K.; Takeuchi, T. Dual role of vitamin C in an oxygen-sensitive system: Discrepancy between DNA damage and cell death. *Free Radic Res.* **2005**, *39*, 213–220. [CrossRef] [PubMed]
78. Chakraborthy, A.; Ramani, P.; Sherlin, H.J.; Premkumar, P.; Natesan, A. Antioxidant and pro-oxidant activity of Vitamin C in oral environment. *Indian J. Dent. Res.* **2014**, *25*, 499–504. [CrossRef] [PubMed]
79. Fujisawa, S.; Atsumi, T.; Kadoma, Y.; Sakagami, H. Antioxidant and prooxidant action of eugenol-related compounds and their cytotoxicity. *Toxicology* **2002**, *177*, 39–54. [CrossRef]
80. Kim, D.O.; Lee, C.Y. Comprehensive study on vitamin C equivalent antioxidant capacity (VCEAC) of various polyphenolics in scavenging a free radical and its structural relationship. *Crit. Rev. Food Sci. Nutr.* **2004**, *44*, 253–273. [CrossRef] [PubMed]
81. Mahboub, R.; Memmou, F. Antioxidant activity and kinetics studies of eugenol and 6-bromoeugenol. *Nat. Prod. Res.* **2015**, *29*, 966–971. [CrossRef] [PubMed]

6

Effect of Sulforaphane and 5-Aza-2′-Deoxycytidine on Melanoma Cell Growth

Tung-chin Chiang [1,*], Brian Koss [2], L. Joseph Su [3], Charity L. Washam [2,4], Stephanie D. Byrum [2,4], Aaron Storey [2] and Alan J. Tackett [2,4,*]

1 Department of Environmental and Occupational Health, University of Arkansas for Medical Sciences, Little Rock, AR 72205, USA
2 Department of Biochemistry & Molecular Biology, University of Arkansas for Medical Sciences, Little Rock, AR 72205, USA
3 Winthrop P. Rockefeller Cancer Institute, Cancer Prevention and Population Sciences Program & Department of Epidemiology, University of Arkansas for Medical Sciences, Little Rock, AR 72205, USA
4 Arkansas Children's Research Institute, Little Rock, AR 72202, USA
* Correspondence: tchiang@uams.edu (T.-c.C.); ajtackett@uams.edu (A.J.T.);

Abstract: Background: UV exposure-induced oxidative stress is implicated as a driving mechanism for melanoma. Increased oxidative stress results in DNA damage and epigenetic dysregulation. Accordingly, we explored whether a low dose of the antioxidant sulforaphane (SFN) in combination with the epigenetic drug 5-aza-2′-deoxycytidine (DAC) could slow melanoma cell growth. SFN is a natural bioactivated product of the cruciferous family, while DAC is a DNA methyltransferase inhibitor. **Methods:** Melanoma cell growth characteristics, gene transcription profiles, and histone epigenetic modifications were measured after single and combination treatments with SFN and DAC. **Results:** We detected melanoma cell growth inhibition and specific changes in gene expression profiles upon combinational treatments with SFN and DAC, while no significant alterations in histone epigenetic modifications were observed. Dysregulated gene transcription of a key immunoregulator cytokine—C-C motif ligand 5 (CCL-5)—was validated. **Conclusions:** These results indicate a potential combinatorial effect of a dietary antioxidant and an FDA-approved epigenetic drug in controlling melanoma cell growth.

Keywords: sulforaphane; epigenetic; 5-aza-2′-deoxycytine; melanoma

---

1. Introduction

While the incidence of certain cancer types has declined, the number of diagnosed melanoma cases has increased sharply over the past three decades [1,2]. Ultraviolet (UV) exposure is one of the most apparent risk factors for melanoma [3]. There are many types of photosensitizers, such as DNA, melanin, and tryptophan, that can receive UV energy and result in direct DNA damage and ROS accumulation [4–6]. UVB affects DNA by forming cyclobutane pyrimidine dimers (CPDs), which lead to DNA mutation [7]. UVA directly induces oxidative stress through the accumulation of 8-oxo-7,8-dihydroguanine (8-oxo-G) and other photoproducts [4]. UV also induces melanin synthesis [8]. There are two types of melanin, eumelanin, and pheomelanin. The ratio of the two types of melanin is dependent on the polymorphism of the melanocortin-1 receptor (MC1R) gene and results in differential pigmentation [6,9]. Synthesis of eumelanin leads to scavenges of reactive oxygen species (ROS) while the synthesis of pheomelanin leads to depletion of antioxidants and results in ROS accumulation [10–12]. This is in concert with the determination that people with pale skin and red hair have low eumelanin and high pheomelanin and are known to have a higher risk of melanoma [13].

Many studies have identified another photosensitizer, tryptophan, which utilizes the energy from UVA and UVB to form a tryptophan photoproduct, 6-formylindolo(3,2-b) carbazole (FICZ) [14,15]. FICZ has a high affinity to the aryl hydrocarbon receptor (AhR) and activates AhR response genes, including cyclooxygenase-2 (Cox2), a melanoma prognostic marker gene [16], and cytochrome P4501A1, which increases ROS accumulation [17]. It has been shown that UVB activates AhR responses that decrease the tumor suppressor gene p27 and impairs nucleotide excision repair (NER) resulting in DNA mutation [18]. In addition to UV exposure, other environmental factors such as cigarette smoking, environmental dioxin 2,3,7,8-tetrachlorodibenzo-p-dioxin (TCDD), and arsenic exposure also induce melanogenesis [3,19–22]. Accumulated ROS from UVA and UVB via different photosensitizers, as well as environmental exposures, have many impacts on cell growth and defense. These impacts include inhibition of p27, cell cycle regulation, increased cytokines, decreased antioxidant glutathione s-transferase, increased 8-oxoG, activation of mitogen-activated protein kinase/extracellular signal-regulated kinases1/2 (MAPK/ERK1/2), increased cell proliferation and decreased tumor suppressor gene p16 [5]. These findings support the fact that melanoma patients have a higher level of oxidative stress and that this stress is associated with the progression of the disease [23].

Studies have shown that environmental exposure-induced DNA damage and oxidative stress can also result in epigenetic changes [24–27]. Elevated ROS is associated with DNA methylation and histone post-translational modifications (PTMs) [25–27]. DNA hypermethylation at promoter CpG sites, especially at tumor suppressor gene promoters, is associated with silencing gene expression in a variety of cancers, including melanoma [28,29]. Many tumor suppressor genes related to cell cycle progression, DNA repair, and apoptosis are methylated in different stages of melanoma [5,24,30–33]. Whole genome DNA methylation profiles from advanced melanoma patients have uncovered a differential methylation pattern that is correlated with survival rates [34]. In addition to aberrant DNA methylation, histone PTMs play critical roles in cancer development independently, in combination with other histone PTMs, and interactively with DNA methylation [24]. Our lab identified the elevation of trimethylation of lysine 27 on histone H3 (H3K27me3) in metastatic melanoma relative to primary melanoma [35]. H3K27me3 is catalyzed by the protein Enhancer of Zeste 2 (EZH2), a member of the Polycomb-group (PcG) family. EZH2 can recruit DNA methyltransferase (DNMT1) to chromatin to form a multisubunit protein complex that suppresses gene expression [36].

Epigenetic therapy using 5-aza-2'-deoxycytidine (DAC), an FDA-approved DNA demethylation agent, has been successfully used to treat myelodysplastic syndromes (MDSs) either alone or in combination with other drugs [37–39]. DAC is a deoxycytidine analog with the replacement of nitrogen at position 5 of the pyrimidine ring [40]. DAC interferes with normal DNA methylation by forming an irreversible covalent bond with DNMT1 [41]. The subsequent DNA-DNMT adducts play a role in controlling cancer cells depending on the dose of DAC. At high doses, DAC induces cytotoxicity by accumulated DNA–DNMT1 adduct-induced apoptosis and DNA synthesis arrest. At low doses, DNA synthesis is continued, while DNA–DNMT1 adduct bonds are being degraded and repaired, resulting in systematically hypomethylated DNA [41,42]. Studies show that DAC has effects on melanoma via decreasing cell growth and invasion [43] as well as alerting gene expression, includes tumor suppressor genes [44].

Regulating oxidative stress via the consumption of antioxidant-rich cruciferous vegetables (e.g., broccoli and Brussels sprouts) has been well-studied in cancer prevention [45–47]. One of the common compounds from cruciferous vegetables with cancer prevention characteristics is glucosinolate. Glucosinolate is not bioactivated until the enzyme myrosinase is released from the plant cell, by chewing or through denaturing by cooking, to catalyze a hydrolytic reaction to form isothiocyanates (ITCs) [48]. Sulforaphane (SFN) is one of the promising anticancer ITCs and can induce biphasic biological impact via generating different level of ROS depending on their doses [48,49]. At a dietary dose, SFN-derived ROS stimulate antioxidant protein expression to balance the ROS level induced from UV exposure. SFN activates nuclear erythroid 2-related factor 2 (Nrf2) to bind to the antioxidant response element at the promoter region of Nrf2-regulated genes. Those genes are phase-II detoxification enzymes (e.g., glutathione S-transferase, quinone reductase, and glucuronosyltransferase). By doing this, SFN increases antioxidant capacity. Furthermore, phase-I enzymes such as P450s, which activate toxic chemical compounds, are reduced by SFN at dietary doses [50–52]. In this way, SFN delivers chemopreventive effects through strengthening cell defense systems by increasing antioxidant enzymes and reducing carcinogen toxicity. Studies have shown that SFN acts as a cell-killing agent at high doses. At a high concentration of SFN, elevated amounts of SFN-derived ROS accumulate in the cells, mitochondrial function is disrupted [49], cell proliferation is blocked, cell cycle G2/M is arrested, and caspase-mediated apoptosis is induced [48,52–55]. High concentrations of SFN also induce epigenetic modification. Studies show that high doses of SFN enhance global histone acetylation by inhibiting histone deacetylase (HDAC) activity and reducing cell growth in prostate cancer [56,57]. The dual roles of SFN in cytoprotection and slowed tumor growth, as well as the low toxicity, are cell-specific [48]. Where and how the ROS is formed by SFN and the impact of surrounding molecular environments has gained great interest in research either with SFN alone or in combination with other chemotherapy drugs in many cancers [58–60].

The research reported here seeks to determine whether combining DAC and SFN can synergistically slow melanoma cell growth. We aimed to utilize a dietary dose of SFN as a natural antioxidant, while at the same time suppressing gene transcription with a low dose of the clinically approved epigenetic modifier DAC. We rationalized that with lower oxidative stress, the low dose of DAC could deliver its epigenetic effect without inducing cytotoxicity. This study is the first step in testing the combined effect of DAC and SFN in a mouse melanoma cell line. Cell growth characteristics, gene expression profiles, and histone PTMs are compared between single and combination treatments of DAC and SFN using mouse melanoma cells. Our data show cell growth inhibition, dysregulation of gene transcription, and increased cytokine production with combination treatment compared to individual treatments. Histone PTMs were identified but did not show differences following treatment. This in-vitro data provides a path to investigate the role of target gene sets and the potential role of the dietary antioxidant SFN in melanoma treatment and prevention.

2. Materials and Methods

2.1. Cell Culture and Treatment

Mouse melanoma B16F10 cells were obtained from ATCC and maintained in Dulbecco's Modified Eagle Medium (DMEM) (ThermoFisher, Waltham, MA, USA) supplemented with 10% FBS (ThermoFisher, Waltham, MA, USA) and 1% penicillin/streptomycin (ThermoFisher, Waltham, MA, USA). Cells were checked for mycoplasma contamination by MycoAler PLUS Mycoplasma Detection Kit (Lonza Walkersville, Walkersville, MD, USA) before experiments.

IC50s for both drugs were determined by using CellTiter 96 AQ_{ueous} One Solution Cell Proliferation Kit (Promega, Madison, WI, USA), following the manufacturer's protocols. In brief, cells were seeded at 1500 cells/well in a 96-well plate for 24 h. Cells were then treated with 5-aza-2′-deoxycytidine (DAC) (Sigma Aldrich, St. Louis, MO, USA) dissolved in dimethyl sulfoxide (DMSO) at concentrations ranging from 25 μM to 6.1 nM (4-fold dilutions from 25 μM, 6.25 μM, 1.56 μM, 390 nM, 97.7 nM, 24.4 nM, to 6.1 nM) for 72 h; and sulforaphane (LKT labs, St Paul, MN, USA) dissolved in water at concentrations ranging from 352 μM to 86 nM (4-fold dilutions ranging from 352 μM, 88.1 μM, 22 μM, 5.5 μM, 1.37 μM, 344 nM, to 86 nM) for 48 h. Dimethyl sulfoxide (DMSO) (Sigma Aldrich, St. Louis, MO, USA) was used as a control in the DMSO wells, at 0.00025%, equivalent to the highest amount of DMSO in the highest dose of treatment (10 mM DAC in DMSO was freshly diluted 400,000 times to 25 nM in culture medium).

Preliminary tests with different doses and duration were performed, based on the results from IC50 measurements, in 6-well plates. The optimal doses and duration of treatments were chosen based on the number of viable cells with greater than 50% of cell survival at single treatment for

DAC and SFN, with fewer cells surviving with combination treatment. SFN at 5 μM and DAC 25 nM were determined to be an optimal dose in the preliminary tests. Cells were seeded in 6-well plates at 4×10^4 cells/well and were allowed to attach for 24 h. For combinatorial drug treatment, cells were treated with DAC at 25 nM for 24 h, the medium was removed, and fresh medium with 25 nM DAC and 5 μM SFN was added. Cells were then incubated for another 48 h. For DAC or SFN single treatment, cells were treated with only DAC or SFN following the same operations as a combination treatment. All treatment groups were harvested at the same time for different target analysis, which included cell number counting and measurements of apoptosis, cell cycle, and gene transcription. Three independent biological repeats were performed.

For cytokine analysis, cells were seeded in 10 cm dishes at 3×10^5 cells/dish and were treated with SFN and DAC as described above in 10% serum-containing medium. Culture medium was replaced from 10% to 1% serum-containing medium with the same dosing scheme at the last 24 h of treatment. The purpose is to reduce potential background. Also, the final culture medium was reduced from 10 mL to 5 mL to increase the concentration of cytokine in the supernatant. The supernatant of each dish was collected for cytokines array analysis. The cell number is calculated to adjust the final amount of supernatant to be loaded from even amount of cells for cytokine analysis.

For CCL5 enzyme-linked immunosorbent assay (ELISA) analysis, cells were grown and treated as described for cytokine array analysis, except the initial cell density is at 2×10^5 cells per10 cm dish, and the final culture medium was reduced from 10 mL to 5 mL.

For histone analysis, cells were seeded in 10 cm dishes at 2×10^5 cells/dish and were treated with SFN and DAC as described above. Additionally, EZH2 inhibitor EPZ6438 (Med Chem Express, Monmouth Junction, NJ, USA), was used at 5 μM to treat cells for 48 h for analysis of histone epigenetic post-translational modifications. The dose of EPZ6438 was selected for optimal inhibition of the catalytic output of EZH2, histone H3K27me3, and was used as a positive control for histone analysis. DMSO at 0.05%, equivalent to the highest amount of DMSO in the treatment (10 mM EPZ6438 in DMSO was freshly diluted 2000 time to 5 μM in culture medium) was used in the control plates. Three independent biological repeats were performed.

2.2. *Assays for Characteristics of Cell Growth*

2.2.1. Viable Cell Count

Cell number was counted with Trypan blue solution (0.4%) using a hemocytometer. The number of the cell count was controlled to within 20–50 cells/square via dilution of cells before mixing with trypan blue.

2.2.2. Cell Cycle Arrest Analysis

Cells cycle was analyzed by fixing cells in 70% ethanol overnight and staining with propidium iodide (PI)/RNase Staining Buffer (BD Biosciences, San Jose, CA, USA). The stained DNA was analyzed at the University of Arkansas for Medical Sciences (UAMS) flow cytometry core with an LSRFortessa Flow cytometer (BD Biosciences, San Jose, CA, USA). Flow cytometry data were analyzed with Flow Jo (Ashland, OR, USA) and Dean-Jett Fox (DJF) model (BD, Franklin Lakes, NJ, USA).

2.2.3. Apoptotic Analysis

Apoptosis was measured by Annexin V and 4′,6-diamidino-2-phenylindole (DAPI) staining using the annexin V-FITC apoptosis detection kit (BD Pharmigen, San Jose, CA, USA), following the manufacturer's protocol. Cells were analyzed at the UAMS flow cytometry core with an LSRFortessa Flow cytometer (BD Biosciences, San Jose, CA, USA). Flow cytometry data were analyzed with Flow Jo (Ashland, OR, USA).

2.3. RNA-Seq Analysis

2.3.1. RNA Extraction and Targeted Gene Expression Analysis

RNA was extracted with the RNeasy Mini Kit (Qiagen, Germantown, MD, USA) following the manufacturer's protocols and eluted in water. RNA was reversed transcribed into cDNA with the One Step iScript kit (BioRad, Hercules, CA, USA) following the manufacturer's protocol.

Targeted genes of interest were amplified with 20 ng of cDNA, SYBR green Supermix (Bio-Rad, Hercules, CA, USA) and primers (final concentration at 750 nM). The PCR cyclic conditions used were 95 °C for 3 min, followed by 39 cycles of 98 °C for 15 s and 57 °C for 30 s. The following primer pairs (Integrated DNA Technologies, Coralville, IA, USA) were used for real-time analysis (Table 1):

Table 1. Primers.

Ccl5-Forward	ACCATATGGCTCGGACACCA
Ccl5-Reverse	TCTCTGGGTTGGCACACACTT
IL33-Forward	GGGGCTCACTGCAGGAAAGT
IL33-Reverse	ATTTTGCAAGGCGGGACCAG
Dusp15-Forward	TATCCACGAATCACCCCA
Dusp15-Reverse	AAGCAGTGCACAAGGCA
UBC-forward	GCCCAGTGTTACCACCAAGAGCC
UBC-Reverse	CCCATCACACCCAAGAACAGTT

Ccl5: (C-C motif) ligand 5 (Gene ID:20304); IL33: interleukin 33 (Gene ID:77125); Dusp15: dual specificity phosphatase-like 15 (Gene ID:252864); UBC: Ubiquitin C (Gene ID: 22190).

2.3.2. RNA-Seq Sample Preparation

cDNA libraries were constructed using Illumina's TruSeq stranded mRNA sample preparation kit according to the manufacturer's protocol. Briefly, 500 ng of total RNA was polyA selected, chemically fragmented, and converted to single-stranded cDNA using random hexamer-primed reverse transcription. Second strand synthesis was then performed to generate double-stranded cDNA, followed by fragment end repair and the addition of a single A base to each end of the cDNA. Adapters, including a 3′ adapter and a 5′ adapter containing 1 of 48 unique indexes, were then ligated to the fragment ends to enable attachment to the sequencing flow cell and sample pooling. Next, library DNA was PCR amplified and validated for fragment size and quantity using an Advanced Analytical Fragment Analyzer (AATI) and Qubit fluorometer (Life Technologies), respectively. Equal amounts (5 μL of 4 nM dilutions) of each library were pooled and 5 μL of the pool was denatured for 5 min by the addition of 5 μL of 0.2 N NaOH, incubated at room temperature for 5 min, neutralized by the addition of 5 μL 200 mM Tris pH 7.0, and diluted to a loading concentration of 1.8 pM; 1.3 mL of the denatured, diluted library was added to a NextSeq reagent cartridge V2.0 for sequencing on a NextSeq 500 platform using a high output flow cell to generate approximately 25 million 75-base reads per sample. All sequencing was conducted by the Center for Translational Pediatric Research Genomics Core Lab at Arkansas Children's Research Institute (Little Rock, AR, USA).

2.3.3. RNA-Seq Data Analysis

RNA reads were checked for quality of sequencing using FastQC v.0.11.7 (http://www.bioinformatics.babraham.ac.uk/projects/fastqc/). The adaptors and low-quality bases ($Q < 20$) were trimmed to a minimum of 36 base pairs using Trimmomatic v0.38 [61]. Reads that passed quality control were aligned to the mouse (mm10) (GCA_000001305.2) reference genome using TopHat v2.1.1 [62]. Sample alignment files (.bam) were then imported into Blast2GO v5.1.13, and gene level expression counts quantified using htseq [63,64]. Only reads uniquely aligned to known genes were retained and counted. Multimapped reads were discarded. Genes with low counts were then removed before downstream analysis. To retain the maximum number of interesting features genes with a minimum of 1 counts-per-million (CPM) values in at least 3 libraries were retained for further investigation. The filtered dataset was then normalized for compositional bias using a trimmed mean of M values (TMM) and $\log_2$ transformed [65]. For each comparison, edgeR quasi-likelihood method (glmQLFTest) correcting for batch effect was used to identify differentially expressed genes between experimental groups [2]. Genes with multiple tests corrected (FDR) *p*-values of 0.05 [66] and a fold change > 2 were selected for further comparisons between treatments and analyzed by Ingenuity Pathway Analysis (IPA) for biological involvement.

2.4. Chemokines Analysis

The supernatant of control and combination treated groups was spun at 10,000 g for 5 min to remove the cell debris. The supernatant was added to the membrane of Proteome Profiler mouse XL Cytokine array kit (R&D system Inc, Minneapolis, MN, USA). The manufactural protocol was followed with modification at the final film developing. Western Lightning Plus-ECL (PerkinElmer, Waltham, MA, USA) was applied at the end of film developing to have clear signals.

For ELISA, the supernatant was spun at 10,000 g for 5 min to remove the cell debris and further diluted 10 times in 1 × PBS. Duplicate diluted supernatant from each group and the serially diluted standards (ranging from 7.8 pg/mL to 500 pg/mL) were tested for the level of CCL5 according to the manufacturer's instructions (R&D Systems Inc., Minneapolis, MN, USA). The cell number is also calculated and applied in data analysis to reflect the level of CCL5 in the supernatant is from the same amount of cells.

2.5. Histone PTM Mass Spectrometry

Histones were purified from approximately 5 million cells by acid extraction, as described by Taverna, SD et al. [67]. The amount of protein was quantified by BCA Protein Assay Kit (ThermoFisher, Waltham, MA, USA). Extracted histones (5 µg), were resolved on a 4–20% gradient SDS-PAGE gel. Histone bands were visualized by staining with GelCode Blue (Thermo). Histones were excised from the gel, destained, and treated with 20 µL/band of 30% d6-acetic anhydride in 50 mM ammonium bicarbonate. Histones were then digested in-gel with 125 ng/band sequencing-grade trypsin at 37 °C overnight. Acidified tryptic peptides were separated using a 2.5 µm Waters XSelect CSH resin on a 150 mm × 0.075 mm column using a nanoAcquity UPLC system (Waters, Milford, MA, USA). Peptides were separated using a 60-min chromatography gradient, with a 40-min linear separation gradient from 97% buffer A (0.1% formic acid in water (v/v)), 3% buffer B (0.1% formic acid (v/v), 99.9% acetonitrile (v/v)), to 80% of buffer A, 20% buffer B. Eluted peptides were ionized by electrospray (2150 V) and analyzed on an Orbitrap Fusion Lumos mass spectrometer (Thermo Fisher, Waltham, MA, USA) using data-dependent acquisition. A full-scan MS was acquired in profile mode at 120,000 resolution from 375 to 1500 m/z (AGC target 5×10^5, max injection time 100 ms), followed by data-dependent MS/MS analysis with a 3 second duty cycle time. Peptides with a determined monoisotopic peak, intensity threshold greater than 2×10^4 counts, and charge state of 2–7 were selected for HCD fragmentation at 30% collision energy, AGC target of 1×10^4, maximum injection time 35 milliseconds, and analyzed in the ion trap with scan speed set to rapid.

Raw data files were analyzed using Mascot (Matrix Science, London, UK) using a custom Uniprot database which included only mouse histones (Table 2). Files were searched with a precursor tolerance of 3 ppm and fragment ion tolerance of 0.5 Da. Fixed modifications included carbamidomethylation of cysteine. Variable modifications to lysine included monomethylation, dimethylation, trimethylation, acetylation, deuterated acetylation, and methylation and deuterated acetylation. Variable modifications to arginine included monomethylation and dimethylation. Variable modifications to serine and threonine were phosphorylation. Up to four missed trypsin cleavages were permitted. Mascot search results were loaded into Scaffold, and filtered for a protein FDR of 1%, a peptide score probability of

80%, and a minimum of 5 peptides per protein. Spectral count data was exported in tabular format and analyzed using R [68].

Table 2. List of mouse histones used for analysis.

Mouse Histones					
H10	H1FOO	H2A2B	H2AX	H2B1H	H2B3B
H11	H1T	H2A2C	H2AY	H2B1K	H31
H12	H2A1	H2A3	H2AZ	H2B1M	H32
H13	H2A1F	H2AB1	H2B1A	H2B1P	H33
H14	H2A1H	H2AJ	H2B1B	H2B2B	H3C
H15	H2A1K	H2AV	H2B1C	H2B2E	H4
H1FNT	H2A2A	H2AW	H2B1F	H2B3A	

3. Results

3.1. *SFN and DAC Single and Combination Treatment Result in Growth Inhibition*

The IC50 for SFN was calculated to be approximately 22 μM for SFN and 44 nM for DAC (Figure 1A). For cell growth inhibition, a dose of 5 μM of SFN and 25 nM of DAC were chosen based on cell viability assays with more than 50% cells surviving from a single treatment of SFN and DAC respectively. Viable cell counts were calculated in the single and combination treatment of DAC and SFN compared to control (Figure 1B). There was 58% ± 4% and 56% ± 7% viable cells compared to control for the single treatment with DAC and SFN, respectively and only 33% ± 5% of viable cells in SFN and DAC combination treatment. The combination treatment induced significant growth inhibition compared to any single treatment ($p < 0.03$, Student's *t*-test).

3.2. *SFN and DAC Single and Combination Treatment Result in Minimal Apoptosis*

Apoptosis analysis showed that most of the cells were noted as alive by negative stain for annexin V and DAPI in all treatments and control (Figure 1C,D). The percentage of viable cells not in apoptosis with DAC and SFN single treatments, was 99% ± 0.2% ($p < 0.01$) and 97% ± 1%($p < 0.01$), respectively, compared to control. Combination treatment of DAC and SFN results in 95% ± 1% ($p < 0.004$) of viable cells compared to control. The percentage of viable cells not in apoptosis with combination treatments was slightly lower than any single treatment of SFN ($p < 0.03$) and DAC ($p < 0.01$).

3.3. *SFN and DAC Single and Combination Treatment Result in No Cell Cycle Arrest*

Cell cycle analysis indicated that all treated and control cells were in normal distributions for different cell cycles with G1 as dominant, followed by S phase and G2 phase, as shown in representative figures (Figure 1E). There was no significant difference between treatments in the G2/M phase (Figure 1F).

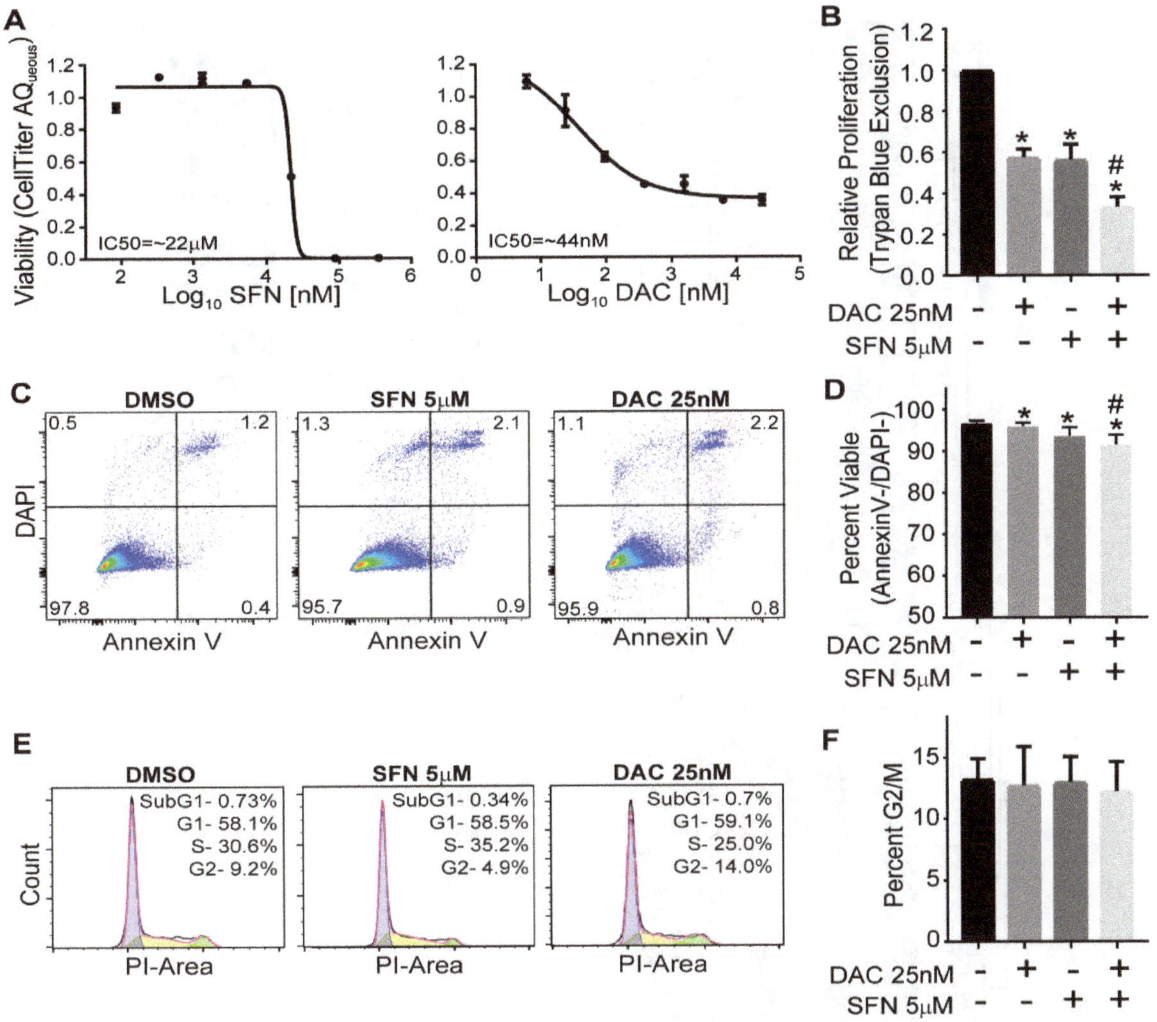

Figure 1. Impact of SFN and DAC single and combination treatment on the growth of B16 melanoma. (**A**) The IC50 of SFN and DAC single treatment is approximately 22 μM and 44 nM, respectively. Cell viability was determined using the CellTiter 96 AQ_{ueous} One Solution Cell Proliferation kit. The data were analyzed by nonlinear regression to determine the IC50. (**B**) Growth inhibition induced from single and combination treatment of SFN and DAC. Viable cells were measured by trypan blue staining and analyzed by Student's *t*-test. (**C**) Representative apoptosis analysis (AnnexinV/DAPI) by flow cytometry from control, SFN, and DAC single treatment. (**D**) The percentage of viable cells with DAC and SFN single and combination treatments were compared to control. (**E**) Representative cell cycle analysis from control and SFN and DAC single treatment. Data were analyzed with Flow Jo /Dean-Jett Fox (DJF) model. (**F**) The percent G2/M phase in DAC and SFN single and combination treatments were compared to control with Student's *t*-test. * Significantly different from control, # Single treatment is significantly different from combinational treatment (Student's *t*-test).

3.4. *SFN Induced Dysregulated Gene Transcription*

RNAseq data analysis revealed a differential gene expression profile by SFN single treatment compared to control. There were 126 genes with greater than 2-fold change compared to control. The data have been deposited in NCBI's Gene Expression Omnibus [69]. The top genes with greater than 2.5-fold change ($p < 0.001$) are shown in the heatmap (Figure 2A). The biological roles of genes responding to SFN single treatment with greater than 2-fold change were analyzed with IPA. The top canonical pathways analysis, with a negative log p-value greater than 2, indicated many important biological pathways dysregulated in response to SFN single treatment (Figure 2B).

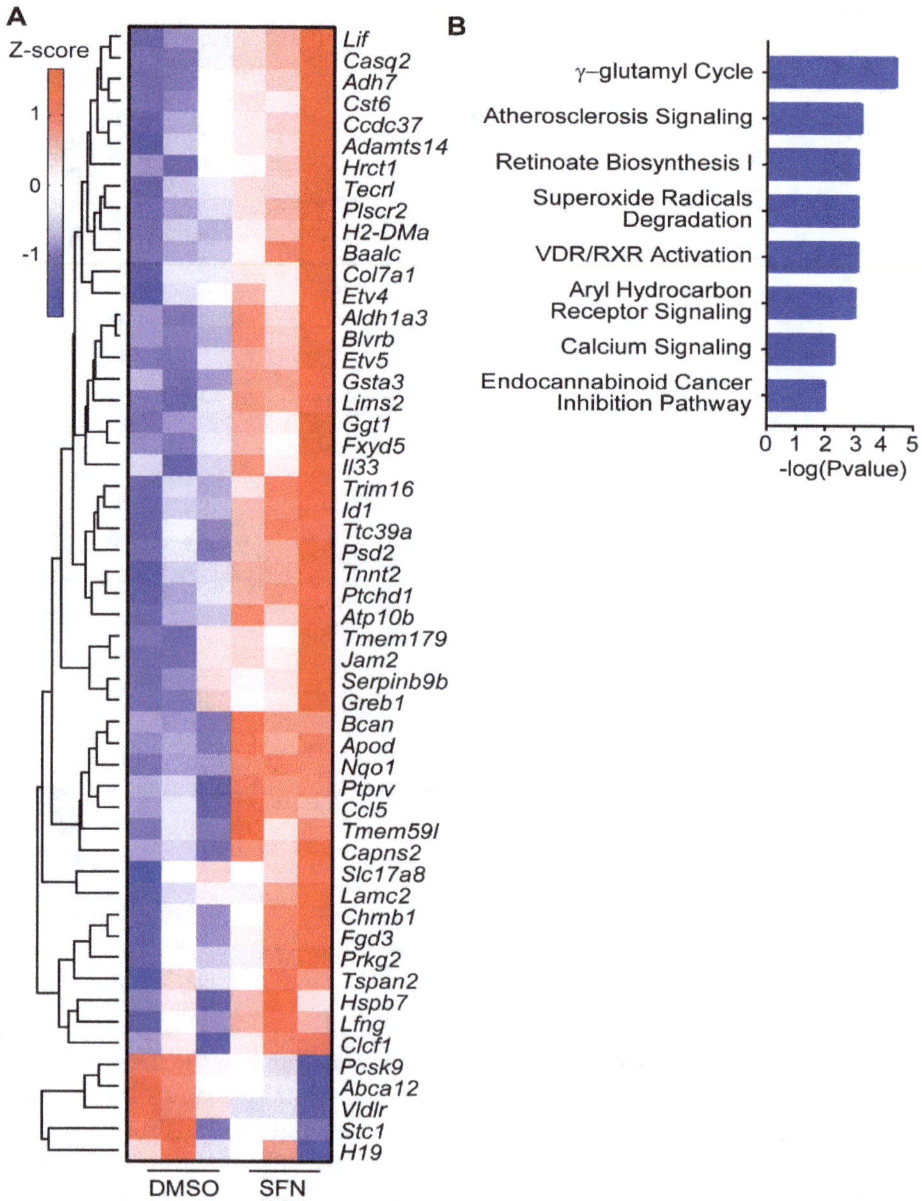

Figure 2. Differential gene expression induced by SFN single treatment and the related biological pathways. (**A**) Differentially expressed genes from SFN single treatment compared to control. Genes with greater than 2.5 fold changes ($p < 0.001$) were analyzed with unsupervised clustering (Z score shown in the color key). (**B**) Top canonical pathways from SFN single treatment. Genes greater than two-fold change relative to control were analyzed with Ingenuity Pathway Analysis (IPA) for their biological significance. The top eight pathways are shown here.

3.5. SFN and DAC Uniquely Induced Dysregulated Gene Transcription

DAC single treatment induced 19 genes to greater than 2-fold change compared to control ($p < 0.05$), and this number is too low for canonical pathway analysis by IPA. However, SFN and DAC combination treatment induced more genes than any single treatment. There were 261 genes with greater than a 2-fold change from the combination treatment of SFN and DAC compared to control ($p < 0.05$). The data from DAC single and SFN and DAC combination treatment have been deposited in NCBI's Gene Expression Omnibus [69] as described above for SFN single treatment with the same accession number GSE12752. The top genes with greater than 3-fold change ($p < 0.001$) induced from SFN and DAC combination treatment are shown in the heatmap (Figure 3A). The biological roles of genes responded to SFN and DAC combination treatment compared to control with greater than 2-fold change were analyzed with IPA. The top canonical pathways analysis, with a negative log p-value greater than 3.5, showed many biological pathways involvement (Figure 3B). The role of vitamin D receptor/retinoid X receptor (VDR/RXR) activation and aryl hydrocarbon receptor signaling were listed as the top two canonical pathways from SFN and DAC combination treatment with a negative log p-value greater than 5.5. These two pathways were also detected in SFN single treatment with a negative log p-value approximately 3.0 (Figure 2B).

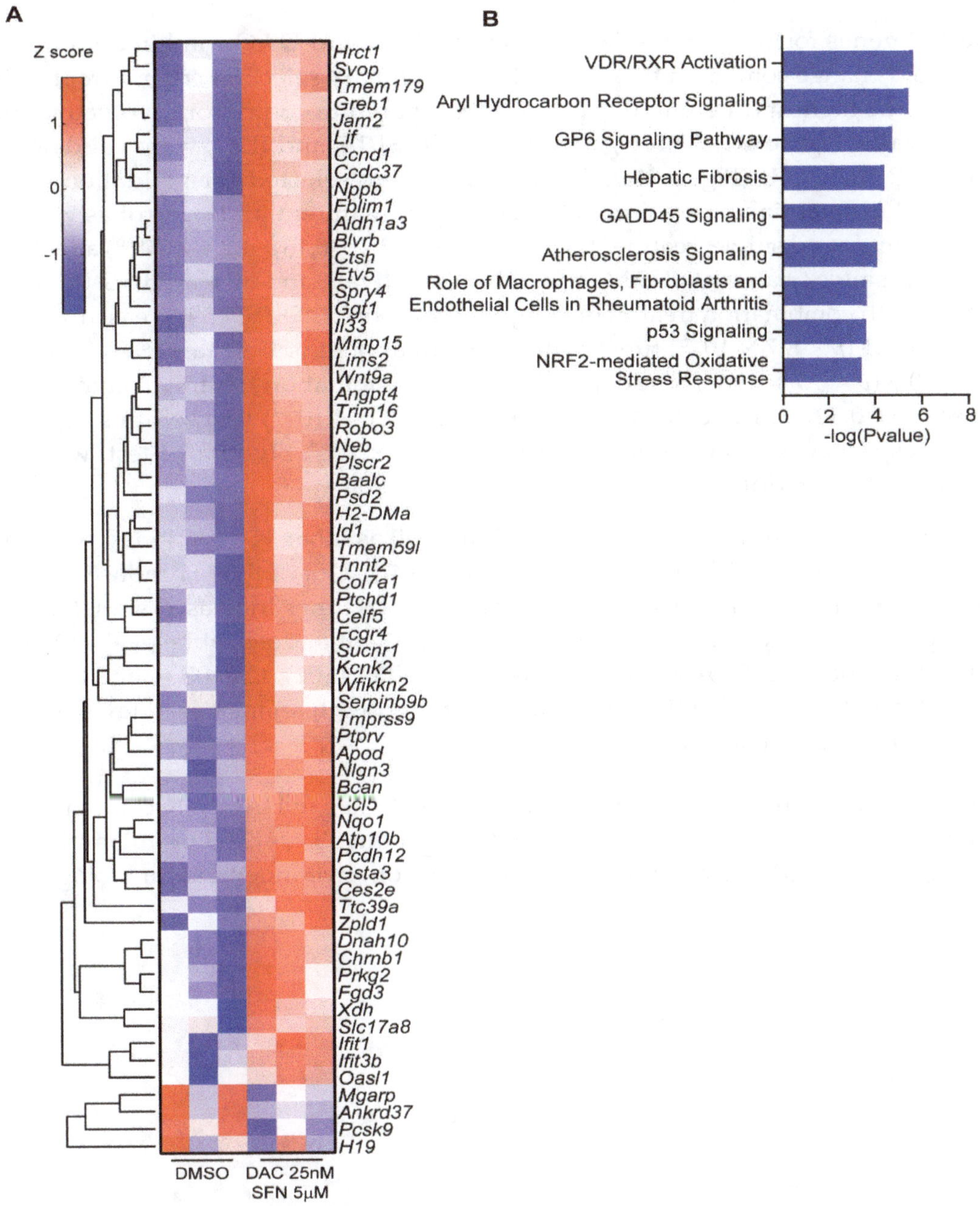

Figure 3. Differential gene expression induced by SFN and DAC combination treatment and the involved biological pathways. (**A**) Differentially expressed genes from the combination treatment of SFN and DAC compared to control treatments. Genes with greater than 3-fold change ($p < 0.001$) were analyzed with unsupervised clustering (Z score shown in the color key). (**B**) Top canonical pathways from the combination treatment of SFN and DAC. Genes greater than 2-fold change than the control with the combination treatment of SFN and DAC were analyzed with IPA for their biological significance. The top nine pathways are shown here.

3.6. Validation of Dysregulated Gene Transcription Induced by SFN and DAC Combination Treatment

There were 261 genes with greater than 2-fold change ($p < 0.05$) of gene expression (either increased or decreased) with DAC plus SFN combination treatments compared to control. The number of genes with expression changes greater than 2-fold ($p < 0.05$), compared to control, from the single treatment were 19 and 126 genes for DAC and SFN, respectively (Figure 4A). Furthermore, there were 150 unique genes from combination treatment compared to control (Figure 4B).

We selected genes for further validation from the SFN and DAC combination treatment with greater than 2-fold change compared to control. The preliminary selection criteria from RNA-seq data were genes with the highest differential expression compared to control or involved in multiple top biological pathways (Figure 4C). Three genes, CCL5, DUSP15, and IL33, were validated by reverse transcription PCR (RT-PCR) (Figure 4D). These genes were selected for validation on the criteria that they showed differential expression between single treatment and control as well as between combination treatment and single treatment. CCL5 increased 2 ± 0.1 ($p < 2.4 \times 10^{-6}$) and 3 ± 0.2 ($p < 1.5 \times 10^{-5}$) times with single treatment of DAC and SFN, respectively, and increased 5 ± 0.2 ($p < 1.3 \times 10^{-7}$, Student's t-test) with combination treatment compared to control. DUSP15 increased 1.7 ± 0.2 ($p < 6.2 \times 10^{-3}$) and 1.9 ± 0.1 ($p < 8.7 \times 10^{-6}$) times with single treatment of DAC and SFN, respectively, and increased 3.6 ± 0.3 ($p < 1.7 \times 10^{-5}$, Student's t-test) with combination treatment compared to control. IL33 increased 1.6 ± 0.3 ($p < 4.2 \times 10^{-2}$) and 2.2 ± 0.2 ($p < 2.0 \times 10^{-4}$) times with single treatment of DAC and SFN, respectively, and increased 3.0 ± 0.3 ($p < 2.1 \times 10^{-4}$, Student's t-test) with combination treatment compared to control.

The level of secreted cytokines CCL5 and IL33, as well as other 111 cytokines, were measured in the supernatant using a mouse XL cytokines array (Figure 4E). Out of the 111 mouse cytokines probes on the membrane, CCL5 was detected with greater than two times increased signal in combination treatment compared to the control group. IL33 was not present at detectable levels. Other cytokines, such as CXCL10 (Gene ID 15945), angiopoietin-2 (Gene ID 11601), CD105 (Gene ID 13805), VEGF (Gene ID 22339), and CCN4 (Gene ID 22402), were detected with an increased level of expression in combination treatment than control.

Specific CCL5 ELISA further confirmed the increase in CCL 5 in DAC/SFN combination treatment, as indicated in Figure 4F. The level of CCL5 in control is about 55 +/− 22.3 pg/mL and is increased to 348 +/− 92.2 pg/mL in SFN/DAC combination treatment from two independent biological runs.

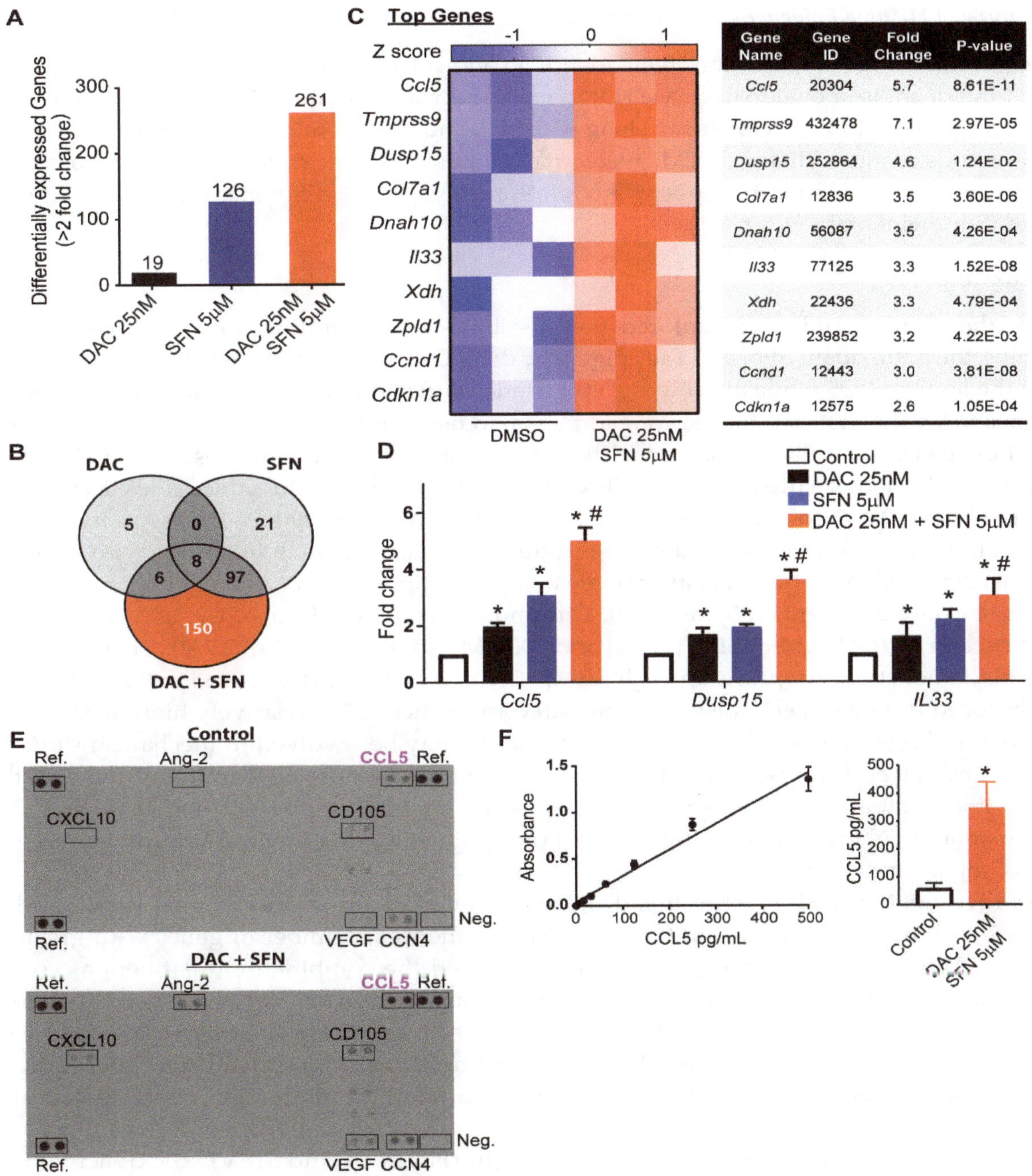

Figure 4. Validation of combination effects from SFN and DAC. (**A**) The number of differentially expressed genes induced by different treatments. (**B**) The number of unique genes responding to single and combination treatment. All genes were selected from greater than 2-fold change compared to control with $p < 0.05$. (**C**) A heatmap and list of top selected genes from SFN and DAC combination treatments (Z score shows in the color key). (**D**) Relative gene expression validation by rtPCR of Ccl5, Dusp15, and IL33 between treatments. * Significantly different from control, $p < 0.05$, # Single treatment is significantly different from combinational treatment, $p < 0.05$ (Student's t-test). (**E**) Expression of cytokines detected by cytokine array. Ref indicates reference spots. Neg: negative control. Arrays were performed in duplicate. (**F**) Specific CCL5 ELISA further confirmed the increase in CCL 5 in DAC/SFN combination treatment. The left side indicated the standard curve of CCL5, ranged from 7.8 pg/mL to 500 pg/mL. The right side indicates the concentration of CCL5 in the supernatant is increased from 55pg/mL in control to 348 pg/mL in DAC/SFN combination treated group. All data were from two independent biological runs.

3.7. Analysis of Histone Epigenetic Post-Translational Modifications (PTMs)

Post-translational modifications were identified and subsequently quantified on histones H3 and H4. EPZ treatment is known to decrease H3K27me3, and was consequently used as a positive control. We treated cells with EPZ6438 for 48 hrs along with SFN and DAC combination treatments as described in the methods section. Histone PTMs were analyzed using lysine derivatization and a bottom-up proteomic workflow. Aside from positive control, no significant differences in histone PTMs were detected (Supplementary Figure S1).

4. Discussion

For the current study, we explored the possibility of controlling melanoma cell growth by combining the antioxidant SFN and the epigenetic drug DAC. The rationale behind this work was to control the level of ROS while altering the epigenetic status with a relatively low dose of each drug. The aim is to lay the first step for our long term goal in using a dietary dose of an antioxidant to help epigenetic drugs in controlling melanoma. Therefore, we aimed to use a low dose of each drug to allow the future application of a dietary dose of SFN and a low dose of DAC to reduce side effects. We chose 5 μM of SFN and 25 nM of DAC, which are equal to or lower than half of the respective IC50 from our test (Figure 1A). These doses of the drugs induce significant growth inhibition with combination treatment compared to control and either single treatment (Figure 1B). We did not find apoptosis or cell cycle arrest in any treatments (Figure 1C–F). This finding is different from other studies using a higher dose of each drug (6–25 μM of SFN [70,71] and 200 nM–0.5 μM of DAC [72,73]). These higher-dose studies all demonstrate apoptosis and cell arrest effects. At the low doses used in this study, the two drugs induced different mechanisms as compared to studies using relatively high doses of SFN or DAC. Our findings suggest that the growth inhibition may be involved in mechanisms other than apoptosis and cell cycle arrest. A combination treatment of low-dose SFN and DAC reduced the cell growth without initiating cell cycle arrest or apoptosis. These data indicate that attenuating ROS with the antioxidant SFN may enhance the utility of the epigenetic drug DAC in controlling cell growth, with less impact on the host.

We investigated the impact of this drug combination at the transcriptional level by RNAseq (Figures 2 and 3). There was a significant increase in the total number of genes with greater than 2-fold ($p < 0.05$) expression change in cells that received the combination treatment as compared to those that received either single treatment and as compared to control (Figure 4A). The absolute number of genes altered by 25 nM of DAC is very low at 19, and those altered by SFN alone is higher at 126. This may be attributed to the low dose treatment with limited impact. Interestingly, the number of altered genes increased to 261 when SFN and DAC combination treatment was applied. The top differentially-expressed genes and canonical pathways showed different distributions between single SFN and combination SFN and DAC treatment (Figures 2 and 3). VDR/RXR activation and aryl hydrocarbon receptor signaling (AhR receptor) are two top-listed pathways from combination treatments. Both pathways are known to be associated with UV exposure [5,15,74–76]. We validated select genes involved in more than one canonical pathway or listed as top differentially-expressed genes (Figure 4C). The transcription level of the three genes (CCL5, IL33, and DUSP15) were significantly higher in the combination treatment than either of the single treatments (Figure 4D). Two (CCL5 and IL33) of the three genes are secreted proteins. We further validated secreted proteins with cytokine arrays and ELISA on CCL5 (Figure 4E,F). CCL5 was validated to have increased levels, both in transcription level and detected extracellularly after combination treatment as compared to control. CCL5 is also known as RANTES (regulated on activation, normal T cell expressed and secreted). It is one of the cytokines which functions as a chemoattractant for natural killer (NK) cells [77], which do not efficiently infiltrate solid tumors such as melanoma [78]. CCL5 is the main factor in inhibiting melanoma growth by bringing NK cells to the tumor site, while autophagy is suppressed [79]. Activated NK cells could stimulate the immune checkpoint programmed cell death protein 1 (PD-1) [80] and cytotoxic T lymphocytes (CTL)-associated antigen 4 (CTLA4) [81] to deliver immunoregulatory effects. Increased expression of CCL5 involves the phosphorylation of the MAPK8/JNK-JUN/c-Jun signaling pathway, which is initiated by decreased expression of protein phosphatase 2 A (PP2A), while autophagy is suppressed [82,83]. Clinically, a high level of CCL5 is positively associated with the NK cell marker NKp46 as well as with melanoma patients' survival [79,84].

We also investigated whether low dose treatments of SFN and DAC have an impact on histone PTMs. There was no differential PTMs detected when control and combination of SNF and DAC treated cells were analyzed (Supplementary Figure S1). This suggests that under the conditions of our treatments, the differential gene expression and cell inhibition may not be associated with histone epigenetic reprogramming, but rather the direct effects of SFN and DAC.

In summary, our data suggest that attenuating ROS through the use of the antioxidant SFN can help the epigenetic drug DAC control cell growth. This control is not via direct cell killing with apoptosis, cell cycle arrest or histone modifications, but, more directly, by changing gene transcription and cytokine production, which may increase the immune defense system by recruiting natural killer cells.

5. Conclusions

Melanoma patients not only have high oxidative stress [23], but also have a high frequency of recurrence of the disease [85,86]. It is apparent that melanoma patients are susceptible to daily UV- and environmental exposure-induced ROS [5]. Managing the level of ROS via natural antioxidants has demonstrated beneficial effects in controlling melanoma [5], but does not eliminate the tumor. Our study aimed to attenuate ROS by a low dose of the antioxidant SFN and allow the epigenetic drug DAC to control melanoma at a lower dose. The current study clearly demonstrates that SFN could have combinational effects with the commonly used, FDA-approved demethylation agent DAC in significantly inhibiting melanoma cell growth. The next goal is to apply our findings to animal studies. The long term goal is for the clinical application of controlling melanoma with a dietary dose of SFN and target drugs (e.g., epigenetic and immunotherapeutic drugs) at lower doses that may have fewer side effects for patients.

Author Contributions: Conceptualization: T.-c.C., L.J.S., and A.J.T.; Methodology: T.-c.C., B.K., L.J.S., C.L.W., S.D.B., A.S., and A.J.T.; Formal analysis: T.-c.C., B.K., C.L.W., and S.D.B.; Resources: L.J.S. and A.J.T. Data curation: T.-c.C., C.L.W., A.S., and B.K.; Writing; T.-c.C., B.K., S.D.B., A.S., L.J.S., and A.J.T.; Visualization: B.K.; Supervision: T.-c.C., L.J.S., and A.J.T.; Project administration: T.-c.C. and A.J.T; Funding acquisition: L.J.S. and A.J.T.

Acknowledgments: Rosalind B Penny for critical editing and review; Hui-Yi Lin for data analysis consultation; Jun Nakamura for idea generation and critical review; Winthrop P. Rockefeller Cancer Institute, University of Arkansas for Medical Science; Department of Biochemistry and Molecular Biology, University of Arkansas for Medical Science; and the Chancellor's Challenge Initiative of the University of Arkansas: Global Expression Pathway Analysis Training: Target Obesity.

References

1. Sandru, A.; Voinea, S.; Panaitescu, E.; Blidaru, A. Survival rates of patients with metastatic malignant melanoma. *J. Med. Life* **2014**, *7*, 572–576. [PubMed]
2. Chen, Y.; Lun, A.T.; Smyth, G.K. From reads to genes to pathways: Differential expression analysis of RNA-Seq experiments using Rsubread and the edgeR quasi-likelihood pipeline. *F1000Research* **2016**, *5*, 1438. [PubMed]
3. Berwick, M.; Buller, D.B.; Cust, A.; Gallagher, R.; Lee, T.K.; Meyskens, F.; Pandey, S.; Thomas, N.E.; Veierød, M.B.; Ward, S. Melanoma Epidemiology and Prevention. *Cancer Treat. Res.* **2016**, *167*, 17–49. [PubMed]
4. Cadet, J.; Wagner, J.R. DNA base damage by reactive oxygen species, oxidizing agents, and UV radiation. *Cold Spring Harb. Perspect. Biol.* **2013**, *5*, a012559. [CrossRef] [PubMed]
5. Venza, M.; Visalli, M.; Beninati, C.; Gaetano, G.V.D.; Teti, D.; Venza, I. Cellular Mechanisms of Oxidative Stress and Action in Melanoma. *Oxid. Med. Cell. Longev.* **2015**, *2015*, 1–11. [CrossRef] [PubMed]

6. Videira, I.F.; Moura, D.F.; Magina, S. Mechanisms regulating melanogenesis. *Bras. Derm.* **2013**, *88*, 76–83. [CrossRef] [PubMed]
7. Drouin, R.; Therrien, J.P. UVB-induced cyclobutane pyrimidine dimer frequency correlates with skin cancer mutational hotspots in p53. *Photochem. Photobiol.* **1997**, *66*, 719–726. [CrossRef]
8. Abdel-Malek, Z.; Swope, V.; Smalara, D.; Babcock, G.; Dawes, S.; Nordlund, J. Analysis of the UV-induced melanogenesis and growth arrest of human melanocytes. *Pigment Cell Res.* **1994**, *7*, 326–332. [CrossRef]
9. Latreille, J.; Ezzedine, K.; Elfakir, A.; Ambroisine, L.; Gardinier, S.; Galan, P.; Hercberg, S.; Gruber, G.; Rees, J.; Tschachler, E.; et al. MC1R gene polymorphism affects skin color and phenotypic features related to sun sensitivity in a population of French adult women. *Photochem. Photobiol.* **2009**, *85*, 1451–1458. [CrossRef]
10. Morgan, A.M.; Lo, J.; Fisher, D.E. How does pheomelanin synthesis contribute to melanomagenesis?: Two distinct mechanisms could explain the carcinogenicity of pheomelanin synthesis. *Bioessays* **2013**, *35*, 672–676. [CrossRef]
11. Hsiao, J.J.; Fisher, D.E. The roles of microphthalmia-associated transcription factor and pigmentation in melanoma. *Arch. Biochem. Biophys.* **2014**, *563*, 28–34. [CrossRef] [PubMed]
12. Samokhvalov, A.; Hong, L.; Liu, Y.; Garguilo, J.; Nemanich, R.J.; Edwards, G.S.; Simon, J.D. Oxidation potentials of human eumelanosomes and pheomelanosomes. *Photochem. Photobiol.* **2005**, *81*, 145–148. [CrossRef] [PubMed]
13. Sulem, P.; Gudbjartsson, D.F.; Stacey, S.N.; Helgason, A.; Rafnar, T.; Magnusson, K.P.; Manolescu, A.; Karason, A.; Palsson, A.; Thorleifsson, G.; et al. Genetic determinants of hair, eye and skin pigmentation in Europeans. *Nat. Genet.* **2007**, *39*, 1443–1452. [CrossRef] [PubMed]
14. Syed, D.N.; Mukhtar, H. FICZ: A Messenger of Light in Human Skin. *J. Investig. Derm.* **2015**, *135*, 1478–1481. [CrossRef] [PubMed]
15. Fritsche, E.; Schäfer, C.; Calles, C.; Bernsmann, T.; Bernshausen, T.; Wurm, M.; Hübenthal, U.; Cline, J.E.; Hajimiragha, H.; Schroeder, P.; et al. Lightening up the UV response by identification of the arylhydrocarbon receptor as a cytoplasmatic target for ultraviolet B radiation. *Proc. Natl. Acad. Sci. USA* **2007**, *104*, 8851–8856. [CrossRef] [PubMed]
16. Becker, M.R.; Siegelin, M.D.; Rompel, R.; Enk, A.H.; Gaiser, T. COX-2 expression in malignant melanoma: A novel prognostic marker? *Melanoma Res.* **2009**, *19*, 8–16. [CrossRef] [PubMed]
17. Furue, M.; Takahara, M.; Nakahara, T.; Uchi, H. Role of AhR/ARNT system in skin homeostasis. *Arch. Derm. Res.* **2014**, *306*, 769–779. [CrossRef] [PubMed]
18. Pollet, M.; Shaik, S.; Mescher, M.; Frauenstein, K.; Tigges, J.; Braun, S.A.; Sondenheimer, K.; Kaveh, M.; Bruhs, A.; Meller, S.; et al. The AHR represses nucleotide excision repair and apoptosis and contributes to UV-induced skin carcinogenesis. *Cell Death Differ.* **2018**, *25*, 1823–1836. [CrossRef]
19. Delijewski, M.; Wrześniok, D.; Otręba, M.; Beberok, A.; Rok, J.; Buszman, E. Nicotine impact on melanogenesis and antioxidant defense system in HEMn-DP melanocytes. *Mol. Cell. Biochem.* **2014**, *395*, 109–116. [CrossRef]
20. Haresaku, S.; Hanioka, T.; Tsutsui, A.; Watanabe, T. Association of lip pigmentation with smoking and gingival melanin pigmentation. *Oral Dis.* **2007**, *13*, 71–76. [CrossRef]
21. Mimura, J.; Fujii-Kuriyama, Y. Functional role of AhR in the expression of toxic effects by TCDD. *Biochim. Biophys. Acta* **2003**, *1619*, 263–268. [CrossRef]
22. Granstein, R.D.; Sober, A.J. Drug- and heavy metal—Induced hyperpigmentation. *J. Am. Acad. Derm.* **1981**, *5*, 1–18. [CrossRef]
23. Bisevac, J.P.; Djukic, M.; Stanojevic, I.; Stevanovic, I.; Mijuskovic, Z.; Djuric, A.; Gobeljic, B.; Banovic, T.; Vojvodic, D. Association Between Oxidative Stress and Melanoma Progression. *J. Med. Biochem.* **2018**, *37*, 12–20. [CrossRef] [PubMed]
24. Sarkar, D.; Leung, E.Y.; Baguley, B.C.; Finlay, G.J.; Askarian-Amiri, M.E. Epigenetic regulation in human melanoma: Past and future. *Epigenetics* **2015**, *10*, 103–121. [CrossRef] [PubMed]
25. Tokarz, P.; Kaarniranta, K.; Blasiak, J. Inhibition of DNA methyltransferase or histone deacetylase protects retinal pigment epithelial cells from DNA damage induced by oxidative stress by the stimulation of antioxidant enzymes. *Eur. J. Pharm.* **2016**, *776*, 167–175. [CrossRef] [PubMed]
26. Donkena, K.V.; Young, C.Y.; Tindall, D.J. Oxidative stress and DNA methylation in prostate cancer. *Obs. Gynecol. Int.* **2010**, *2010*, 1–14. [CrossRef]
27. Wachsman, J.T. DNA methylation and the association between genetic and epigenetic changes: Relation to carcinogenesis. *Mutat. Res.* **1997**, *375*, 1–8. [CrossRef]

28. Sigalotti, L.; Covre, A.; Fratta, E.; Parisi, G.; Colizzi, F.; Rizzo, A.; Danielli, R.; Nicolay, H.J.; Coral, S.; Maio, M. Epigenetics of human cutaneous melanoma: Setting the stage for new therapeutic strategies. *J. Transl. Med.* **2010**, *8*, 56. [CrossRef]
29. Furuta, J.; Umebayashi, Y.; Miyamoto, K.; Kikuchi, K.; Otsuka, F.; Sugimura, T.; Ushijima, T. Promoter methylation profiling of 30 genes in human malignant melanoma. *Cancer Sci.* **2004**, *95*, 962–968. [CrossRef]
30. Hoon, D.S.; Spugnardi, M.; Kuo, C.; Huang, S.K.; Morton, D.L.; Taback, B. Profiling epigenetic inactivation of tumor suppressor genes in tumors and plasma from cutaneous melanoma patients. *Oncogene* **2004**, *23*, 4014–4022. [CrossRef]
31. Shen, L.; Kondo, Y.; Guo, Y.; Zhang, J.; Zhang, L.; Ahmed, S.; Shu, J.; Chen, X.; Waterland, R.A.; Issa, J.P. Genome-wide profiling of DNA methylation reveals a class of normally methylated CpG island promoters. *PLoS Genet.* **2007**, *3*, 2023–2036. [CrossRef] [PubMed]
32. Muthusamy, V.; Duraisamy, S.; Bradbury, C.M.; Hobbs, C.; Curley, D.P.; Nelson, B.; Bosenberg, M. Epigenetic silencing of novel tumor suppressors in malignant melanoma. *Cancer Res.* **2006**, *66*, 11187–11193. [CrossRef] [PubMed]
33. Koga, Y.; Pelizzola, M.; Cheng, E.; Krauthammer, M.; Sznol, M.; Ariyan, S.; Narayan, D.; Molinaro, A.M.; Halaban, R.; Weissman, S.M. Genome-wide screen of promoter methylation identifies novel markers in melanoma. *Genome Res.* **2009**, *19*, 1462–1470. [CrossRef] [PubMed]
34. Sigalotti, L.; Covre, A.; Fratta, E.; Parisi, G.; Sonego, P.; Colizzi, F.; Coral, S.; Massarut, S.; Kirkwood, J.M.; Maio, M. Whole genome methylation profiles as independent markers of survival in stage IIIC melanoma patients. *J. Transl. Med.* **2012**, *10*, 185. [CrossRef] [PubMed]
35. Sengupta, D.; Byrum, S.D.; Avaritt, N.L.; Davis, L.; Shields, B.; Mahmoud, F.; Reynolds, M.; Orr, L.M.; Mackintosh, S.G.; Shalin, S.C.; et al. Quantitative Histone Mass Spectrometry Identifies Elevated Histone H3 Lysine 27 (Lys27) Trimethylation in Melanoma. *Mol. Cell. Proteom.* **2016**, *15*, 765–775. [CrossRef] [PubMed]
36. Vire, E.; Brenner, C.; Deplus, R.; Blanchon, L.; Fraga, M.; Didelot, C.; Morey, L.; Van Eynde, A.; Bernard, D.; Vanderwinden, J.M.; et al. The Polycomb group protein EZH2 directly controls DNA methylation. *Nature* **2006**, *439*, 871–874. [CrossRef]
37. Malik, P.; Cashen, A.F. Decitabine in the treatment of acute myeloid leukemia in elderly patients. *Cancer Manag. Res.* **2014**, *6*, 53–61.
38. Young, C.S.; Clarke, K.M.; Kettyle, L.M.; Thompson, A.; Mills, K.I. Decitabine-Vorinostat combination treatment in acute myeloid leukemia activates pathways with potential for novel triple therapy. *Oncotarget* **2017**, *8*, 51429–51446. [CrossRef]
39. Momparler, R.L.; Côté, S.; Momparler, L.F.; Idaghdour, Y. Epigenetic therapy of acute myeloid leukemia using 5-aza-2-deoxycytidine (decitabine) in combination with inhibitors of histone methylation and deacetylation. *Clin. Epigenetics* **2014**, *6*, 19. [CrossRef]
40. Sorm, F.; Vesely, J. Effect of 5-aza-2-deoxycytidine against leukemic and hemopoietic tissues in AKR mice. *Neoplasma* **1968**, *15*, 339–343.
41. Christman, J.K. 5-Azacytidine and 5-aza-2-deoxycytidine as inhibitors of DNA methylation: Mechanistic studies and their implications for cancer therapy. *Oncogene* **2002**, *21*, 5483–5495. [CrossRef] [PubMed]
42. Issa, J.P.; Garcia-Manero, G.; Giles, F.J.; Mannari, R.; Thomas, D.; Faderl, S.; Bayar, E.; Lyons, J.; Rosenfeld, C.S.; Cortes, J.; et al. Phase 1 study of low-dose prolonged exposure schedules of the hypomethylating agent 5-aza-2-deoxycytidine (decitabine) in hematopoietic malignancies. *Blood* **2004**, *103*, 1635–1640. [CrossRef] [PubMed]
43. Rajaii, F.; Asnaghi, L.; Enke, R.; Merbs, S.L.; Handa, J.T.; Eberhart, C.G. The demethylating agent 5-Aza reduces the growth, invasiveness, and clonogenicity of uveal and cutaneous melanoma. *Invest. Ophthalmol. Vis. Sci.* **2014**, *55*, 6178–6186. [CrossRef] [PubMed]
44. El Baroudi, M.; La Sala, D.; Cinti, C.; Capobianco, E. Pathway landscapes and epigenetic regulation in breast cancer and melanoma cell lines. *Theor. Biol. Med. Model.* **2014**, *11*, S8. [CrossRef] [PubMed]
45. Herr, I.; Buchler, M.W. Dietary constituents of broccoli and other cruciferous vegetables: Implications for prevention and therapy of cancer. *Cancer Treat. Rev.* **2010**, *36*, 377–383. [CrossRef]
46. Higdon, J.V.; Delage, B.; Williams, D.E.; Dashwood, R.H. Cruciferous vegetables and human cancer risk: Epidemiologic evidence and mechanistic basis. *Pharm. Res.* **2007**, *55*, 224–236. [CrossRef]
47. Durko, L.; Malecka-Panas, E. Lifestyle Modifications and Colorectal Cancer. *Curr. Colorectal Cancer Rep.* **2014**, *10*, 45–54. [CrossRef]

48. Sestili, P.; Fimognari, C. Cytotoxic and Antitumor Activity of Sulforaphane: The Role of Reactive Oxygen Species. *Biomed. Res. Int.* **2015**, *2015*, 1–9. [CrossRef]
49. Xiao, D.; Powolny, A.A.; Antosiewicz, J.; Hahm, E.R.; Bommareddy, A.; Zeng, Y.; Desai, D.; Amin, S.; Herman-Antosiewicz, A.; Singh, S.V. Cellular responses to cancer chemopreventive agent D,L-sulforaphane in human prostate cancer cells are initiated by mitochondrial reactive oxygen species. *Pharm. Res.* **2009**, *26*, 1729–1738. [CrossRef]
50. Prochaska, H.J.; Santamaria, A.B.; Talalay, P. Rapid detection of inducers of enzymes that protect against carcinogens. *Proc. Natl. Acad. Sci. USA* **1992**, *89*, 2394–2398. [CrossRef]
51. Riedl, M.A.; Saxon, A.; Diaz-Sanchez, D. Oral sulforaphane increases Phase II antioxidant enzymes in the human upper airway. *Clin. Immunol.* **2009**, *130*, 244–251. [CrossRef] [PubMed]
52. Fimognari, C.; Hrelia, P. Sulforaphane as a promising molecule for fighting cancer. *Mutat. Res.* **2007**, *635*, 90–104. [CrossRef] [PubMed]
53. Cho, S.D.; Li, G.; Hu, H.; Jiang, C.; Kang, K.S.; Lee, Y.S.; Kim, S.H.; Lu, J. Involvement of c-Jun N-terminal kinase in G2/M arrest and caspase-mediated apoptosis induced by sulforaphane in DU145 prostate cancer cells. *Nutr. Cancer* **2005**, *52*, 213–224. [CrossRef] [PubMed]
54. Choi, S.; Singh, S.V. Bax and Bak are required for apoptosis induction by sulforaphane, a cruciferous vegetable-derived cancer chemopreventive agent. *Cancer Res.* **2005**, *65*, 2035–2043. [CrossRef] [PubMed]
55. Pledgie-Tracy, A.; Sobolewski, M.D.; Davidson, N.E. Sulforaphane induces cell type-specific apoptosis in human breast cancer cell lines. *Mol. Cancer Ther.* **2007**, *6*, 1013–1021. [CrossRef] [PubMed]
56. Myzak, M.C.; Hardin, K.; Wang, R.; Dashwood, R.H.; Ho, E. Sulforaphane inhibits histone deacetylase activity in BPH-1, LnCaP and PC-3 prostate epithelial cells. *Carcinogenesis* **2006**, *27*, 811–819. [CrossRef]
57. Myzak, M.C.; Tong, P.; Dashwood, W.M.; Dashwood, R.H.; Ho, E. Sulforaphane retards the growth of human PC-3 xenografts and inhibits HDAC activity in human subjects. *Exp. Biol. Med.* **2007**, *232*, 227–234.
58. Wang, X.; Li, Y.; Dai, Y.; Liu, Q.; Ning, S.; Liu, J.; Shen, Z.; Zhu, D.; Jiang, F.; Zhang, J.; et al. Sulforaphane improves chemotherapy efficacy by targeting cancer stem cell-like properties via the miR-124/IL-6R/STAT3 axis. *Sci. Rep.* **2016**, *6*, 36796. [CrossRef]
59. Bose, C.; Awasthi, S.; Sharma, R.; Beneš, H.; Hauer-Jensen, M.; Boerma, M.; Singh, S.P. Sulforaphane potentiates anticancer effects of doxorubicin and attenuates its cardiotoxicity in a breast cancer model. *PLoS ONE* **2018**, *13*, e0193918. [CrossRef]
60. Fan, P.; Zhang, Y.; Liu, L.; Zhao, Z.; Yin, Y.; Xiao, X.; Bauer, N.; Gladkich, J.; Mattern, J.; Gao, C.; et al. Continuous exposure of pancreatic cancer cells to dietary bioactive agents does not induce drug resistance unlike chemotherapy. *Cell Death Dis.* **2016**, *7*, e2246. [CrossRef]
61. Bolger, A.M.; Lohse, M.; Usadel, B. Trimmomatic: A flexible trimmer for Illumina sequence data. *Bioinformatics* **2014**, *30*, 2114–2120. [CrossRef] [PubMed]
62. Trapnell, C.; Pachter, L.; Salzberg, S.L. TopHat: Discovering splice junctions with RNA-Seq. *Bioinformatics* **2009**, *25*, 1105–1111. [CrossRef] [PubMed]
63. Anders, S.; Pyl, P.T.; Huber, W. HTSeq—A Python framework to work with high-throughput sequencing data. *Bioinformatics* **2015**, *31*, 166–169. [CrossRef] [PubMed]
64. Gotz, S.; García-Gómez, J.M.; Terol, J.; Williams, T.D.; Nagaraj, S.H.; Nueda, M.J.; Robles, M.; Talón, M.; Dopazo, J.; Conesa, A. High-throughput functional annotation and data mining with the Blast2GO suite. *Nucleic Acids Res.* **2008**, *36*, 3420–3435. [CrossRef] [PubMed]
65. Robinson, M.D.; Oshlack, A. A scaling normalization method for differential expression analysis of RNA-seq data. *Genome Biol.* **2010**, *11*, R25. [CrossRef] [PubMed]
66. Benjamini, Y.; Hochberg, Y. Controlling The False Discovery Rate-A Practical And Powerful Approach To Multiple Testing. *J. R. Stat. Soc. Ser. B* **1995**, *57*, 289–300. [CrossRef]
67. Taverna, S.D.; Ueberheide, B.M.; Liu, Y.; Tackett, A.J.; Diaz, R.L.; Shabanowitz, J.; Chait, B.T.; Hunt, D.F.; Allis, C.D. Long-distance combinatorial linkage between methylation and acetylation on histone H3 N termini. *Proc. Natl. Acad. Sci. USA* **2007**, *104*, 2086–2091. [CrossRef]
68. El Kennani, S.; Crespo, M.; Govin, J.; Pflieger, D. Proteomic Analysis of Histone Variants and Their PTMs: Strategies and Pitfalls. *Proteomes* **2018**, *6*, 29. [CrossRef]
69. Chiang, T.; Koss, B.; Su, L.; Washam, C.; Byrum, S.; Storey, A.; Tackett, A. Effect of sulforaphane and 5-aza-2′-deoxycytidine on melanoma cell growth. *NCBI: Gene Expression Omnibus*, accession number GSE127252,

2019. Available online: https://www.ncbi.nlm.nih.gov/geo/query/acc.cgi?acc=GSE127252 (accessed on 26 June 2019).

70. Parnaud, G.; Li, P.; Cassar, G.; Rouimi, P.; Tulliez, J.; Combaret, L.; Gamet-Payrastre, L. Mechanism of sulforaphane-induced cell cycle arrest and apoptosis in human colon cancer cells. *Nutr. Cancer* **2004**, *48*, 198–206. [CrossRef]
71. Cheng, Y.M.; Tsai, C.C.; Hsu, Y.C. Sulforaphane, a Dietary Isothiocyanate, Induces G(2)/M Arrest in Cervical Cancer Cells through CyclinB1 Downregulation and GADD45beta/CDC2 Association. *Int. J. Mol. Sci.* **2016**, *17*, 1530. [CrossRef]
72. Alcazar, O.; Achberger, S.; Aldrich, W.; Hu, Z.; Negrotto, S.; Saunthararajah, Y.; Triozzi, P. Epigenetic regulation by decitabine of melanoma differentiation in vitro and in vivo. *Int. J. Cancer* **2012**, *131*, 18–29. [CrossRef] [PubMed]
73. Vijayaraghavalu, S.; Labhasetwar, V. Efficacy of decitabine-loaded nanogels in overcoming cancer drug resistance is mediated via sustained DNA methyltransferase 1 (DNMT1) depletion. *Cancer Lett.* **2013**, *331*, 122–129. [CrossRef] [PubMed]
74. Park, S.L.; Justiniano, R.; Williams, J.D.; Cabello, C.M.; Qiao, S.; Wondrak, G.T. The Tryptophan-Derived Endogenous Aryl Hydrocarbon Receptor Ligand 6-Formylindolo[3,2-b]Carbazole Is a Nanomolar UVA Photosensitizer in Epidermal Keratinocytes. *J. Investig. Derm.* **2015**, *135*, 1649–1658. [CrossRef] [PubMed]
75. Tran, T.T.; Schulman, J.; Fisher, D.E. UV and pigmentation: Molecular mechanisms and social controversies. *Pigment Cell Melanoma Res.* **2008**, *21*, 509–516. [CrossRef] [PubMed]
76. Reichrath, J.; Rass, K. Ultraviolet damage, DNA repair and vitamin D in nonmelanoma skin cancer and in malignant melanoma: An update. *Adv. Exp. Med. Biol.* **2014**, *810*, 208–233. [PubMed]
77. Loetscher, P.; Seitz, M.; Clark-Lewis, I.; Baggiolini, M.; Moser, B. Activation of NK cells by CC chemokines. Chemotaxis, Ca2+ mobilization, and enzyme release. *J. Immunol.* **1996**, *156*, 322–327. [PubMed]
78. Sconocchia, G.; Arriga, R.; Tornillo, L.; Terracciano, L.; Ferrone, S.; Spagnoli, G.C. Melanoma cells inhibit NK cell functions. *Cancer Res.* **2012**, *72*, 5428–5429. [CrossRef]
79. Mgrditchian, T.; Arakelian, T.; Paggetti, J.; Noman, M.Z.; Viry, E.; Moussay, E.; Van Moer, K.; Kreis, S.; Guerin, C.; Buart, S.; et al. Targeting autophagy inhibits melanoma growth by enhancing NK cells infiltration in a CCL5-dependent manner. *Proc. Natl. Acad. Sci. USA* **2017**, *114*, E9271–E9279. [CrossRef]
80. Norris, S.; Coleman, A.; Kuri-Cervantes, L.; Bower, M.; Nelson, M.; Goodier, M.R. PD-1 expression on natural killer cells and CD8(+) T cells during chronic HIV-1 infection. *Viral Immunol.* **2012**, *25*, 329–332. [CrossRef]
81. Stojanovic, A.; Fiegler, N.; Brunner-Weinzierl, M.; Cerwenka, A. CTLA-4 is expressed by activated mouse NK cells and inhibits NK Cell IFN gamma production in response to mature dendritic cells. *J. Immunol.* **2014**, *192*, 4184–4191. [CrossRef]
82. Noman, M.Z.; Berchem, G.; Janji, B. Targeting autophagy blocks melanoma growth by bringing natural killer cells to the tumor battlefield. *Autophagy* **2018**, *14*, 730–732. [CrossRef] [PubMed]
83. Noman, M.Z.; Paggetti, J.; Moussay, E.; Berchem, G.; Janji, B. Driving Natural Killer cells toward the melanoma tumor battlefield: Autophagy as a valuable therapeutic target. *Oncoimmunology* **2018**, *7*, e1452583. [CrossRef] [PubMed]
84. Bottcher, J.P.; Bonavita, E.; Chakravarty, P.; Blees, H.; Cabeza-Cabrerizo, M.; Sammicheli, S.; Rogers, N.C.; Sahai, E.; Zelenay, S.; Reis e Sousa, C. NK Cells Stimulate Recruitment of cDC1 into the Tumor Microenvironment Promoting Cancer Immune Control. *Cell* **2018**, *172*, 1022–1037. [CrossRef] [PubMed]
85. Benvenuto-Andrade, C.; Oseitutu, A.; Agero, A.L.; Marghoob, A.A. Cutaneous melanoma: Surveillance of patients for recurrence and new primary melanomas. *Derm. Ther.* **2005**, *18*, 423–435. [CrossRef] [PubMed]
86. Faries, M.B.; Steen, S.; Ye, X.; Sim, M.; Morton, D.L. Late recurrence in melanoma: Clinical implications of lost dormancy. *J. Am. Coll. Surg.* **2013**, *217*, 27–34. [CrossRef] [PubMed]

7

Targeting Histone Deacetylases with Natural and Synthetic Agents: An Emerging Anticancer Strategy

Amit Kumar Singh [1], Anupam Bishayee [2] and Abhay K. Pandey [1,*]

1 Department of Biochemistry, University of Allahabad, Allahabad 211 002, Uttar Pradesh, India; amitfbs21@gmail.com
2 Department of Pharmaceutical Sciences, College of Pharmacy, Larkin University, Miami, FL 33169, USA; abishayee@ULarkin.org or abishayee@gmail.com
* Correspondence: akpandey23@rediffmail.com;

Abstract: Cancer initiation and progression are the result of genetic and/or epigenetic alterations. Acetylation-mediated histone/non-histone protein modification plays an important role in the epigenetic regulation of gene expression. Histone modification is controlled by the balance between histone acetyltransferase and (HAT) and histone deacetylase (HDAC) enzymes. Imbalance between the activities of these two enzymes is associated with various forms of cancer. Histone deacetylase inhibitors (HDACi) regulate the activity of HDACs and are being used in cancer treatment either alone or in combination with other chemotherapeutic drugs/radiotherapy. The Food and Drug Administration (FDA) has already approved four compounds, namely vorinostat, romidepsin, belinostat, and panobinostat, as HDACi for the treatment of cancer. Several other HDACi of natural and synthetic origin are under clinical trial for the evaluation of efficiency and side-effects. Natural compounds of plant, fungus, and actinomycetes origin, such as phenolics, polyketides, tetrapeptide, terpenoids, alkaloids, and hydoxamic acid, have been reported to show potential HDAC-inhibitory activity. Several HDACi of natural and dietary origin are butein, protocatechuic aldehyde, kaempferol (grapes, green tea, tomatoes, potatoes, and onions), resveratrol (grapes, red wine, blueberries and peanuts), sinapinic acid (wine and vinegar), diallyl disulfide (garlic), and zerumbone (ginger). HDACi exhibit their antitumor effect by the activation of cell cycle arrest, induction of apoptosis and autophagy, angiogenesis inhibition, increased reactive oxygen species generation causing oxidative stress, and mitotic cell death in cancer cells. This review summarizes the HDACs classification, their aberrant expression in cancerous tissue, structures, sources, and the anticancer mechanisms of HDACi, as well as HDACi that are either FDA-approved or under clinical trials.

Keywords: cancer; histone deacetylases; histone deacetylase inhibitors; vorinostat; natural HDACi; apoptosis

---

1. Introduction

Cancer is the second leading cause of death worldwide and caused 8.8 million deaths in 2015. Globally, 1 out of 6 deaths is because of cancer. Low and middle-income countries are the hotspot of cancer deaths, accounting for approximately 70% of deaths. Lung cancer is the most common cause of cancer death worldwide. According to the National Center for Health Statistics about 1.73 million new cancer cases and 0.6 million cancer deaths are projected to occur in the United States in 2018 [1]. Cancer results from altered cell physiology leading to self-sufficient growth potential, loss of cell cycle control, extended angiogenesis, delay in replicative senescence, dysregulated apoptosis, invasion, and metastasis [2,3]. Progression of the disease is not only governed by genomic and genetic changes, such as translocation, amplification, deletion and point mutation, it also involves epigenetic changes; i.e., alteration in the pattern of gene expression without changing underlying DNA sequence.

Methylation of DNA, histone protein modifications and non-coding RNA-mediated gene silencing are the major epigenetic changes, reversible in nature [4].

Chromatin is a compact and highly ordered structure comprised of DNA and histone protein. Nucleosome, the basic unit of chromatin, is made up of 147 bp of DNA superhelix wrapped around histone core protein containing two copies each of H2A, H2B, H3 and H4. H1 is the linker histone. The core plays an important role in establishing interactions between the nucleosomes and within the nucleosome particle itself. N-terminals (histone tails) of core histones are flexible and unstructured while the rest of histone proteins are basically globular and highly ordered. Depending on the epigenetic changes in histone tail, chromatin undergoes various conformational changes responsible for upregulation or downregulation of respective genes [5,6]. The common posttranslational modifications occurring in histones are acetylation, methylation, phosphorylation, sumoylation, ubiquitinylation, and ADP ribosylation.

Acetylation of a lysine residue of histone was discovered by Vincent Allfrey and colleagues in 1964 and based on the finding it has been proposed that acetylation of ε-amino group of lysine residues could play a role in gene expression [7,8]. Acetylation and deacetylation of N-terminal ε-amino group of lysine residues are regulated by two enzymes, namely histone acetyltransferase (HAT) and histone deacetylase (HDAC) (Figure 1). Acetylation neutralizes the positive charge and decreases the affinity between the histone and DNA helix responsible for relaxation of conformation and greater accessibility to transcription machinery [4,9]. Therefore, acetylation is generally associated with gene activation, however, deacetylation catalyzed by HDAC induces chromatin condensation and downregulation of gene expression. N-terminal acetylation of lysine residue also occurs in non-histone proteins, such as cytoplasmic proteins, transcription factors responsible for alteration in gene expression and other cellular processes [10].

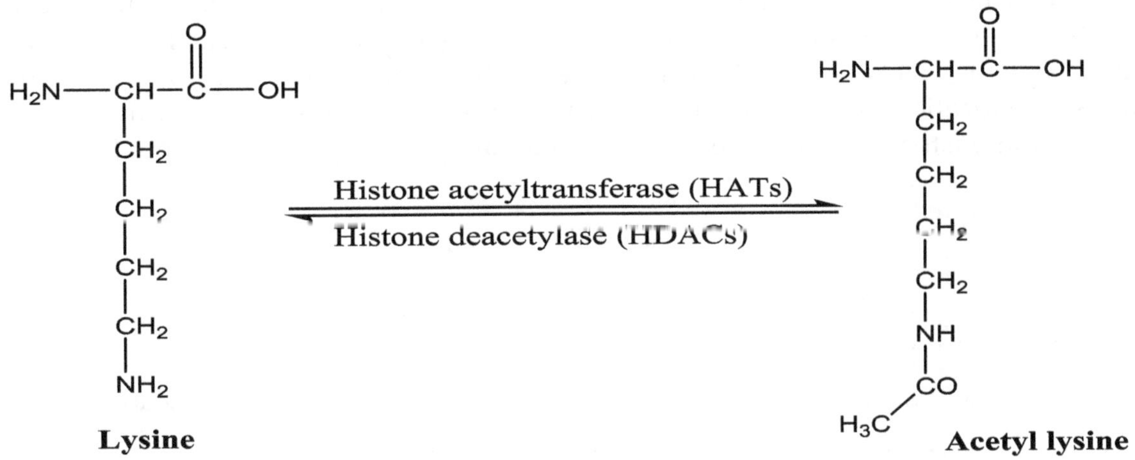

Figure 1. Histone acetylation at the N-terminus lysine by histone acetyltransferases (HATs) and deacetylation by histone deacetylases (HDACs).

Imbalance in the activities of enzymes HATs and HDACs is responsible for the development and progression of wide variety of cancers [2]. Histone deacetylase inhibitors (HDACi) increase the level of acetylated lysine residues of core histone which in turn restarts the expression of silenced regulatory genes in the cancerous cell and therefore, HDACi are now emerging as anticancer agents [11].

Epidemiological studies have suggested that vegetables, fruits, whole grains, microorganism-derived bioactive components, and fatty acids provide protection against some forms of cancer and other diseases without detectable side effects [12–14]. Many dietary compounds that have been identified as having HDAC-inhibitory activities implicated in therapeutic potential in the context of a whole food [11,15]. In the present review an effort has been made to highlight the role of HDACs in the tumor initiation and progression and their inhibitors from natural (dietary and non-dietary) as well as synthetic sources in the management of cancer either alone or in combination with other chemotherapeutic drugs/radiotherapy.

2. Classification of HDACs

In humans, 18 HDACs have been identified so far and are divided into two families and four classes based on their sequence homology to *Saccharomyces cerevisiae* HDACs (Figure 2) [16]. One of the family group members are zinc-dependent, they require Zn^{++} as a cofactor for their deacetylase activity and include HDAC 1 to HDAC 11. HDACs 1, 2, 3 and 8 are grouped into class 1 having a sequence similarity with yeast reduced potassium dependency-3 (Rpd3) and class II HDACs are subdivided into class IIA and Class IIB that include HDACs 4, 5, 6, 7, 9 and 10 which are reported to have sequence homology with yeast histone deacetylase-1 (hda-1) while HDAC 11 of class IV share sequence similarity with both classes of yeast deacetylase Rpd3 and hda-1.

Another group of the family requires nicotinamide adenine dinucleotide (NAD) as a cofactor for deacetylase activity classified as class III, has sequence similarity to yeast deacetylase silent information regulator-2 (Sir2) and includes seven members from sirtuins (SIRTs) 1 to 7. Sirtuins are known to regulate several cellular processes; e.g., survival, aging, stress response, and various metabolic processes. The members of class I and IV are located in the nucleus while class IIA is mainly located into the cytoplasm and class IIB is found shuttling between the nucleus and cytoplasm. Cellular localization of class III HDACs are nucleus, cytoplasm, and mitochondria [11,17]. Nomenclature of class I, II and IV HDACs are based on their chronological order of discovery; for example, both HDAC 1 and 2 were discovered in 1996 while HDAC 2 was discovered a few months after HDAC 1 [18,19]. Later on, HDAC 3 was discovered in the subsequent years [20]. While HDACs 4, 5, and 6 were first reported in 1999, the HDAC 7 was discovered in early 2000 and so on [21,22]. Table 1 summarizes the HDACs classification, number of amino acids, cellular and chromosomal locations, biological functions, relevant histone/non-histone target proteins, and their expression pattern [6,23,24].

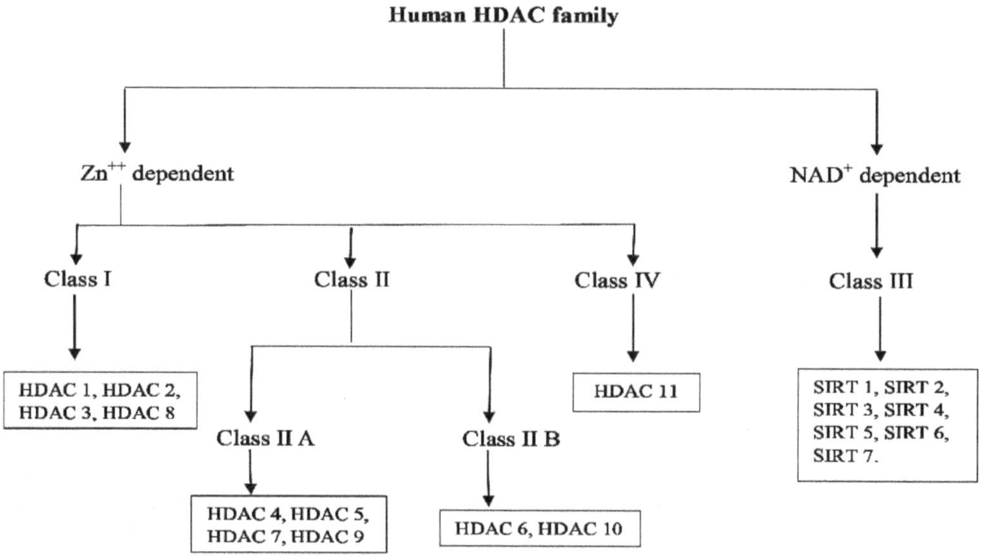

Figure 2. Classification of HDAC family.

Table 1. Histone deacetylase (HDAC) enzymes classification, number of amino acids, localization, function, protein targets and expression pattern.

Class	HDACs	Number of Amino Acid	Cellular Location	Chromosomal Location	Biological Function	Histone/Non-Histone Protein Target	Pattern of Expression of Gene
I	HDAC 1	483	Nucleus	1p35.2-p35.1	Proliferation and survival of cells	Histones, pRb, SHP, BRCA1, MECP2, ATM, MEF2, MyoD, p53, NF-κB, AR, DNMT1	Ubiquitous expression
	HDAC 2	488		6q21	Proliferation of cell and insulin resistance	Histones, BRCA1, NF-κB, MECP, GATA 2, pRb	
	HDAC 3	428		5q31.3	Proliferation and survival of cells	Histones, HDAC (4, 5, 7, 9), GATA 1, NF-κB, pRb	
	HDAC 8	377		Xq13.1	Proliferation of cell	HSP70	
IIA	HDAC 4	1084	Nucleus/Cytoplasm	2q37.3	Regulation of cytoskeleton dynamics and cell mobility	Histones, HDAC 3, 14-3-3, CaM, MEF 2	Tissue restricted expression
	HDAC 5	1122		17q21.31	Helps in endothelial cell function, gluconeogenesis, cardiac myocyte growth and function		
	HDAC 7	912		12q13.11	Helps in endothelial cell function and glyconeogenesis.		
	HDAC 9	1069		7p21.1	Helps in thymocyte differentiation, homologous recombination, cardiac cell function		
IIB	HDAC 6	1215	Cytoplasm	Xp11.23	Regulation of cytoskeleton dynamics and cell mobility	HDAC 11, SHP, HSP 90, α tubulin	Tissue restricted expression
	HDAC 10	669		2q13-33	Regulation of autophagy, homologous recombination.	LcoR, PP1	
III	SIRT 1	747	Nucleus/Cytoplasm	10q21.3	Autoimmunity, aging, redox balance, and cell survival	Histones, NF-κB, p53, p300	Variable expression
	SIRT 2	389	Nucleus	19q13.2	Survival, migration, and invasion of cell	Histone H4, PPAR-Υ, p53, p300, α-tubulin, FOXO	

Table 1. *Cont.*

Class	HDACs	Number of Amino Acid	Cellular Location	Chromosomal Location	Biological Function	Histone/Non-Histone Protein Target	Pattern of Expression of Gene
	SIRT 3	399	Mitochondria	11p15.5	Regulate ATP production and metabolism, cell signaling, apoptosis, urea cycle	Complex I of ETC, PGC-1α, p53, Ku70, Acetyl-CoA Synthetase, FOXO	
	SIRT 4	314		12q24.31	Energy metabolism, Urea cycle, cell signaling	Glutamate dehydrogenase	
	SIRT 5	310		6p23	Regulate ATP production and metabolism, cell signaling, apoptosis, urea cycle	Carbamoyl phosphate synthetase I, Cytochrome c	
	SIRT 6	355	Nucleus	19p13.3	Regulate metabolism	Histone H3, TNF-α	
	SIRT 7	400		17q25.3	Apoptosis	p53, RNA polymerase I	
IV	HDAC 11	347	Nucleus	3p25.1	DNA replication, Immunomodulation	HDAC 6	Ubiquitous in nature

AR, androgen receptor; ATM, ataxia-telangiectasia-mutated; BRCA, breast cancer; CaM, calmodulin; CoA, co-enzyme A; DNMT, DNA methyltransferase; FOXO, forkhead box O; GATA, GATA binding protein; HIF, hypoxia-inducible factor; HSP, heat shock protein; LcoR, ligand-dependent receptor co-repressor; MECP, methyl-CpG-binding domain protein; MEF, myocyte enhancer factor; NF-κB, nuclear factor-kappa B; PGC, peroxisome proliferator-activated receptor gamma coactivator; PP1, protein phosphatase; PPAR, peroxisome proliferator-activated receptor; pRb, retinoblastoma protein; SHP, Src homology region 2-domain-containing phosphatase; SIRT, sirtuin; TNF, tumor necrosis factor.

3. Cellular Targets of Histone/Non-Histone Protein Acetylation

The acetylation or deacetylation status of histone proteins and transcription factors modulate the gene expression pattern. Hyperacetylation of lysine residues of histone proteins promotes the relaxed state of chromatin and activates gene expression [25]. Besides this, acetylation of transcription factors affects their cellular localization. For example, signal transducer and activator of transcription 1 (STAT 1) and nuclear factor-κB (NF-κB) are internalized into the nucleus from cytosol after the acetylation of specific lysine residues where they activate transcription of respective genes. The activity of other transcription factors, such as p53 and FOXO, is also positively regulated by the acetylation process. Acetylation process also affects the stability of proteins, i.e., acetylation of p53, p73, and mothers against decapentaplegic homolog 7 (SMAD 7) prevents their ubiquitinylation and degradation. Interestingly, cell mobility is also affected by the acetylation pattern of α-tubulin and cortactin. It has been reported that HDAC 6 and SIRT2 cause deacetylation of α-tubulin, which promotes microtubule depolymerization and therefore increases microtubule dynamics and cell mobility. Acetylation also affects the activity of retinoblastoma protein (pRB) by blocking its cyclin E-cdk2 dependent phosphorylation so acetylation-dependent hypophosphorylation causes cell cycle arrest [26,27].

4. HDAC Mutations in Cancer

Mutations of HDACs have also been observed. HDAC2 mutation in human epithelial cancer resulted in microsatellite instability. Interestingly, a truncating mutation of HDAC2 in human cancers confers resistance to HDACi. These findings suggest that the HDAC2 mutational status of patients should be assessed before therapies using HDACi [28]. HDAC3 are associated with DNA damage control response. Inactivation of HDAC3 causes genomic instability. HDAC4 acts s transcriptional repressor and its mutations have been identified at significant frequency in breast and colorectal cancers. SIRT 2 acts as a tumor suppressor and mutation in its catalytic domain eliminates its enzymatic activity, which compromises the mitotic checkpoint, contributing to genomic instability and tumorigenesis. HDAC9 and 10 are reported to be involved in homologous recombination, and depletion in HDAC 9 and 10 resulted in inhibition of homologous recombination [11].

5. HDACs and Cancer: Expression Pattern and Function

Altered acetylation level and mutation/or aberrant expression of various HDACs have been observed frequently in numerous human diseases including cancer, hence making them an important drug target [2]. Fraga et al. (2005) reported that change in genome-wide patterns of acetylation may lead to the initiation and progression of cancer by demonstrating that cancer cells undergo a loss of acetylation at lysine 16 of H4 [29]. HDACs have various histone and non-histone protein targets that not only regulate the chromatin activity, but also control apoptosis, cell cycle progression and differentiation. Association of HDACs with regulatory processes reflects their involvement in cancer phenotypes [30].

5.1. Class I HDACs

5.1.1. HDAC 1

HDAC 1 overexpression has been reported in Hodgkin's lymphoma (HL), gastric, ovarian, and prostate cancers [11,23]. Choi and co-workers (2001) have shown the overexpression of HDAC 1 in 60% cases compared with normal tissue [31]. This study was further validated by a recent study including 293 gastric cancer samples showing upregulation in expression of HDACs 1, 2, and 3 [32,33]. Elevated level of expression of HDAC 1, 2, and 3 was reported in pancreatic cancer involving 192 samples and this overexpression was responsible for dedifferentiation and enhanced proliferation of pancreatic cancer cell [34]. Overexpression of HDAC 1, 2, and 3 is associated with mortality rate in colorectal cancer. Expression of HDAC 2 has emerged as an independent prognostic marker in colorectal cancer [35]. Furthermore, overexpression of HDAC 1 is reported in hepatocellular carcinoma [36], lung cancer [37] and breast cancer [38]. Direct correlation between HDAC 1, 3 expression and estrogen and progesterone receptor expression have been reported by Krusche et al. [39].

HDAC 1 induces cell proliferation and inhibition of differentiation and apoptosis [23,38]. HDAC 1 and 3 knockdowns (KD) resulted in the inhibition of cell proliferation in Hela cells [40]. HDAC 1 KD has been shown to result in cell cycle arrest either at the G1 phase or at the G2/M transition phase, causing loss of mitotic cells, inhibition of cell growth, and an increase in the number of apoptotic cells in osteosarcoma and breast cancer cells. However, HDAC 2 KD showed no such effects in these cells [41]. HDAC1 might also be involved in multidrug resistance as they showed overexpression in a pattern in chemotherapeutically resistant neuroblastoma cells [42].

5.1.2. HDAC 2

Overexpression of HDAC2 reported in uterine, cervical, gastric, cutaneous T cell lymphoma (CTCL), HL, prostate and colorectal cancers [38]. Elevated expression of HDAC 2 along with HDAC 1 and 3 are associated with advance stage of disease and prognosis of gastric, colorectal, and prostate cancers [33–35].

Knockdown of HDAC2 in cervical cancer causes increased apoptosis and the differentiated phenotype of cells associated with increased $p21^{Cip1/WAF1}$ expression that was independent of p53 [43]. In breast carcinoma cells, HDAC 2 KD results into the increased DNA binding activity of tumor suppressor protein p53, which causes the inhibition of cell proliferation and induction of cellular senescence [44]. HDAC 2 KD also causes decreased viability, growth arrest, and increased apoptosis in colorectal and breast cancer cells [45].

5.1.3. HDAC 3

HDAC 3 overexpression has been reported in HL, ovarian and lung cancers, colon cancer, and chronic lymphocyte leukemia (CLL) [11,38,46]. An upregulated expression of HDAC1 along with HDAC3 was paradoxically related to disease-free survival in invasive breast cancer patients [24]. HDAC3 elevated expression together with HDAC 1 and 2 significantly causes poor prognosis in gastric, colon, and prostate cancers [33–35]. Decreased expression of HDAC 3 has been observed in liver cancer [45].

HDAC 3 KD in acute promyelocytic leukemia (APL) cells causes restoration of expression of a retinoic acid-dependent gene whose transcription repression was caused by promyelocytic leukemia retinoic acid receptor alpha (PML-RARα) [47]. While HDAC3 KD in colon cancer causes a decrease in the viability of cell by increasing the rate of apoptosis [45].

5.1.4. HDAC 8

Expression of HDAC 8 has been reported to increase in childhood neuroblastoma. HDAC KD shows reduction in proliferation of lung, colon, and cervical cancer. In childhood neuroblastoma cell HDAC 8 KD causes cell cycle arrest, reduction in cell proliferation [48,49]. HDAC 8 has also been reported in controlling telomerase activity [50].

5.2. Class IIA HDACs

5.2.1. HDAC4

A breast cancer sample showed overexpressed genotype of HDAC 4 [51]. However, lung and colon cancer analysis showed downregulated expression of HDAC 4 [11].

In APL, HDAC 4 was found to repress the expression of differentiation-associated genes by interacting with a leukemic fusion protein, PLZF-RARa [52]. HDAC 4 also regulates the activity of hypoxia inducing factor-1α (HIF-1α). HDAC4 has also been shown to help prostate cancer cells overcome hypoxic conditions by stabilizing HIF-1α. The binding of HDAC4 to HIF-1α generates a complex that regulates glycolysis and the cytotoxic stress of cell adaptation to hypoxic conditions [53]. HDAC4 KD in colon and glioblastoma cells causes an increased apoptosis rate and reduced growth rate [54].

5.2.2. HDAC 5

HDAC 5 overexpression has been reported in medulloblastoma [55] and colon cancer [51] while interestingly, the lung cancer sample showed a downregulated genotypic expression of HDAC5 [11]. HDAC 5 traverses from the nucleus to the cytosol upon interacting with transcription factor GATA-1 during differentiation of mouse erythroleukemia cells [56]. Knock down of HDAC 5 has been shown to cause reduced growth and viability of medulloblastoma cells [55].

5.2.3. HDAC 7

They are highly expressed in ALP, CLL, and colon cancer [46,51] and downregulated expression is reported in lung cancer samples [45,57]. HDAC 7 silencing in endothelial cells altered their morphology, their migration, and their capacity to form capillary tube-like structures in vitro but did not affect cell adhesion, proliferation, or apoptosis, suggesting that HDAC7 may represent a rational target for anti-angiogenesis in cancer [58].

5.2.4. HDAC 9

Elevated expression of HDAC 9 was reported in ALL and medulloblastoma [59,60] and in cervical cancer [31]. Silencing HDAC 9 results into inhibition of homologous recombination, sensitivity towards DNA damage and decreased viability and growth of medulloblastoma [45].

5.3. Class IIB HDACs

5.3.1. HDAC 6

A significantly higher expression of HDAC 6 was reported in oral squamous cell carcinoma, hepatocellular carcinoma, acute myeloid leukemia, CLL, breast cancer, CTCL and ovarian cancer, whereas its expression increased in the advanced stages of cancer compared to the early stages of cancer [5,61].

HDAC 6 overexpression causes increased migration of the fibroblast cell while the inhibition of HDAC 6 results in decreased fibroblast cell migration [62]. HDAC 6 targeted inhibition causes HSP 90 protein acetylation and disruption of its chaperone activity resulting in decreased viability of K562 leukemic cell [63]. HDAC4/6 has the potential to help prostate cancer cells overcome hypoxic conditions by stabilizing HIF-1 α [53]. HDAC 6 is also involved in metastasis, epithelial to mesenchymal transition in lung cancer cells by compromising TGF-β SMAD 3 pathway [64].

5.3.2. HDAC 10

Osada and colleague [57] described the potential role of HDAC 10 in cancer initiation and progression and reported the downregulated expression of HDAC 10 in non-small lung carcinoma cells and this is related with poor prognosis in lung cancer patients. Its role in gastric cancer and CLL is also reported [65].

HDAC 10 are shown to regulate the production of reactive oxygen species in gastric cancer cells [66]. HDAC 10 KD causes reduced vascular endothelial growth factor of receptor 1 and 2 (VEGF 1 and 2) and increased sensitivity towards DNA damage in cancer cells [67].

5.4. Class III HDACs

Sirtuins

Growing evidence supports the relation between cancer and sirtuins. As other HDACs they are also both tumor suppressors as well as pro-oncogenic in nature. SIRT 1 expression was shown to be upregulated in acute myeloid leukemia (AML), non-melanoma skin cancer and prostate cancer [68–70] while downregulated in colorectal cancer [51]. SIRT 2 expression decreased in glioma and gastric cancer [71]. However, a mutation in the catalytic domain of SIRT 2 has also been reported [72]. Expression pattern of SIRT 3 has been found to increase or decrease in different kinds of breast cancer tissues [73]. SIRT 6 expression was reported to decrease in liver cancer while increased expression pattern in CLL [46]. SIRT 7 shows an upregulated expression pattern in breast cancer [73].

SIRT 2 functions as a tumor suppressor protein and the mutation in its catalytic domain results in compromised cell cycle checkpoints leading to genomic instability and tumorigenesis [74]. In many cancerous cells, increased expression of SIRT 1 induces the p-glycoprotein expression responsible for chemotherapeutically resistant cancer cells whereas siRNA-mediated SIRT 1 KD causes a reversal of drug-resistant phenotype [75]. SIRT 3 functions both as a tumor suppressor and a tumor promoter protein. Higher expression of SIRT 3 was responsible for preventing bladder cancer cells from p53-mediated cell growth arrest [76]. SIRT 7 was shown to stabilize cancer cell phenotypes. SIRT 7 KD results in the tumorigenic potential of human cancer xenograft in mice [77].

5.5. Class IV HDACs

HDAC 11

The involvement of HDAC 11 in cancer is not well understood. However aberrant expression of HDAC 11 were reported in HL and Philadelphia-negative chronic myeloproliferative neoplasms (CMPN) [78].

siRNA-mediated HDAC 11, KD results in an increased apoptosis rate in HL, colon, prostate, breast, and ovarian cell lines [45,79]. Selective inhibition of HDAC 11 with histone deacetylase inhibitor (HDACi) reduces the chance of splenomegaly and other metabolic disorders reported in CMPN affected people [78].

6. Histone Deacetylase Inhibitors as an Anticancer Agent

The aberrant or altered expression of HDACs or their functions is frequently observed in a variety of cancer types and is the reason for targeting HDACs in cancer therapy. The availability of HDACi not only has accelerated our understanding of HDAC functions and its mechanism of actions but also presented a promising new class of compounds for cancer treatment. HDACi belong to a large and diverse family of both natural and synthetic compounds and can be categorized into four groups; i.e., hydroximic acid, benzamides, cyclic peptides, and aliphatic fatty acids [80]. Several natural or synthetic compounds are isolated and characterized for their potential as histone deacetylase inhibitors. The first significant compound identified as HDACi was *n*-butyrate, responsible for the accumulation of hyperacetylated histone inside the nucleus [81]. Subsequently, trichostatin A (TSA) and trapoxin A were found to be reversible and irreversible inhibitors of HDACs, respectively [11,82]. Schreiber et al. (1996) were first to discover and clone the human HDAC by using trapoxin A [80]. While developing these compounds as anticancer agents, parameters like their specificity, efficiency, pharmacokinetic and toxicological properties were analyzed [83]. Some HDACi, such as TSA, lycorine and zerumbone, are pan-HDAC inhibitors since they act on all isoform of zinc-dependent HDAC classes, while others are class specific.

HDCAs can reversibly modify the acetylation pattern of histone/non-histone protein resulted in abnormal gene expression without changing the DNA sequence. HDACi can overcome this problem and can resume the expression of tumor the suppressor genes responsible for apoptosis, cell cycle arrest, and the inhibition of angiogenesis and metastasis. Ungerstedt and co-workers [84] reported that cancerous cells are more sensitive than normal cells towards HDACi-induced apoptosis.

6.1. Natural HDACi

Altogether natural compounds provide pleiotropic and potent inhibitors of all hallmarks of cancer. Many of the HDACi discovered to date are of natural origin; for example in 1976, Tsuji et al. [85] isolated a naturally occurring HDACi, TSA from *Streptomyces hygroscopicus*. FK322, a cyclic peptide isolated from *Chromobacterium violaceum* selectively inhibits the activity of HDAC 1 and 2. TSA causes differentiation of cell and arrests the cell cycle of both normal and cancerous cells, resulting in the accumulation of acetylated histones [86]. Depudecin and trapoxin A and B are also the examples of naturally occurring HDACi extracted from a fungus. Marine organisms are also the source of natural HDACi, such as largazole and azumamides, and they are reported to be active even at nanomolar concentrations [11]. Other well-characterized naturally occurring HDACi, such as butein, kaempferol, protocatechuic aldehyde, sinapinic acid, resveratrol and zerumbone, are isolated from plant, fruits or vegetables (Table 2). Molecular modelling studies revealed the HDACi like activity of other dietary compounds; i.e., vitamin E, α-lipoic acid, and biotin [48]. For the first time, the clinical validation of natural HDACi was done by Riggs and colleague [81] in 1977. They analyzed the effect of butyrate on histone modificationin HeLa and Friend erythroleukemia cell lines [80]. Later in 1980, McKnight et al. [87] reported the effect of propionate on histone deacetylation in chick oviduct and showed it to have lesser activity than butyrate. Both these compounds were active at millimolar concentrations and synthesized by colonic bacteria. Valproic acid, a longer chain aliphatic fatty acid, also reported to have significant HDACi activity. Valproic acid inhibits HDACs activity by binding to its active site [87]. Detailed features of other natural histone deacetylase inhibitors and their sources are shown in Table 2.

Table 2. Examples of the natural compound with histone deacetylase inhibitory activity.

S.N	Class of Compounds	Name of the Compound	HDAC Target	Source (Species/Family)	Structure	Reference
1.	Phenolics	Aceroside VIII	HDAC6	*Betula platyphylla*	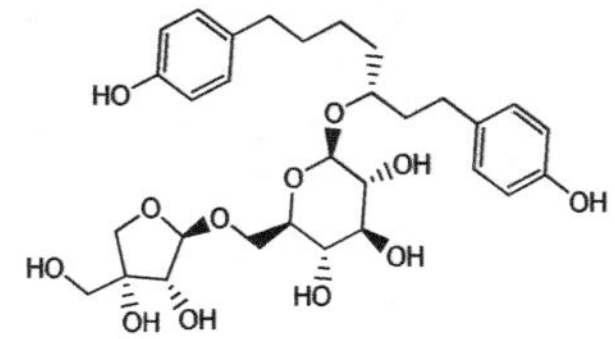	[87]
		Homobutein	Class I, II and IV	*Butea frondosa*	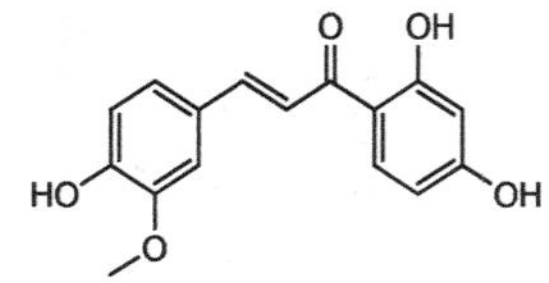	[88]
		Isoliquiritigenin	Class I, II and IV	*Glycyrhiza glabra*	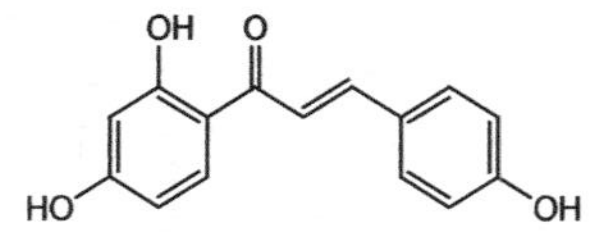	[89]
		Butein	Class I, II and IV	*Toxicodendron vernicifluum*	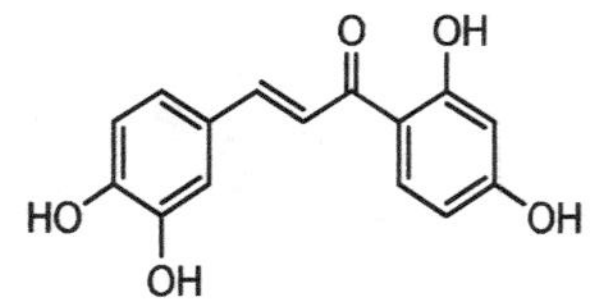	[88]
		Kaempferol	Class I, II and IV	*Aloe vera*	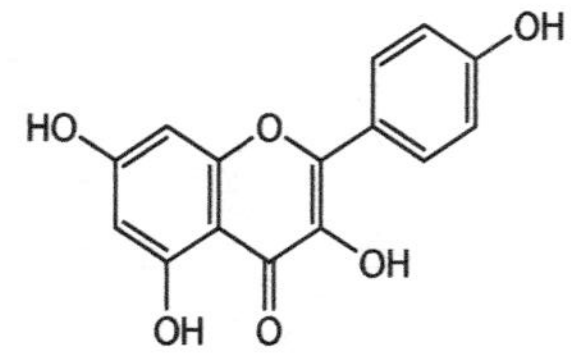	[89]
		Marein	Class I, II and IV	*Coreopsis maritima*	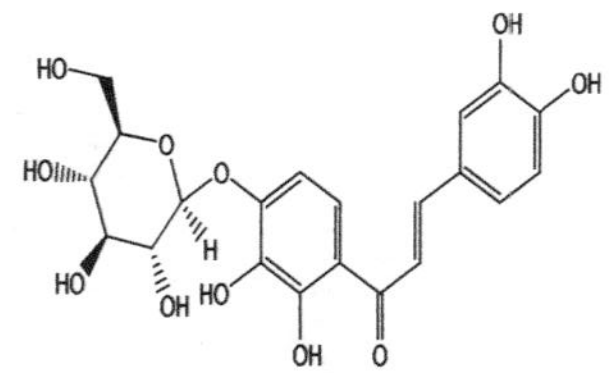	[88]
		Protocatechuic aldehyde	HDAC2	*Hordeum vulgare*	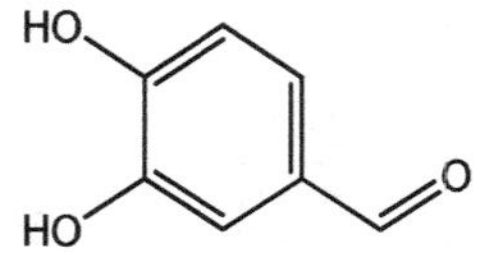	[23]

Table 2. *Cont.*

S.N	Class of Compounds	Name of the Compound	HDAC Target	Source (Species/Family)	Structure	Reference
		Psammaplin A	Class I	*Poecillastra* spp. and *Jaspis* spp.	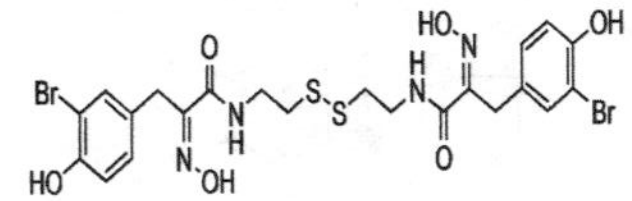	[23]
		Sinapinic acid	Pan-HDAC	*Hydnophytum formicarum Jack*	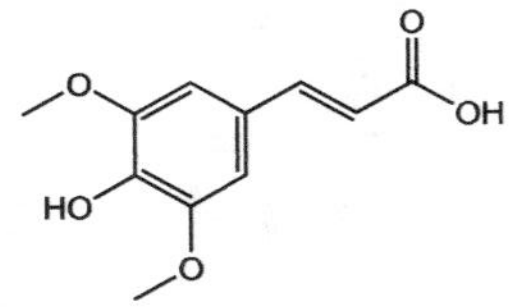	[90]
		Resveratrol	Class I, II and IV	*Vitis vinifera*	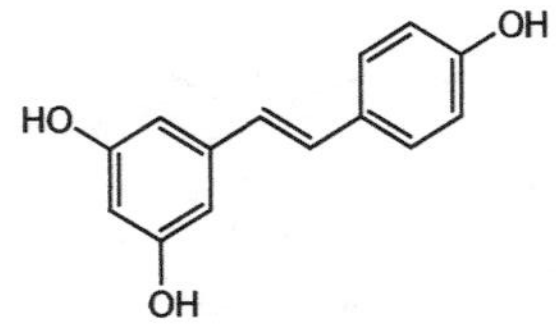	[91]
2.	Polyketides	Depudecin	HDAC 1	*Alternaria brassicicola*	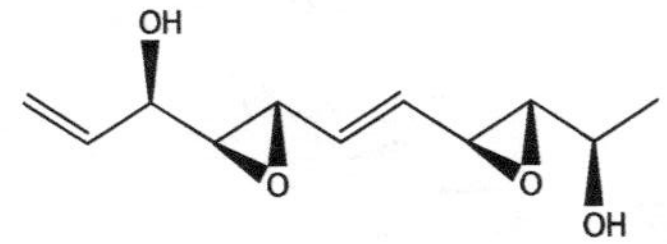	[92]
3.	Tetrapeptide	Apicidin	Class I HDAC	*Fusarium* spp.	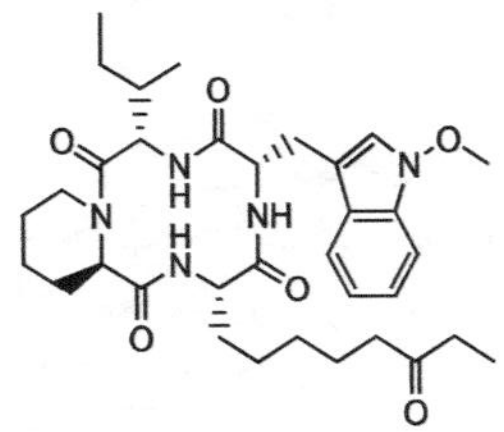	[93]
		Azumamide E	Class I	*Mycale izuensis*	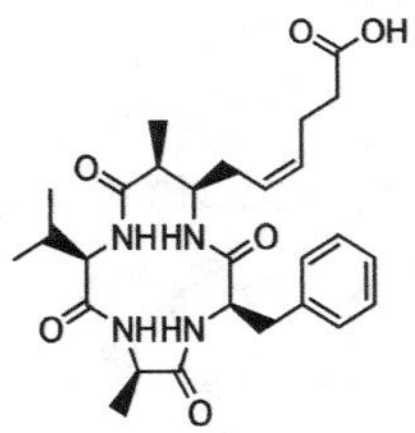	[94]

Table 2. *Cont.*

S.N	Class of Compounds	Name of the Compound	HDAC Target	Source (Species/Family)	Structure	Reference
		Chlamydocin	HDAC 1, 6	*Diheterospora chlamydosporia*	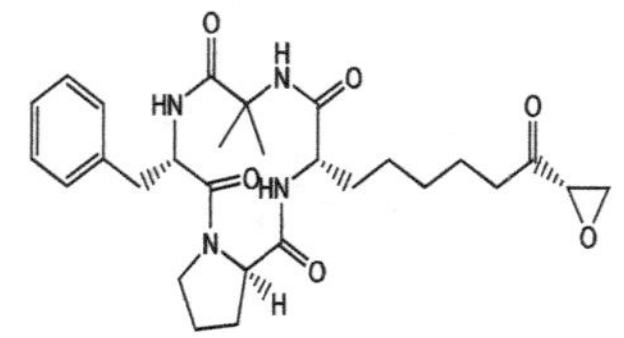	[95]
		Trapoxin A	Class I	*Helicoma ambiens* RF-1023	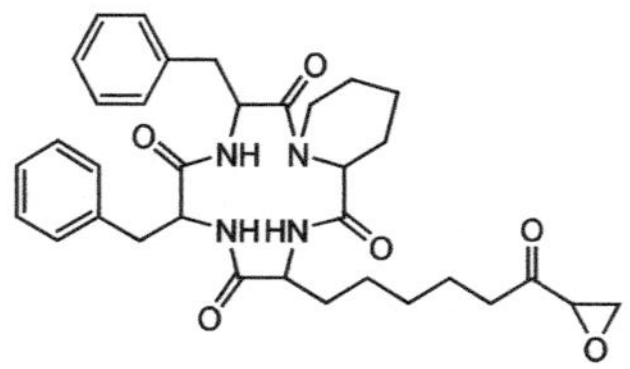	[96]
4.	Terpenoids	Zerumbone	Pan HDAC	*Zingiber zerumbet*	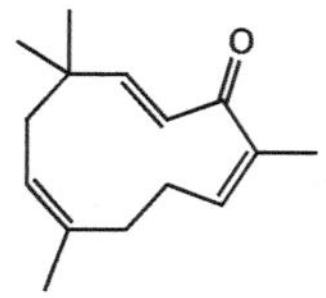	[23]
		β-Thujaplicin	HDAC 2	*Cupressaceae* spp.	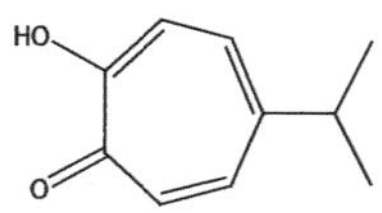	[23]
		6-methoxy-2*E*,9*E*-humuladien-8-one	Pan HDAC	*Zingiber zerumbet*	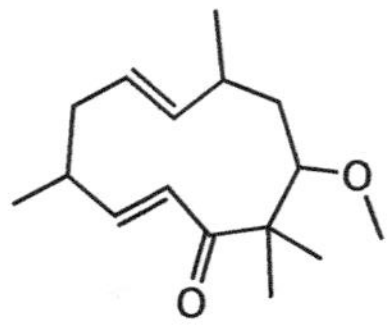	[23]
5.	Alkaloid	Lycorine	Pan HDAC	*Amaryllidaceae*	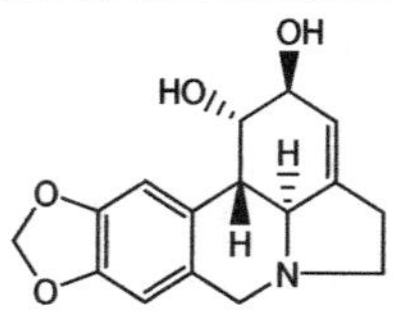	[97]
6.	Fatty acid	9-Hydroxystearic acid	Class I	Lipid peroxidation product	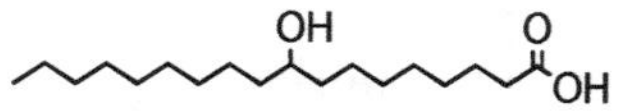	[98]

Table 2. *Cont.*

S.N	Class of Compounds	Name of the Compound	HDAC Target	Source (Species/Family)	Structure	Reference
7.	Organosulphur compounds	Diallyl disulfide	Acetylation Level increased	*Allium sativum*	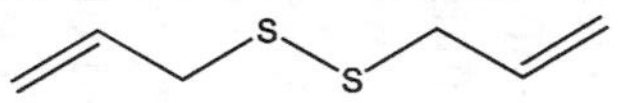	[99,100]
		(*S*)-allylmercaptocysteine		*Allium sativum*	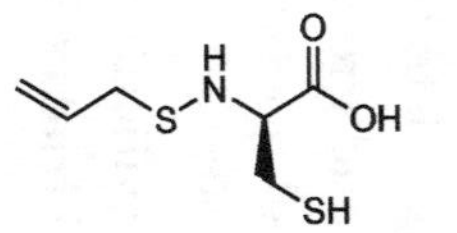	[101]
8.	Hydroxamic acid	Trichostatin A	Class I and II	*Streptomyces hygroscopicus*	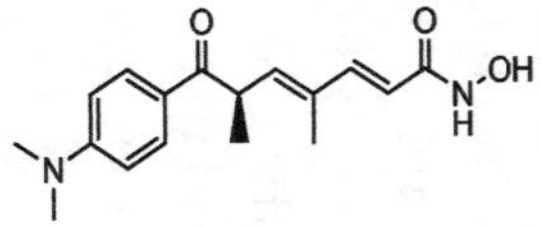	[2,11]
9.	Desipeptides	FK228	HDAC 1, 2	*Chromobacterium violaceum*	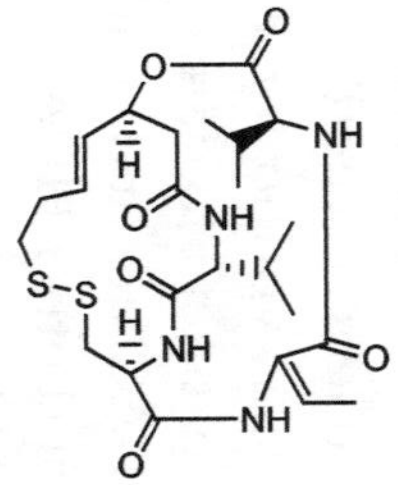	[11]
		Largazole	Class I	*Symploca* spp.	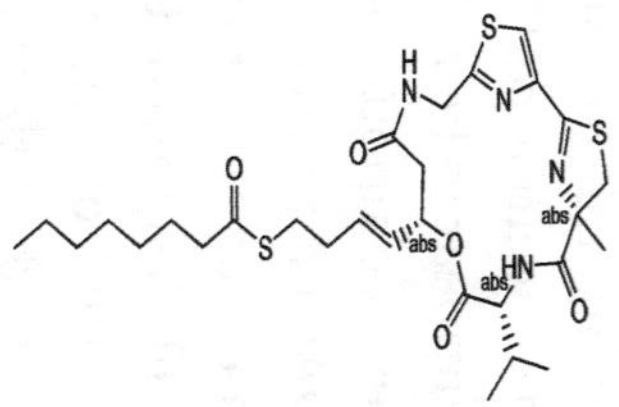	[99]

6.2. FDA-Approved and Under Clinical Trial HDACi

Aberrant expression of HDACs gene is reported in various cancer types. So, the scientists across the globe are searching for a therapeutic alternative, which not only can inhibit the increased activity of HDACs, but also reverse the malignant phenotype. The histone deacetylase inhibitors chiefly cause the gene to be in a hyperacetylated state, which in turn restarts the gene expression, and are also involved in chromatin stability, mitosis, and the DNA repair mechanism [23]. However, it has been reported that both normal and cancerous cells show accumulation of acetylated histone after treatment with HDACi, but healthy cells appear to be much less susceptible to apoptosis and growth inhibition than a cancerous cell. Four synthetic compounds, viz., vorinostat, romidepsin, belinostat, and panobinostat have been approved as HDACi for cancer treatment to date by the United States Food and Drug Administration (FDA). In addition, many other HDACi are under clinical trials in patients suffering from various types of cancer [101,102]. FDA-approved and other HDACi under clinical trials are presented in Table 3.

Vorinostat, a hydroximic acid-based drug, is also known as suberanilohydroxamic acid (SAHA) and is marketed with different names. Zolinza was the first FDA-approved vorinostat drug for cutaneous T cell lymphoma treatment (CTCL). It inhibits the HDACs except class III sirtuins and was developed by Merck & Co. (Kenilworth, NJ, USA). In phase II clinical trial study (NCT00958074) on 74 CTCL patients with a daily oral dose of vorinostat (400 mg), an objective response rate (ORR) of 30% was observed [11]. Vorinostat is also reported to be useful in other cancer types, such as brain metastasis, refractory colorectal, advanced solid tumors, melanoma, pancreatic, lung cancer and multiple myeloma [6]. A combinatorial therapy of vorinostat with temozolomide and radiotherapy is under clinical trial for the treatment of early stage of glioblastoma multiformae (NCT00731731).

Romidepsin, a cyclic tetrapeptide, was the second FDA-approved drug for treatment of CTCL in 2009 and in 2011, for treatment of peripheral T cell lymphoma (PTCL) with the response rate of 34% and 25%, respectively. However, romidepsin treatment was associated with side effects, such as nausea, vomiting, cardiac toxicity, and myelotoxicity [11,37]. Romidepsin has been evaluated for treatment of T-cell lymphoma either as a single agent (NCT00426764) or in combination with other drugs (NCT03141203) in 30 clinical trials. Romidepsin intake produced fatigue, nausea, vomiting, diarrhea, constipation, phlebitis, headache, and dyspnea as side effects [6]. Romidepsin either singly or in combination with paclitaxel exhibited elimination of both primary tumors and a metastatic lesion at multiple sites formed by the SUM149 IBC cell line in the Mary-X preclinical model [103].

In 2014, belinostat was the third drug approved by the FDA for PTCL treatment. It is a hydroxamate that inhibits the activity of class I and II HDACs. Clinical trial study (NCT00865969) on 120 PTCL patients showed an ORR of 26% [6]. Belinostat is now being investigated in more than 15 clinical trials for the treatment of CTCL (NCT00274651), multiple myeloma (NCT00431340), Burkitt lymphoma (NCT00303953), and solid tumors as in fallopian tube cancer (NCT00301756) [23].

Panobinostat was approved by the FDA in 2015 for the treatment of multiple myelomas [37]. It is a hydroxamate derivative causing the inhibition of class I, II, and IV HDACs. An ORR of 27% was reported for panobinostat. Diarrhoea and cardio-toxicity are side effects associated with Panobinostat. It has been used for treating other cancer types, such as CTCL (NCT00490776), AML (NCT01613976), Hodgkin's lymphoma (NCT00742027), MDS (NCT00594230), thyroid carcinoma (NCT01013597), and colorectal and prostate cancers (NCT00663832) in more than 50 clinical trials [23].

In contrast to the above mentioned clinical trials and studies reporting efficacy of HDACi in the treatment of various lymphomas, leukemia and myeloma, solid tumors have shown limited response against HDACi. The study conducted by Paller and colleagues [104] reported that HDACi VPA and vorinostat in combination with AMG 900, a pan-aurora kinase inhibitor, significantly enhanced cellular senescence, polyploidy, and apoptosis in prostate cancer cell lines (DU-145, LNCaP and PC3) as compared with a single agent treatment. Combination therapy with Janus kinase (JAK) inhibitor INCB018424 has been shown to improve the clinical efficacy of vorinostat in triple-negative breast cancer patients [105]. Similarly, combination therapies targeting HDACs and IκB kinase have shown potential against ovarian cancer [106].

Table 3. FDA approved and under clinical trials histone deacetylase inhibitors (HDACi).

S.N	Chemical Class	Name of the Compounds	HDAC Target	Cancer Specificity	Trial Stage	Structure of the Compound	Reference
1.	Hydroxamic acid	SAHA (Vorinostat)	Class I, II and IV	CTCL	FDA approved (2006)	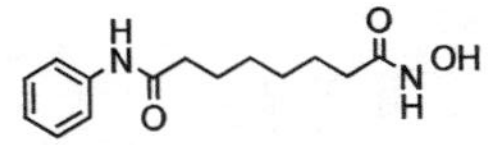	[107]
		Belinostat	Class I, II and IV	PTCL	FDA approved (2014)	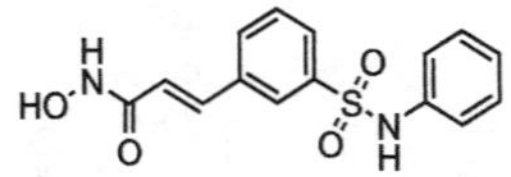	[108]
		Panobinostat	Class I, II and IV	MM	FDA approved in 2015	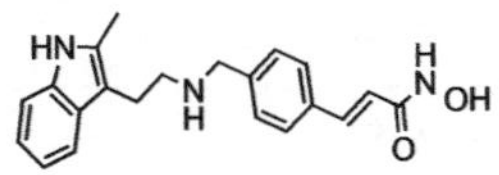	[109]
		Resminostat	Class I and II	Colorectal, HCC, HL	Phase II trial	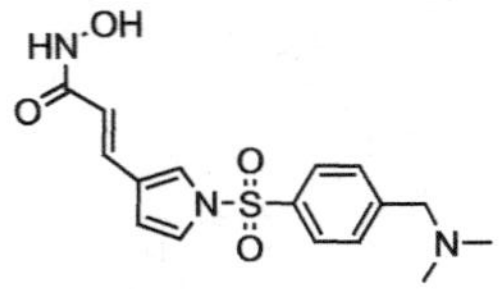	[6]
		Givinostat	Class I and II	CLL, HL, MM	Phase II trial	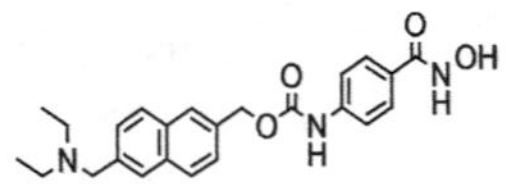	[110]
		Pracinostat	Classes I, II and IV	AML	Phase II trial	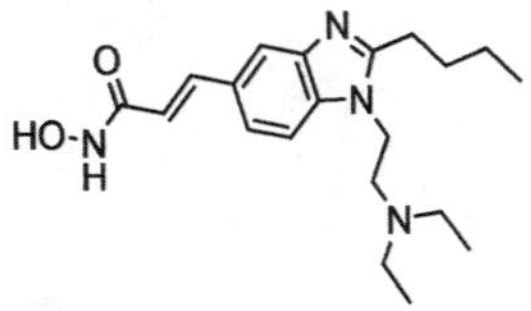	[111]
		Abexinostat	Class I and II	CLL, HL, Non-HL, Solid tumors	Phase I trial	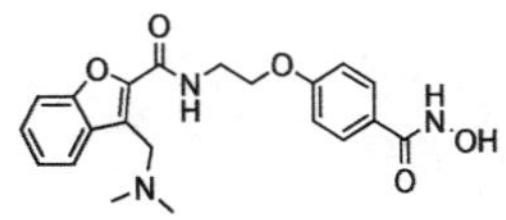	[45]
		Quisinostat	Class I and II	Solid tumor, CTCL	Phase I and II trial	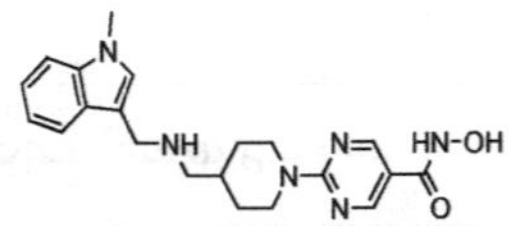	[45]

Table 3. *Cont.*

S.N	Chemical Class	Name of the Compounds	HDAC Target	Cancer Specificity	Trial Stage	Structure of the Compound	Reference
		MPT0E028	HDAC 1, 2 and 6	Solid tumor, B-cell lymphoma	Phase I trial	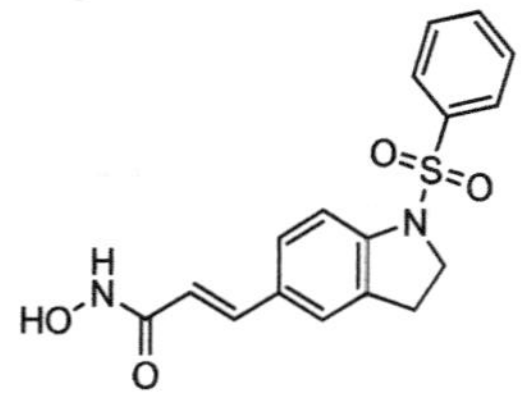	[112]
		CHR 3996	Class I	Solid tumors	Phase I trial	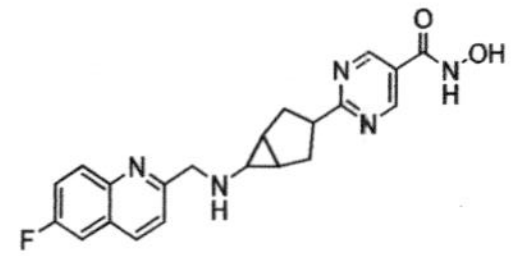	[113]
		CUDC 101	Class I and II	Solid tumor	Phase I trial	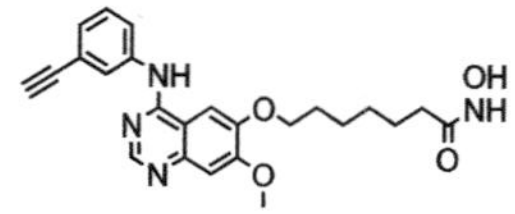	[6]
		CUDC 907	Class I and II	MM; lymphoma; solid tumor	Phase I trial	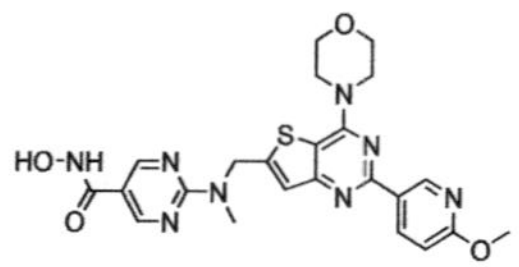	[6]
2.	Benzamides	Entinostat	Class I	Solid tumors	Phase I and II trial	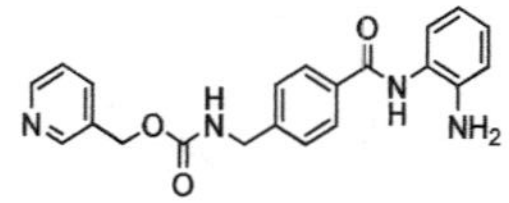	[113]
		Chidamide	HDAC 1, 2,3 and 10	Breast cancer	Phase II and III trial	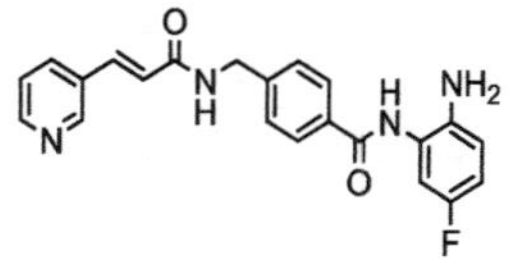	[114]
		Ricolinostat	HDAC 6	MM, Lymphoma	Phase I and II trial	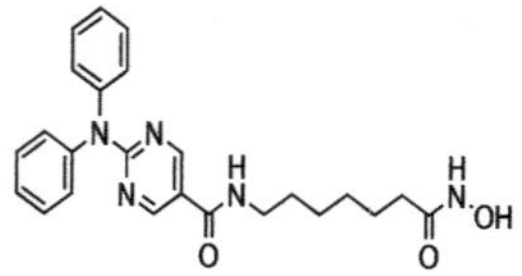	[115]

Table 3. *Cont.*

S.N	Chemical Class	Name of the Compounds	HDAC Target	Cancer Specificity	Trial Stage	Structure of the Compound	Reference
		Tacedinaline	Class I	Lung and pancreatic cancer, MM	Phase II and III trial	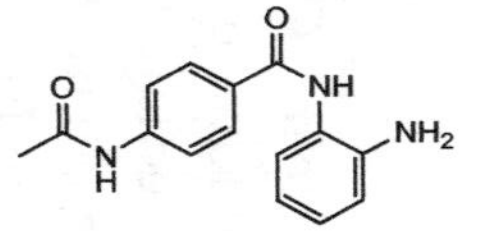	[6]
		Mocetinostat	Class I and IV	Solid malignancies	Phase I and II trial	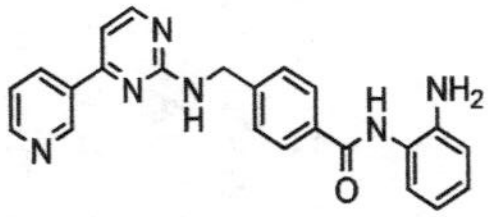	[116]
3.	Cyclic peptides	Romidepsin	Class I	CTCL, PTCL	FDA approved in 2009	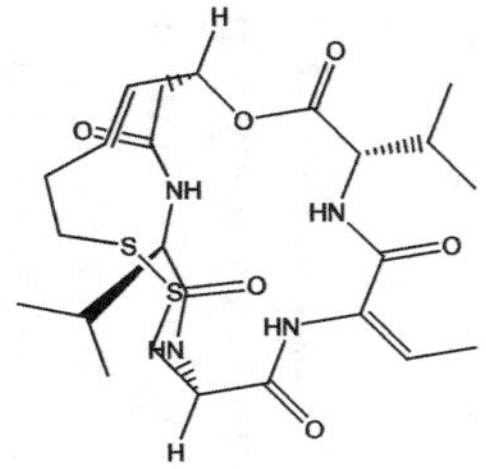	[6,117]
4.	Fatty acids	Valproic acid	Class I and II	Solid and hematological tumors	Phase I and II trial	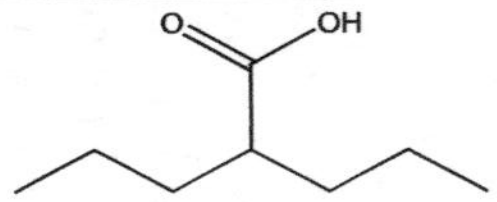	[118]
		AR-42	Class I and IIb	AML	Phase I trial	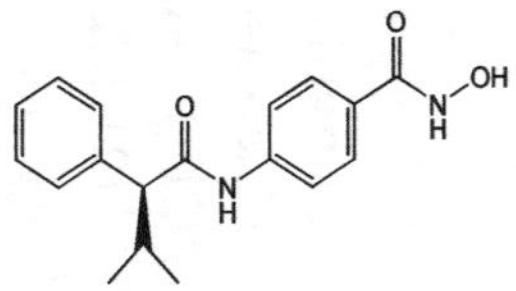	[45]
		Phenyl butyrate	Class I and II	Solid and hematological tumors	Phase I and II trial	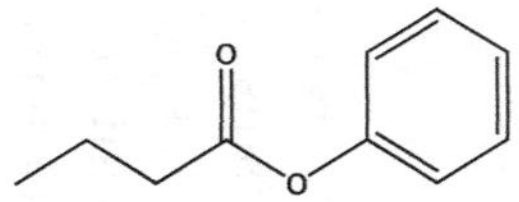	[118]
		Pivanex	Class I and II	NSCLC, Myeloma, CLL	Phase II trial	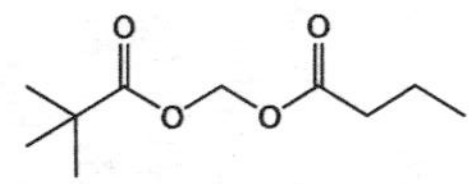	[113]

CTCL, cutaneous T cell lymphoma treatment; PTCL, peripheral T cell lymphoma; MM, multiple myeloma; HCC, hepatocellular Carcinoma; HL, Hodgkin lymphoma; CLL, chronic lymphocyte leukemia; AML, acute myeloid leukemia; NSCLC, non-small cell lung cancer.

7. Mechanisms of Action of HDACi

HDACi induces cell cycle arrest, differentiation, and apoptosis as well as inhibits angiogenesis [119]. The mechanism of the anticancer effect of HDACi depends upon the cancer type, individual, stage of cancer, dose, and some other factors [120]. The antiproliferative mechanisms of HDACi action are described below.

7.1. Cell Cycle Arrest

Various mechanisms are involved in HDACi-mediated cell cycle arrest. One of the most important mechanisms is the increased expression of the cyclin-dependent kinase (CDK) inhibitor gene CDKN1A (p21, WAF1/CIP1). An interesting fact is that the HDACi-mediated overexpression of p21 is independent of p53 [121,122]. The concentration-dependent cell cycle inhibitory effects of HDACi have been observed. At lower concentrations HDACi predominately induces G1 arrest while at higher concentrations induces both G1 and G2/M arrest [123]. p21 is mainly associated with G1 and G2/M arrest, inhibits the activity of CDKs (i.e., CDK 4/6), which regulates the progression of the G1 stage of cell cycle, CDK 2 responsible for G1/S transition and cdc2/CDK 1 causes G2/M transition. The p21 mutation abolishes the HDACi induced G1 arrest [124]. However, HDACi-mediated G1 arrest is also observed in a cell without p21. Hitomi et al. [125] reported that TSA causes G1 arrest in human colon p21 mutant cell by induction of p15 (INK4b), which subsequently causes inhibition of cyclin D-dependent kinases resulting in the absence of CDK 2. Protein p53 interacts with the p21 promoter by competing with HDAC1 and alters the expression of the p21 gene. HDAC1 is the transcriptional repressor of p21, which gets detached from the Sp1 (promoter-specific RNA polymerase II transcription factor) after HDACi treatment, resulting in increased p21 expression. Moreover, HDACi also causes an increase in the half-life of protein p53 thereby improving its interaction with p21 and increased levels of p21 inside the cell mediates cell cycle arrest and apoptosis [126]. HDACi treatment also compromises the CDK activity, which may account for the dephosphorylation of the retinoblastoma protein (Rb), which blocks the elongation factor, E2F function in the transcription of genes for G1 progression and G1/S transition [118].

7.2. Induction of Apoptosis in Transformed Cell

HDACi induces the rate of apoptosis in a transformed cell by regulating both pro-apoptotic and anti-apoptotic genes (Figure 3) and this involves the activation of both extrinsic and intrinsic apoptotic pathways. HDACi induced extrinsic pathway initiation involves the binding of death receptor such as Fas (Apo-1 or CD95), tumor necrosis factor (TNF) receptor-1 (TNFR-1), TNF-related apoptosis-inducing ligand (TRAIL) receptors (DR-4 and DR-5), DR-3 (Apo3) and DR-6 to their ligand FasL, TNF, TRAIL, and TL1A resulting into activation of caspase 8 and 10. In vitro and in vivo studies suggest that HDACi upregulates the expression of both death receptor and their ligand in transformed cells but no such effect is observed in normal cells [127]. Upregulated expression of Fas and FasL have been reported in the treatment of human neuroblastoma cells with m-carboxycinnamic acid bihydroxamide, nude mice xenograft of osteocarcinoma with FK228, acute promyelocytic leukemia model of a rat with valproic acid, and so on [128,129]. FK228 also induces the expression of TNF α in HL 60 and K562 cells. cFLIP, an inhibitor of the activity of the death receptor has been reported to be downregulated after HDACi treatment in cancer cells [127]. HDACi-mediated apoptosis also involves the activation of the intrinsic apoptotic pathway, which causes the release of inter mitochondrial membrane protein, such as cytochrome c, Smac, apoptosis-inducing factor (AIF), and the subsequent activation of caspase. HDACi activate the intrinsic apoptotic pathways by regulating the transcription of pro-apoptotic genes; i.e., Bid (BH3 interacting domain death agonist protein), Bad (Bcl-2 associated agonist of cell death protein), and Bim [130]. The mechanism of HDACi-mediated intrinsic pathway activation is not well understood, but it is suggested that HDACi causes leaking of mitochondrial intermembrane proteins, cytochrome c, AIF and Smac. The release of cytochrome c from mitochondria in turn causes activation of caspase-9 [131,132]. The intrinsic apoptotic pathway is regulated by changing the HDACi-mediated expression of factors. It can be concluded that HDACi upregulate the expression of proapoptotic genes and pathways (BAX, Apaf1 and BAK) and downregulate the expression of the antiapoptotic Bcl-2 family proteins, Bcl-2, Bcl-XL and Mcl-1 [133].

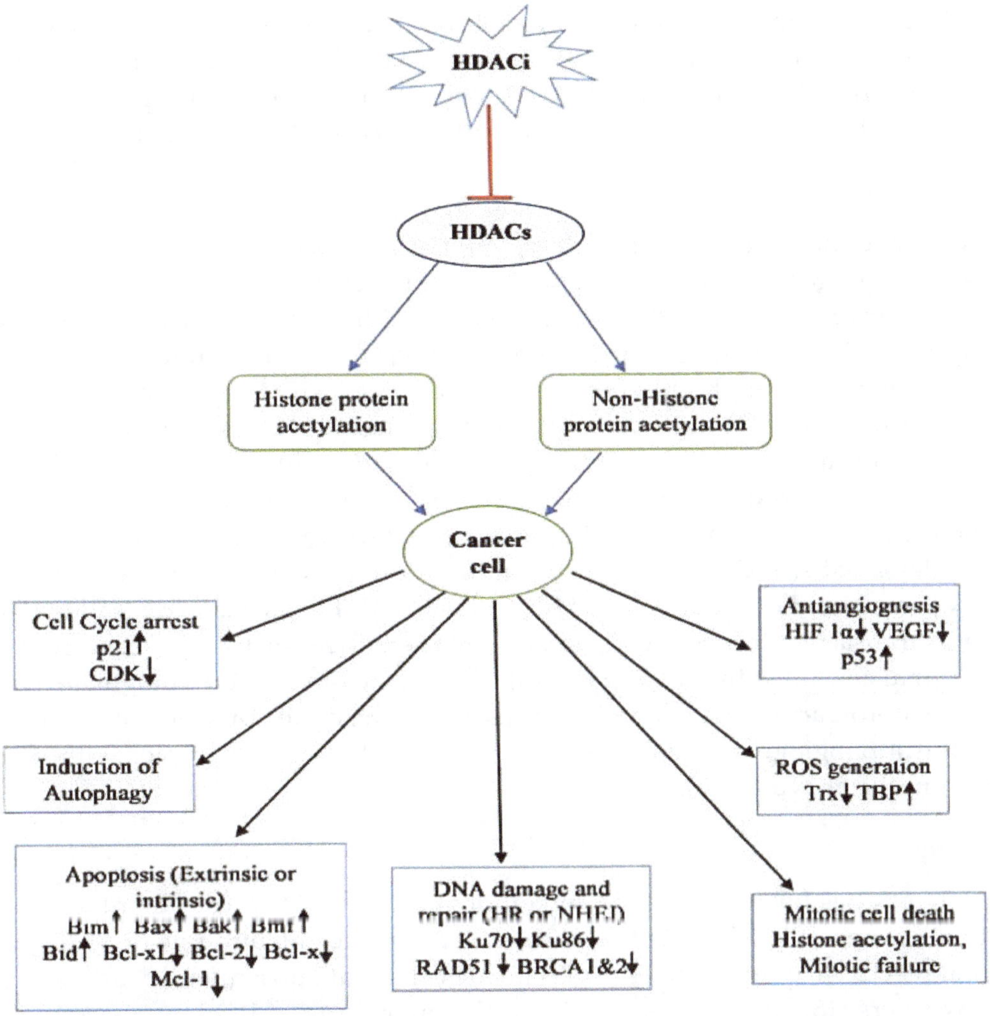

Figure 3. Multiple anti-tumor pathways such as, cell cycle arrest, induction of autophagy and apoptosis, DNA damage repair, ROS generation, angiogenesis inhibitor and mitotic cell death are activated by the action of HDACi in cancer cells. Arrows (↑ and ↓) indicates the increase and decrease, respectively, in the obtained variables. HIF, Hypoxia inducing factor; VEGF, Vascular endothelial growth factor; HR, homologous recombination; NHEJ, Non-homologous end joining; Trx, Thioredoxin; TBP, Thioredoxin binding protein.

7.3. Autophagic Cell Death

The role of HDACi in autophagy is not well understood. Recent findings suggest that autophagy serves as cell death mechanism, therefore, autophagy inhibitors or knockdown of autophagy-related gene decreases the anticancer effect of HDACi. When HeLa cell line having an Apaf-1 knockout or Bcl-XL overexpression was cultured with vorinostat or butyrate, it undergoes autophagic cell death by forming autophagosome inside cytoplasm [134]. Treatment of a colon carcinoma cell HCT116 with vorinostat resulted in the inhibition of cell growth as well as senescence type phenotype [135]. SAHA causes cell death in endometrial stromal sarcoma cell via autophagy [136]. In p53 mutant cancer cells, SAHA induces autophagy and cell death. HDACi-mediated autophagy involves several signaling pathways, one such pathway is the mechanistic target of the rapamycin (mTOR) pathway that is the main suppressor of autophagy via phosphorylation and the inactivation of the Unc51 like autophagy activating kinase 1 (ULK1) complex. SAHA inhibits the activity of mTOR and resumes the activity of ULK1, upstream component of autophagy pathway [137]. SAHA up-regulates the expression of autophagy-related protein by stimulating NF-κβ activity [138]. SAHA also induces autophagy via ROS production in leukemic and hepatocellular carcinoma cells. Romidepsin induces autophagy in HeLa cells [139]. SAHA inhibited the growth of glioblastoma cells xenograft in nude mice by inducing autophagy via downregulation of AKT-mTOR signaling [140]. In some cancer cells showing resistance towards apoptosis, HDACi can induce cell death via the induction of autophagy by bypassing the apoptosis. Hence, HDACi induced autophagy stimulation could be a promising anticancer strategy.

7.4. Inhibition of Angiogenesis

HDACi mediated inhibition of angiogenesis can interfere with the metastasis. HDAC inhibitors downregulate proangiogenic genes, such as the vascular endothelial growth factor gene (VEGF) and endothelial nitric oxide synthase gene [141]. The inhibition of the activity of hypoxia-inducible factor (HIF) by HDACi can block the angiogenesis. Hypoxia is a commonly occurring condition in tumor cells responsible for the overexpression of class I HDACs, except HDAC 8, which in turn causes activation of HIF 1α and promotes angiogenesis [142]. Several compounds viz., TSA, vorinostat, FK228, butyrate and LAQ824, have been reported to inhibit the angiogenesis process and thereby decrease the expression of proangiogenic (HIF 1α and VEGF) factors. Several mechanisms are responsible for the HDACi-mediated degradation of HIF 1α. These include the degradation of HIF 1α by acetylation at Lys532 leading to ubiquitination, class II HDACs associate with HIF 1α and cause siRNA-mediated degradation of HIF 1α [143,144]. HDACi also degrades HIF 1α through compromising its transactivation potential, and also reduces the sensitivity of cancerous cells towards the angiogenic signal generated by VEGF [145,146]. Vorinostat and TSA downregulate the expression of VEGF receptors. Valproic acid impedes angiogenesis by increasing the production of thrombospondin-1 and activin A, the antiangiogenic proteins [147]. Use of combination therapies with VEGF inhibitors finds support from the above reports.

7.5. ROS Generation

Oxidative stress has been implicated in cell death [148–151]. Experimental facts support the treatment of transformed cells with HDACi, such as TSA, vorinostat, butyrate or MS275, leading to the accumulation of reactive oxygen species (ROS) inside cells that subsequently induce cell death [152]. Ruelfi and co-workers [153] in 2001 reported that the quenching of ROS by N-acetylcysteine, a free radical scavenger decreases HDACi induced apoptosis, suggesting the role of HDACi in cell death. Thioredoxin (Trx), a hydrogen ion donor, is a ROS scavenger [154]. It is required in several redox reactions and is responsible for the activity of many protein, such as ribonucleotide reductase, which play an important role in the synthesis of DNA and the transcription factor. HDACi inhibits the activity of Trx by inducing the expression of Trx binding protein 2 (TBP2), which binds to it and inhibits its activity in cancer cells but not in normal cells [155]. Trx binds and inhibits the activity of ASK1. ASK1, an apoptosis signal regulating kinase, increases the rate of apoptosis by the activation of the SET1-JNK and MKK3/MKK6-p38 signaling pathways, and by elevating the expression of pro-apoptotic protein Bim. Therefore, higher expression of TBP2 by HDACi prevents the activity of Trx resulting in the increased expression of ASK1 and ultimately leading to apoptosis [156].

7.6. Mitotic Cell Death

HDACi treatment causes an abnormal acetylation pattern of histone protein in heterochromatin and centromere region. Newly synthesized chromatin contains acetylated histones and TSA treatment in transformed cells causes newly synthesized chromatin to remain acetylated, leading to the structural and functional disorder of centromere and pericentric heterochromatin [157], and this structural disturbance interferes with the phosphorylation of histone as well as disrupts the activity of mitotic spindle checkpoint proteins; i.e., BubR1, hBUB1, CENP-F, and CENP-E [123]. And this causes cell division arrest at the prometaphase stage followed by abnormal mitosis, such as the disaggregation and chromosomal loss leading to cell death either through apoptosis or mitotic cell death [2,124,158].

8. Potential Limitation and Side-Effects of HDACi

There are potential limitations to selective HDACi therapy. The effects of class I HDACi on DNA damage and repair pathways suggest that prolonged exposure to these agents could lead to unacceptable toxicities and secondary malignancies [159]. Class I HDACs may also play an oncogenic role depending on the context. Sontoro et al. [160] reported that in mouse tumor model, a single putative barrier to full transformation is surprisingly provided by HDAC 1 and HDAC2. Knock-down of HDAC 1 resulted in the both blockade of cellular differentiation and the increased genomic instability mediated by PML-RAR in hematopoietic progenitors. Either or both biological deregulations could be sufficient to cooperate with the tumor-promoting activities of oncoproteins, such as PML-RAR and Myc, and would provide a functional explanation for the observed increase in frequency of transformation to leukemia in HDAC1-deficient cells. Epigenetic changes are important for reprogramming somatic cells into pluripotent stem cells. Therefore, several inhibitors of epigenetic-modifying enzymes, including HDACi, are able to reprogram somatic cells into the pluripotent stem cells by modifying a chromatin structure and making it more permissive to transcription factors [119].

9. Conclusions

The present review summarizes the biological activities of HDAC. Further, emphasis has been given on the structural and functional features of the natural and synthetic inhibitors of HDAC as well as on their antitumor potential. HDACs are multisubstrate (histone and non-histone) enzyme involved in many biological processes; i.e., cell proliferation, differentiation, apoptosis, and senescence. According to scientific reports, histone deacetylase inhibitors have shown their efficacy as inhibitors of cancer initiation and progression. Generally, normal cells are resistant to HDACi, which selectively modulates gene expression in cancerous cells. Pan-HDAC inhibitors, such as vorinostat, belinostat, and panobinostat stimulate antitumor pathways, suggesting their therapeutic potential. FDA-approved HDACi are being used for the treatment of several types of cancers. Many HDACi are under clinical trial stages. HDACi show their anticancer action involving various mechanisms; i.e., cell cycle arrest, induction of apoptosis and autophagy in transformed cells, inhibition of angiogenesis, ROS as mediators of cell death, and mitotic cell death. Several natural HDACi are present in our diet: kaempferol (grapes, green tea, tomatoes, potatoes, and onions), resveratrol (grapes, red wine, blueberries and peanuts), sinapinic acid (wine and vinegar), diallyl disulfide (garlic) and zerumbone (ginger). Hence a better understanding of dietary HDACi regarding their target specificity and toxicity may underscore potential health benefits through nutritional intervention. Combination therapy might be another important direction to enhance the therapeutic efficacy of HDACi. Elucidation and validation of the detailed mechanistic aspects of HDACi action will provide a bright future for the use of HDACi as one of the important tools in the fight against cancer.

Author Contributions: A.K.S. and A.K.P. have equally contributed to the structure, preparation, and finalization of manuscript. A.K.S. conducted the literature search and prepared the first draft of the manuscript. A.K.P. and A.B. thoroughly reviewed the manuscript and made desired corrections in the final draft. All the authors have read and approved the final manuscript.

Acknowledgments: A.K.S. acknowledges the CSIR New Delhi for providing financial support in the form of Junior Research Fellowship. A.K.S. and A.K.P. also acknowledge the UGC-SAP and DST-FIST facilities of the Department of Biochemistry, University of Allahabad, Allahabad, India.

References

1. Siegel, R.L.; Miller, K.D.; Jemal, A. Cancer Statistics, 2018. *CA Cancer J. Clin.* **2018**, *68*, 7–30. [CrossRef] [PubMed]

2. Kumar, S.; Ahmad, M.K.; Waseem, M.; Pandey, A.K. Drug Targets for Cancer Treatment: An Overview. *Med. Chem.* **2015**, *5*, 115–123. [CrossRef]
3. Sharma, U.K.; Sharma, A.K.; Pandey, A.K. Medicinal attributes of major phenylpropanoids present in cinnamon. *BMC Complement. Altern. Med.* **2016**, *16*, 156. [CrossRef] [PubMed]
4. Kumar, S.; Pandey, A.K. Oxidative stress-related microRNAs as diagnostic markers: A newer Insight in diagnostics. In *Oxidative Stress: Diagnostic Methods and Applications in Medical Science*; Maurya, P., Chandra, P., Eds.; Springer: Singapore, 2017; pp. 113–125.
5. Zahonero, B.B.; Parra, M. Histone deacetylases and cancer. *Mol. Oncol.* **2012**, *6*, 579–589. [CrossRef] [PubMed]
6. Mottamal, M.; Zheng, S.; Huang, T.L.; Wang, G. Histone Deacetylase Inhibitors in Clinical Studies as Templates for New Anticancer Agents. *Molecules* **2016**, *20*, 3898–3941. [CrossRef] [PubMed]
7. Allfrey, V.G.; Faulkner, R.; Mirsky, A.E. Acetylation and methylation of histones and their possible role in the regulation of Rna synthesis. *Proc. Natl. Acad. Sci. USA* **1964**, *51*, 786–794. [CrossRef] [PubMed]
8. Gershey, E.L.; Vidali, G.; Allfrey, V.G. Chemical studies of histone acetylation. The occurrence of epsilon-N-acetyllysine in the f2a1 histone. *J. Biol. Chem.* **1968**, *243*, 5018–5022. [PubMed]
9. Haberland, M.; Montgomery, R.L.; Olson, E.N. The many roles of histone deacetylases in development and physiology: implications for disease and therapy. *Nat. Rev. Genet.* **2009**, *10*, 32–42. [CrossRef] [PubMed]
10. Peng, L.; Seto, E. Deacetylation of Nonhistone Proteins by HDACs and the Implications in Cancer. In *Histone Deacetylases: The Biology and Clinical Implication*; Yao, T.P., Seto, E., Eds.; Handbook of Experimental Pharmacology; Springer: Berlin/Heidelberg, Germany, 2011; Volume 206, pp. 39–56. ISBN 978-3-642-21631-2.
11. Basset, S.A.; Barnett, M.P. The Role of Dietary Histone Deacetylases (HDACs) Inhibitors in Health and Disease. *Nutrients* **2014**, *6*, 4273–4301. [CrossRef] [PubMed]
12. Miller, P.E.; Snyder, D.C. Phytochemicals and cancer risk: A review of the epidemiological evidence. *Nutr. Clin. Pract.* **2012**, *27*, 599–612. [CrossRef] [PubMed]
13. Hou, I.C.; Amarnani, S.; Chong, M.T.; Bishayee, A. Green tea and the risk of genetic cancer: Epidemiological evidence. *World J. Gastroenterol.* **2013**, *19*, 3713–3722. [CrossRef] [PubMed]
14. Ivey, K.L.; Jensen, M.K.; Hodgson, J.M.; Eliassen, A.H.; Cassidy, A.; Rimm, E.B. Association of flavonoid-rich foods and flavonoids with risk of all-cause mortality. *Br. J. Nutr.* **2017**, *117*, 1470–1477. [CrossRef] [PubMed]
15. Kumar, S.; Pandey, A.K. Chemistry and biological activities of flavonoids: an overview. *Sci. World J.* **2013**, *2013*, 162750. [CrossRef] [PubMed]
16. Kim, H.J.; Bae, S.C. Histone deacetylase inhibitors: Molecular mechanisms of action and clinical trials as anti-cancer drugs. *Am. J. Transl. Res.* **2011**, *3*, 166–179. [PubMed]
17. Lawson, M.; Uciechowska, U.; Schemies, J.; Rumpf, T.; Jung, M.; Sippl, W. Inhibitors to understand molecular mechanisms of NAD^+-dependent deacetylases (sirtuins). *Biochim. Biophys. Acta* **2010**, *1799*, 726–739. [CrossRef] [PubMed]
18. Taunton, J.; Hassig, C.A.; Schreiber, S.L. A mammalian histone deacetylase related to the yeast transcriptional regulator Rpd3p. *Science* **1996**, *272*, 408–411. [CrossRef] [PubMed]
19. Yang, W.M.; Inouye, C.; Zeng, Y.; Bearss, D.; Seto, E. Transcriptional repression by YY1 is mediated by interaction with a mammalian homolog of the yeast global regulator RPD3. *Proc. Natl. Acad. Sci. USA* **1996**, *93*, 12845–12850. [CrossRef] [PubMed]
20. Yang, W.M.; Yao, Y.L.; Sun, J.M.; Davie, J.R.; Seto, E. Isolation and characterization of cDNAs corresponding to an additional member of the human histone deacetylase gene family. *J. Biol. Chem.* **1997**, *272*, 28001–28007. [CrossRef] [PubMed]
21. Grozinger, C.M.; Hassig, C.A.; Schreiber, S.L. Three proteins define a class of human histone deacetylases related to yeast Hda1p. *Proc. Natl. Acad. Sci. USA* **1999**, *96*, 4868–4873. [CrossRef] [PubMed]
22. Kao, H.Y.; Downes, M.; Ordentlich, P.; Evans, R.M. Isolation of a novel histone deacetylase reveals that class I and class II deacetylases promote SMRT-mediated repression. *Genes Dev.* **2000**, *14*, 55–66. [PubMed]
23. Losson, H.; Schnekenburger, M.; Dicato, M.; Diederich, M. Natural Compound Histone Deacetylase Inhibitors (HDACi): Synergy with Inflammatory Signalling Pathway Modulators and Clinical Applications in Cancer. *Molecules* **2016**, *21*, 1608. [CrossRef] [PubMed]
24. Lane, A.A.; Chabner, B.A. Histone deacetylase inhibitors in cancer therapy. *J. Clin. Oncol.* **2009**, *27*, 5459–5468. [CrossRef] [PubMed]
25. Minucci, S.; Pelicci, P.G. Histone deacetylase inhibitors and the promise of epigenetic (and more) treatments for cancer. *Nat. Rev. Cancer* **2006**, *6*, 38–51. [CrossRef] [PubMed]

26. Hubbert, C.; Guardiola, A.; Shao, R.; Kawaguchi, Y.; Ito, A.; Nixon, A.; Yoshida, M.; Wang, X.F.; Yao, T.P. HDAC6 is a microtubule associated deacetylase. *Nature* **2002**, *417*, 455–458. [CrossRef] [PubMed]
27. Seidel, C.; Schnekenburger, M.; Dicato, M.; Diederich, M. Histone deacetylase modulators provided by Mother Nature. *Genes Nutr.* **2012**, *7*, 357. [CrossRef] [PubMed]
28. Ropero, S.; Fraga, M.F.; Ballestar, E.; Hamelin, R.; Yamamoto, H.; Boix-Chornet, M.; Caballero, R.; Alaminos, M.; Setien, F.; Paz, M.F.; et al. A truncating mutation of HDAC2 in human cancers confers resistance to histone deacetylase inhibition. *Nat. Genet.* **2006**, *38*, 566–569. [CrossRef] [PubMed]
29. Fraga, M.F.; Ballestar, E.; Villar-Garea, A.; Boix-Chornet, M.; Espada, J.; Schotta, G.; Bonaldi, T.; Haydon, C.; Ropero, S.; Petrie, K.; et al. Loss of acetylation at Lys16 and trimethylation at Lys20 of histone H4 is a common hallmark of human cancer. *Nat. Genet.* **2005**, *37*, 391–400. [CrossRef] [PubMed]
30. Mai, A.; Massa, S.; Rotili, D.; Cerbara, I.; Valente, S.; Pezzi, R.; Simeoni, S.; Ragno, R. Histone deacetylation in epigenetics: An attractive target for anticancer therapy. *Med. Res. Rev.* **2005**, *25*, 261–309. [CrossRef] [PubMed]
31. Choi, J.H.; Kwon, H.J.; Yoon, B.I.; Kim, J.H.; Han, S.U.; Joo, H.J.; Kim, D.Y. Expression profile of histone deacetylase 1 in gastric cancer tissues. *Jpn. J. Cancer Res.* **2001**, *92*, 1300–1304. [CrossRef] [PubMed]
32. Witt, O.; Deubzer, H.E.; Milde, T.; Oehme, I. HDAC family: What are the cancer relevant targets? *Cancer Letters* **2009**, *277*, 8–21. [CrossRef] [PubMed]
33. Weichert, W.; Roske, V.A.; Gekeler, T.; Beckers, M.P.; Ebert, M.; Pross, M.; Dietel, C.; Denkert, C.; Rocken, C. Association of patterns of class I histone deacetylase expression with patient prognosis in gastric cancer: A retrospective analysis. *Lancet Oncol.* **2008**, *9*, 139–148. [CrossRef]
34. Weichert, W.; Roske, A.; Gekeler, V.; Beckers, T.; Stephan, C.; Jung, K.; Fritzsche, F.R.; Niesporek, S.; Denkert, C.; Dietel, M.; Kristiansen, G. Histone deacetylases 1, 2 and 3 are highly expressed in prostate cancer and HDAC2 expression is associated with shorter PSA relapse time after radical prostatectomy. *Br. J. Cancer* **2008**, *98*, 604–610. [CrossRef] [PubMed]
35. Weichert, W.; Roske, A.; Niesporek, S.; Noske, A.; Buckendahl, A.C.; Dietel, M.; Gekeler, V.; Boehm, M.; Beckers, T.; Denkert, C. Class I histone deacetylase expression has independent prognostic impact in human colorectal cancer: Specific role of class I histone deacetylases in vitro and in vivo. *Clin. Cancer Res.* **2008**, *14*, 1669–1677. [CrossRef] [PubMed]
36. Rikimaru, T.; Taketomi, A.; Yamashita, Y.; Shirabe, K.; Hamatsu, T.; Shimada, M.; Maehara, Y. Clinical significance of histone deacetylase 1 expression in patients with hepatocellular carcinoma. *Oncology* **2007**, *72*, 69–74. [CrossRef] [PubMed]
37. Sasaki, H.; Moriyama, S.; Nakashima, Y.; Kobayashi, Y.; Kiriyama, M.; Fukai, I.; Yamakawa, Y.; Fujii, Y. Histone deacetylase 1 mRNA expression in lung cancer. *Lung Cancer* **2004**, *46*, 171–178. [CrossRef] [PubMed]
38. Yoon, S.; Eom, G.H. HDAC and HDAC Inhibitor: From Cancer to Cardiovascular Diseases. *Chonnam Med. J.* **2016**, *52*, 1–11. [CrossRef] [PubMed]
39. Krusche, C.A.; Wulfing, P.; Kersting, C.; Vloet, A.; Bocker, W.; Kiesel, L.; Beier, H.M.; Alfer, J. Histone deacetylase-1 and -3 protein expression in human breast cancer: A tissue microarray analysis. *Breast Cancer Res. Treat.* **2005**, *90*, 15–23. [CrossRef] [PubMed]
40. Glaser, K.B.; Li, J.; Staver, M.J.; Wei, R.Q.; Albert, D.H.; Davidsen, S.K. Role of class I and class II histone deacetylases in carcinoma cells using siRNA. *Biochem. Biophys. Res. Commun.* **2003**, *310*, 529–536. [CrossRef] [PubMed]
41. Senese, S.; Zaragoza, K.; Minardi, S.; Muradore, I.; Ronzoni, A.S.; Passafaro, L.; Bernard, G.F.; Draetta, M.; Alcalay, C.; Seiser, S.; et al. Role for histone deacetylase 1 in human tumor cell proliferation. *Mol. Cell. Biol.* **2007**, *27*, 4784–4795. [CrossRef] [PubMed]
42. Keshelava, N.; Davicioni, E.; Wan, Z.; Ji, L.; Sposto, R.; Triche, T.J.; Reynolds, C.P. Histone deacetylase 1 gene expression and sensitization of multidrug-resistant neuroblastoma cell lines to cytotoxic agents by depsipeptide. *J. Natl. Cancer Inst.* **2007**, *99*, 1107–1119. [CrossRef] [PubMed]
43. Huang, B.H.; Laban, M.; Leung, C.H.; Lee, L.; Lee, C.K.; Salto-Tellez, M.; Raju, G.C.; Hooi, S.C. Inhibition of histone deacetylase 2 increases apoptosis and p21Cip1/WAF1 expression, independent of histone deacetylase 1. *Cell Death Differ.* **2005**, *12*, 395–404. [CrossRef] [PubMed]
44. Harms, K.L.; Chen, X. Histone deacetylase 2 modulates p53 transcriptional activities through regulation of p53-DNA binding activity. *Cancer Res.* **2007** *67*, 3145–3152. [CrossRef] [PubMed]

45. West, A.C.; Johnstone, R.W. New and emerging HDAC inhibitors for cancer treatment. *J. Clin. Investig.* **2014**, *124*, 30–39. [CrossRef] [PubMed]
46. Wang, J.C.; Kafeel, M.I.; Avezbakiyev, B.; Chen, C.; Sun, Y.; Rathnasabapathy, C.; Kalavar, M.; He, Z.; Burton, J.; Lichter, S. Histone deacetylase in chronic lymphocytic leukemia. *Oncology* **2011**, *81*, 325–329. [CrossRef] [PubMed]
47. Atsumi, A.; Tomita, A.; Kiyoi, H.; Naoe, T. Histone deacetylase 3 (HDAC3) is recruited to target promoters by PML-RARa as a component of the N-CoR co-repressor complex to repress transcription in vivo. *Biochem. Biophys. Res. Commun.* **2006**, *345*, 1471–1480. [CrossRef] [PubMed]
48. Vannini, A.; Volpari, C.; Filocamo, G.; Casavola, E.C.; Brunetti, M.; Renzoni, D.; Chakravarty, P.; Paolini, C.; De Francesco, R.; Gallinari, P.; et al. Crystal structure of a eukaryotic zinc dependent histone deacetylase, human HDAC8, complexed with a hydroxamic acid inhibitor. *Proc. Natl. Acad. Sci. USA* **2004**, *101*, 15064–15069. [CrossRef] [PubMed]
49. Oehme, I.; Deubzer, H.E.; Wegener, D.; Pickert, D.; Linke, J.P.; Hero, B.; Kopp-Schneider, A.; Westermann, F.; Ulrich, S.M.; Von Deimling, A.; Fischer, M.; Witt, O. Histone deacetylase 8 in neuroblastoma tumorigenesis. *Clin. Cancer Res.* **2009**, *15*, 91–99. [CrossRef] [PubMed]
50. Lee, H.; Sengupta, N.; Villagra, A.; Rezai-Zadeh, N.; Seto, E. Histone deacetylase 8 safeguards the human ever-shorter telomeres 1B (hEST1B) protein from ubiquitin-mediated degradation. *Mol. Cell. Biol.* **2006**, *26*, 5259–5269. [CrossRef] [PubMed]
51. Ozdag, H.; Teschendorff, A.E.; Ahmed, A.A.; Hyland, S.J.; Blenkiron, C.; Bobrow, L.; Veerakumarasivam, A.; Burtt, G.; Subkhankulova, T.; Arends, M.J.; et al. Differential expression of selected histone modifier genes in human solid cancers. *BMC Genom.* **2006**, *7*, 90. [CrossRef] [PubMed]
52. Chauchereau, A.; Mathieu, M.; de Saintignon, J.; Ferreira, R.; Pritchard, L.L.; Mishal, Z.; Dejean, A.; Harel-Bellan, A. HDAC4 mediates transcriptional repression by the acute promyelocytic leukaemiaassociated protein PLZF. *Oncogene* **2004**, *23*, 8777–8784. [CrossRef] [PubMed]
53. Geng, H.; Harvey, C.T.; Pittsenbarger, J.; Liu, Q.; Beer, T.M.; Xue, C.; Qian, D.Z. HDAC4 protein regulates HIF1alpha protein lysine acetylation and cancer cell response to hypoxia. *J. Biol. Chem.* **2011**, *286*, 38095–38102. [CrossRef] [PubMed]
54. Wilson, A.J.; Byun, D.S.; Nasser, S.; Murray, L.B.; Ayyanar, K.; Arango, D.; Figueroa, M.; Melnick, A.; Kao, G.D.; Augenlicht, L.H.; et al. HDAC4 promotes growth of colon cancer cells via repression of p21. *Mol. Biol. Cell.* **2008**, *19*, 4062–4075. [CrossRef] [PubMed]
55. Milde, T.; Oehme, I.; Korshunov, A.; Kopp-Schneider, A.; Remke, M.; Northcott, P.; Deubzer, H.E.; Lodrini, M.; Taylor, M.D.; von Deimling, A.; et al. HDAC5 and HDAC9 in medulloblastoma: Novel markers for risk stratification and role in tumor cell growth. *Clin. Cancer Res.* **2010**, *16*, 3240–3252. [CrossRef] [PubMed]
56. Watamoto, K.; Towatari, M.; Ozawa, Y.; Miyata, Y.; Okamoto, M.; Abe, A.; Naoe, T.; Saito, H. Altered interaction of HDAC5 with GATA-1 during MEL cell differentiation. *Oncogene* **2003**, *22*, 9176–9184. [CrossRef] [PubMed]
57. Osada, H.; Tatematsu, Y.; Saito, H.; Yatabe, Y.; Mitsudomi, T.; Takahashi, T. Reduced expression of class II histone deacetylase genes is associated with poor prognosis in lung cancer patients. *Int. J. Cancer* **2004**, *112*, 26–32. [CrossRef] [PubMed]
58. Mottet, D.; Bellahcene, A.; Pirotte, S.; Waltregny, D.; Deroanne, C.; Lamour, V.; Lidereau, R.; Castronovo, V. Histone deacetylase 7 silencing alters endothelial cell migration, a key step in angiogenesis. *Circ. Res.* **2007**, *101*, 1237–1246. [CrossRef] [PubMed]
59. Kotian, S.; Liyanarachchi, S.; Zelent, A.; Parvin, J.D. Histone deacetylases 9 and 10 are required for homologous recombination. *J. Biol. Chem.* **2011**, *286*, 7722–7726. [CrossRef] [PubMed]
60. Moreno, D.A.; Scrideli, C.A.; Cortez, M.A.; de Paula Queiroz, R.; Valera, E.T.; da Silva Silveira, V.; Yunes, J.A.; Brandalise, S.R.; Tone, L.G. Differential expression of HDAC3, HDAC7 and HDAC9 is associated with prognosis and survival in childhood acute lymphoblastic leukaemia. *Br. J. Haematol.* **2010**, *150*, 665–673. [CrossRef] [PubMed]
61. Seidel, C.; Schnekenburger, M.; Dicato, M.; Diederich, M. Histone deacetylase 6 in health and disease. *Epigenomics* **2015**, *7*, 103–118. [CrossRef] [PubMed]
62. Sakuma, T.; Uzawa, K.; Onda, T.; Shiiba, M.; Yokoe, H.; Shibahara, T.; Tanzawa, H. Aberrant expression of histone deacetylase 6 in oral squamous cell carcinoma. *Int. J. Oncol.* **2006**, *29*, 117–124. [CrossRef] [PubMed]

63. Haggarty, S.J.; Koeller, K.M.; Wong, J.C.; Grozinger, C.M.; Schreiber, S.L. Domain-selective small-molecule inhibitor of histone deacetylase 6 (HDAC6)-mediated tubulin deacetylation. *Proc. Natl. Acad. Sci. USA* **2003**, *100*, 4389–4394. [CrossRef] [PubMed]
64. Bali, P.; Pranpat, M.; Bradner, J.; Balasis, M.; Fiskus, W.; Guo, F.; Rocha, K.; Kumaraswamy, S.; Boyapalle, S.; Atadja, P.; et al. Inhibition of histone deacetylase 6 acetylates and disrupts the chaperone function of heat shock protein 90: A novel basis for antileukemia activity of histone deacetylase inhibitors. *J. Biol. Chem.* **2005**, *280*, 26729–26734. [CrossRef] [PubMed]
65. Shan, B.; Yao, T.P.; Nguyen, H.T.; Zhuo, Y.; Levy, D.R.; Klingsberg, R.C.; Palmer, M.L.; Holder, K.N.; Lasky, J.A. Requirement of HDAC6 for TGF-β 1-induced epithelial-mesenchymal transition. *J. Biol. Chem.* **2008**, *283*, 21065–21073. [CrossRef] [PubMed]
66. Lee, J.H.; Jeong, E.G.; Choi, M.C.; Kim, S.H.; Park, J.H.; Song, S.H.; Park, J.; Bang, Y.J.; Kim, T.Y. Inhibition of histone deacetylase 10 induces thioredoxin-interacting protein and causes accumulation of reactive oxygen species in SNU-620 human gastric cancer cells. *Mol. Cell.* **2010**, *30*, 107–112. [CrossRef] [PubMed]
67. Johnson, E.K.; Wilgus, A.T. Vascular endothelial growth factor and angiogenesis in the regulation of cutaneous wound repair. *Adv. Wound Care (New Rochelle)*, **2014**, *3*, 647–661. [CrossRef] [PubMed]
68. Park, J.H.; Kim, S.H.; Choi, M.C.; Lee, J.; Oh, D.Y.; Im, S.A.; Bang, Y.J.; Kim, T.Y. Class II histone deacetylases play pivotal roles in heat shock protein 90-mediated proteasomal degradation of vascular endothelial growth factor receptors. *Biochem. Biophys. Res. Commun.* **2008**, *368*, 318–322. [CrossRef] [PubMed]
69. Bradbury, C.A.; Khanim, F.L.; Hayden, R.; Bunce, C.M.; White, D.A.; Drayson, M.T.; Craddock, C.; Turner, B.M. Histone deacetylases in acute myeloid leukaemia show a distinctive pattern of expression that changes selectively in response to deacetylase inhibitors. *Leukemia* **2005**, *19*, 1751–1759. [CrossRef] [PubMed]
70. Hida, Y.; Kubo, Y.; Murao, K.; Arase, S. Strong expression of a longevity-related protein, SIRT1, in Bowen's disease. *Arch. Dermatol. Res.* **2007**, *299*, 103–106. [CrossRef] [PubMed]
71. Huffman, D.M.; Grizzle, W.E.; Bamman, M.M.; Kim, J.S.; Eltoum, I.A.; Elgavish, A.; Nagy, T.R. SIRT1 is significantly elevated in mouse and human prostate cancer. *Cancer Res.* **2007**, *67*, 6612–6618. [CrossRef] [PubMed]
72. Hiratsuka, M.; Inoue, T.; Toda, T.; Kimura, N.; Shirayoshi, Y.; Kamitani, H.; Watanabe, T.; Ohama, E.; Tahimic, C.G.; Kurimasa, A.; et al. Proteomics-based identification of differentially expressed genes in human gliomas: Down-regulation of SIRT2 gene. *Biochem. Biophys. Res. Commun.* **2003**, *309*, 558–566. [CrossRef] [PubMed]
73. Lennerz, V.; Fatho, M.; Gentilini, C.; Frye, R.A.; Lifke, A.; Ferel, D.; Wolfel, C.; Huber, C.; Wolfel, T. The response of autologous T cells to a human melanoma is dominated by mutated neoantigens. *Proc. Natl. Acad. Sci. USA* **2005**, *102*, 16013–16018. [CrossRef] [PubMed]
74. Ashraf, N.; Zino, S.; Macintyre, A.; Kingsmore, D.; Payne, A.P.; George, W.D.; Shiels, P.G. Altered sirtuin expression is associated with node-positive breast cancer. *Br. J. Cancer* **2006**, *95*, 1056–1061. [CrossRef] [PubMed]
75. Dryden, S.C.; Nahhas, F.A.; Nowak, J.E.; Goustin, A.S.; Tainsky, M.A. Role for human SIRT2 NAD-dependent class II histone deacetylases in a Sin3-independent repression pathway. *Genes Dev.* **2003**, *14*, 45–54.
76. Chu, F.; Chou, P.M.; Zheng, X.; Mirkin, B.L.; Rebbaa, A. Control of multidrug resistance gene mdr1 and cancer resistance to chemotherapy by the longevity gene sirt1. *Cancer Res.* **2005**, *65*, 10183–10187. [CrossRef] [PubMed]
77. Yang, H.; Yang, T.; Baur, J.A.; Perez, E.; Matsui, T.; Carmona, J.J.; Lamming, D.W.; Souza-Pinto, N.C.; Bohr, V.A.; Rosenzweig, A.; et al. Nutrient-sensitive mitochondrial NAD^+ levels dictate cell survival. *Cell* **2007**, *130*, 1095–1107. [CrossRef] [PubMed]
78. Bell, E.L.; Emerling, B.M.; Ricoult, S.J.; Guarente, L. SirT3 suppresses hypoxia inducible factor 1alpha and tumor growth by inhibiting mitochondrial ROS production. *Oncogene* **2011**, *30*, 2986–2996. [CrossRef] [PubMed]
79. Skov, V.; Larsen, T.S.; Thomassen, M.; Riley, C.H.; Jensen, M.K.; Bjerrum, O.W.; Kruse, T.A.; Hasselbalch, H.C. Increased gene expression of histone deacetylases in patients with Philadelphia-negative chronic myeloproliferative neoplasms. *Leuk. Lymphoma* **2012**, *53*, 123–129. [CrossRef] [PubMed]
80. Gao, L.; Cueto, M.A.; Asselbergs, F.; Atadja, P. Cloning and functional characterization of HDAC11, a novel member of the human histone deacetylase family. *J. Biol. Chem.* **2002**, *277*, 25748–25755. [CrossRef] [PubMed]

81. Riggs, M.G.; Whittaker, R.G.; Neumann, J.R.; Ingram, V.M. *n*-Butyrate causes histone modification in HeLa and Friend erythroleukaemia cells. *Nature* **1977**, *268*, 462–464. [CrossRef] [PubMed]
82. Kijima, M.; Yoshida, M.; Sugita, K.; Horinouchi, S.; Beppu, T. Trapoxin, an antitumor cyclic tetrapeptide, is an irreversible inhibitor of mammalian histone deacetylase. *J. Biol. Chem.* **1993**, *268*, 22429–22435. [PubMed]
83. Li, Y.; Seto, E. HDACs and HDAC Inhibitors in Cancer Development and Therapy. *Cold Spring Harb. Perspect. Med.* **2016**, *6*, 10. [CrossRef] [PubMed]
84. Ungerstedt, J.S.; Sowa, Y.; Xu, W.S.; Shao, Y.; Dokmanovic, M.; Perez, G.; Ngo, L.; Holmgren, A.; Jiang, X.; Marks, P.A. Role of thioredoxin in the response of normal and transformed cells to histone deacetylase inhibitors. *Proc. Natl. Acad. Sci. USA* **2005**, *102*, 673–678. [CrossRef] [PubMed]
85. Tsuji, N.; Kobayashi, M.; Nagashima, K.; Wakisaka, Y.; Koizumi, K. A new antifungal antibiotic, trichostatin. *J. Antibiot.* **1976**, *29*, 1–6. [CrossRef] [PubMed]
86. Yoshida, M.; Kijima, M.; Akita, M.; Beppu, T. Potent and specific inhibition of mammalian histone deacetylase both in vivo and in vitro by trichostatin A. *J. Biol. Chem.* **1990**, *265*, 17174–17179. [PubMed]
87. Mcknight, G.S.; Hanger, L.; Palmiter, R.D. Butyrate and related inhibitors of histone deacetylation block the induction of egg white genes by steroid harmones. *Cell* **1980**, *22*, 469–477. [CrossRef]
88. Orlikova, B.; Schnekenburger, M.; Zloh, M.; Golais, F.; Diederich, M.; Tasdemir, D. Natural chalcones as dual inhibitors of HDACs and NF-κB. *Oncol. Rep.* **2012**, *28*, 797–805. [CrossRef] [PubMed]
89. Berger, A.; Venturelli, S.; Kallnischkies, M.; Bocker, A.; Busch, C.; Weiland, T.; Noor, S.; Leischner, C.; Weiss, T.S.; Lauer, U.M.; et al. Kaempferol, a new nutrition-derived pan-inhibitor of human histone deacetylases. *J. Nutr. Biochem.* **2013**, *24*, 977–985. [CrossRef] [PubMed]
90. Senawong, T.; Misuna, S.; Khaopha, S.; Nuchadomrong, S.; Sawatsitang, P.; Phaosiri, C.; Surapaitoon, A.; Sripa, B. Histone deacetylase (HDAC) inhibitory and antiproliferative activities of phenolic-rich extracts derived from the rhizome of Hydnophytum formicarum Jack.: Sinapinic acid acts as HDAC inhibitor. *BMC Complement. Altern. Med.* **2013**, *13*, 232. [CrossRef] [PubMed]
91. Venturelli, S.; Berger, A.; Bocker, A.; Busch, C.; Weiland, T.; Noor, S.; Leischner, C.; Schleicher, S.; Mayer, M.; Weiss, T.S.; et al. Resveratrol as a pan-HDAC inhibitor alters the acetylation status of histone [corrected] proteins in human-derived hepatoblastoma cells. *PLoS ONE* **2013**, *8*, 73097. [CrossRef]
92. Ryu, H.W.; Lee, D.H.; Shin, D.H.; Kim, S.H.; Kwon, S.H. Aeroside VIII is a natural selective HDAC6 inhibitor that synergistically enhances the anticancer activity of HDAC inhibitor in HT29 cells. *Planta Med.* **2015**, *81*, 222–227. [CrossRef] [PubMed]
93. Jones, P.; Altamura, S.; Chakravarty, P.K.; Cecchetti, O.; de Francesco, R.; Gallinari, P.; Ingenito, R.; Meinke, P.T.; Petrocchi, A.; Rowley, M.; et al. A series of novel, potent, and selective histone deacetylase inhibitors. *Bioorg. Med. Chem. Lett.* **2006**, *16*, 5948–5952. [CrossRef] [PubMed]
94. Maulucci, N.; Chini, M.G.; Micco, S.D.; Izzo, I.; Cafaro, E.; Russo, A.; Gallinari, P.; Paolini, C.; Nardi, M.C.; Casapullo, A.; et al. Molecular Insights into Azumamide E Histone Deacetylases Inhibitory Activity. *J. Am. Chem. Soc.* **2007**, *129*, 3007–3012. [CrossRef] [PubMed]
95. De Schepper, S.; Bruwiere, H.; Verhulst, T.; Steller, U.; Andries, L.; Wouters, W.; Janicot, M.; Arts, J.; vanHeusden, J. Inhibition of histone deacetylases by chlamydocin induces apoptosis and proteasome-mediated degradation of survivin. *J. Pharmacol. Exp. Ther.* **2003**, *304*, 881–888. [CrossRef] [PubMed]
96. Itazaki, H.; Nagashima, K.; Sugita, K.; Yoshida, H.; Kawamura, Y.; Yasuda, Y.; Matsumoto, K.; Ishii, K.; Uotani, N.; Nakai, H.; et al. Isolation and structural elucidation of new cyclotetrapeptides, trapoxins A and B, having detransformation activities as antitumor agents. *J. Antibiot.* **1990**, *43*, 1524–1532. [CrossRef] [PubMed]
97. Li, L.; Dai, H.J.; Ye, M.; Wang, S.L.; Xiao, X.J.; Zheng, J.; Chen, H.Y.; Luo, Y.H.; Liu, J. Lycorine induces cell-cycle arrest in the G0/G1 phase in K562 cells via HDAC inhibition. *Cancer Cell Int.* **2012**, *12*, 49. [CrossRef] [PubMed]
98. Parolin, C.; Calonghi, N.; Presta, E.; Boga, C.; Caruana, P.; Naldi, M.; Andrisano, V.; Masotti, L.; Sartor, G. Mechanism and stereoselectivity of HDAC 1 inhibition by (R)-9-hydroxystearic acid in colon cancer. *Biochim. Biophys. Acta* **2012**, *1821*, 1334–1340. [CrossRef] [PubMed]
99. Ghosh, A.K.; Kulkarni, S. Enantioselective total synthesis of (+)-largazole, a potent inhibitor of histone deacetylase. *Org. Lett.* **2008**, *10*, 3907–3909. [CrossRef] [PubMed]

100. Druesne, N.; Pagniez, A.; Mayeur, C.; Thomas, M.; Cherbuy, C.; Duee, P.H.; Martel, P.; Chaumontet, C. Diallyl disulfide (DADS) increases histone acetylation and p21(waf1/cip1) expression in human colon tumor cell lines. *Carcinogenesis* **2004**, *25*, 1227–1236. [CrossRef] [PubMed]
101. Lea, M.A.; Rasheed, M.; Randolph, V.M.; Khan, F.; Shareef, A.; desBordes, C. Induction of histone acetylation and inhibition of growth of mouse erythroleukemia cells by S-allylmercaptocysteine. *Nutr. Cancer* **2002**, *43*, 90–102. [CrossRef] [PubMed]
102. Ververis, K.; Hiong, A.; Karagiannis, T.C.; Licciardi, P.V. Histone deacetylase inhibitors (HDACIs): Multitargeted anticancer agents. *Biologics* **2013**, *7*, 47–60. [CrossRef] [PubMed]
103. Robertson, F.M.; Chu, K.; Boley, K.M.; Ye, Z.; Liu, H.; Wright, M.C.; Moraes, R.; Zhang, X.; Green, T.L.; Barsky, S.H.; et al. The class I HDAC inhibitor romidepsin targets inflammatory breast cancer tumor emboli and synergizes with paclitaxel to inhibit metastasis. *J. Exp. Ther. Oncol.* **2013**, *10*, 219–233. [PubMed]
104. Paller, C.J.; Wissing, M.D.; Mendonca, J.; Sharma, A.; Kim, E.; Kim, H.S.; Kortenhorst, M.S.Q.; Gerber, S.; Rosen, M.; Shaikh, F.; et al. Combining the pan-aurora kinase inhibitor AMG 900 with histone deacetylase inhibitors enhances antitumor activity in prostate cancer. *Cancer Med.* **2014**, *3*, 1322–1335. [CrossRef] [PubMed]
105. Ferrarelli, L.K. HDAC inhibitors in solid tumors and blood cancers. *Sci. Signal.* **2016**, *9*, ec216. [CrossRef]
106. Vancurova, I.; Uddin, M.M.; Zou, Y.; Vancura, A. Combination Therapies Targeting HDAC and IKK in Solid Tumors. *Trends Pharmacol. Sci.* **2018**, *39*, 295–306. [CrossRef] [PubMed]
107. Marks, P.A.; Breslow, R. Dimethyl sulfoxide to vorinostat: Development of this histone deacetylase inhibitor as an anticancer drug. *Nat. Biotechnol.* **2007**, *25*, 84–90. [CrossRef] [PubMed]
108. Giaccone, G.; Rajan, A.; Berman, A.; Kelly, R.J.; Szabo, E.; Lopez-Chavez, A.; Trepel, J.; Lee, M.J.; Cao, L.; Espinoza-Delgado, I.; et al. Phase II study of belinostat in patients with recurrent or refractory advanced thymic epithelial tumors. *J. Clin. Oncol.* **2011**, *29*, 2052–2059. [CrossRef] [PubMed]
109. Duvic, M.; Dummer, R.; Becker, J.C.; Poulalhon, N.; Ortiz Romero, P.; Grazia Bernengo, M.; Lebbé, C.; Assaf, C.; Squier, M.; Williams, D.; et al. Panobinostat activity in both bexarotene- exposed and -naive patients with refractory cutaneous T-cell lymphoma: Results of a phase II trial. *Eur. J. Cancer* **2013**, *49*, 386–394. [CrossRef] [PubMed]
110. Rambaldi, A.; Dummer, R.; Becker, J.C.; Poulalhon, N.; Ortiz, R.P.; Grazia, B.M.; Lebbe, C.; Assaf, C.; Squier, M.; Williams, D.; et al. A pilot study of the Histone-Deacetylase inhibitor Givinostat in patients with JAK2V617F positive chronic myeloproliferative neoplasms. *Br. J. Haematol.* **2010**, *150*, 446–455. [CrossRef] [PubMed]
111. Razak, A.R.; Hotte, S.J.; Siu, L.L.; Chen, E.X.; Hirte, H.W.; Powers, J.; Walsh, W.; Stayner, L.A.; Laughlin, A.; Novotny-Diermayr, V.; et al. Phase I clinical, pharmacokinetic and pharmacodynamic study of SB939, an oral histone deacetylase (HDAC) inhibitor, in patients with advanced solid tumours. *Br. J. Cancer* **2011**, *104*, 756–762. [CrossRef] [PubMed]
112. Pili, R.; Salumbides, B.; Zhao, M.; Altiok, S.; Qian, D.; Zwiebel, J.; Carducci, M.A.; Rudek, M.A. Phase I study of the histone deacetylase inhibitor entinostat in combination with 13-cis retinoic acid in patients with solid tumours. *Br. J. Cancer* **2012**, *106*, 77–84. [CrossRef] [PubMed]
113. Banerji, U.; van Doorn, L.; Papadatos-Pastos, D.; Kristeleit, R.; Debnam, P.; Tall, M.; Stewart, A.; Raynaud, F.; Garrett, M.D.; Toal, M.; et al. A phase I pharmacokinetic and pharmacodynamics study of CHR-3996, an oral class I selective histone deacetylase inhibitor in refractory solid tumors. *Clin. Cancer Res.* **2012**, *18*, 2687–2694. [CrossRef] [PubMed]
114. Dong, M.; Ning, Z.Q.; Xing, P.Y.; Xu, J.L.; Cao, H.X.; Dou, G.F.; Meng, Z.Y.; Shi, Y.K.; Lu, X.P.; Feng, F.Y. Phase I study of chidamide (CS055/HBI-8000), a new histone deacetylase inhibitor, in patients with advanced solid tumors and lymphomas. *Cancer Chemother. Pharmacol.* **2012**, *69*, 1413–1422. [CrossRef] [PubMed]
115. Eckschlager, T.; Plch, J.; Stiborova, M.; Hrabeta, J. Histone Deacetylase Inhibitors as Anticancer Drugs. *Int. J. Mol. Sci.* **2017** *18*, 1414. [CrossRef] [PubMed]
116. Younes, A.; Oki, Y.; Bociek, R.G.; Kuruvilla, J.; Fanale, M.; Neelapu, S.; Copeland, A.; Buglio, D.; Galal, A.; Besterman, J.; et al. Mocetinostat for relapsed classical Hodgkin's lymphoma: An open-label, single-arm, phase 2 trial. *Lancet Oncol.* **2011**, *12*, 1222–1228. [CrossRef]
117. Coiffier, B.; Pro, B.; Prince, H.M.; Foss, F.; Sokol, L.; Greenwood, M.; Caballero, D.; Borchmann, P.; Morschhausér, F.; Wilhelm, M.; et al. Results from a pivotal, open-label, phase II study of romidepsin

in relapsed or refractory peripheral T-cell lymphoma after prior systemic therapy. *J. Clin. Oncol.* **2012**, *30*, 631–636. [CrossRef] [PubMed]
118. Bolden, J.E.; Peart, M.J.; Johnstone, R.W. Anticancer activities of histone deacetylase inhibitors. *Nat. Rev. Drug Discov.* **2006**, *5*, 769–784. [CrossRef] [PubMed]
119. Bao, L.; Diao, H.; Dong, N.; Xu, S.; Wang, B.; Mo, Q.; Yu, H.; Wang, X.; Chen, C. Histone deacetylase inhibitor induces cell apoptosis and cycle arrest in lung cancer cell via mitochondrial injury and p53 up-acetylation. *Cell Biol. Toxicol.* **2016**, *32*, 469–482. [CrossRef] [PubMed]
120. Kretsovali, A.; Hadjimichael, C.; Charmpilas, N. Histone deacetylase inhibitors in cell pluripotency, differentiation, and reprogramming. *Stem Cells Int.* **2012**, *2012*, 184154. [CrossRef] [PubMed]
121. Vrana, J.A.; Decker, R.H.; Johnson, C.R.; Wang, Z.; Jarvis, W.D.; Richon, V.M.; Ehinger, M.; Fisher, P.B.; Grant, S. Induction of apoptosis in U937 human leukemia cells by suberoylanilide hydroxamic acid (SAHA) proceeds through pathways that are regulated by Bcl-2/Bcl-XL, c-Jun, and p21CIP1, but independent of p53. *Oncogene* **1999**, *18*, 7016–7025. [CrossRef] [PubMed]
122. Richon, V.M.; Sandhoff, T.W.; Rifkind, R.A.; Marks, P.A. Histone deacetylase inhibitor selectively induces p21WAF1 expression and gene-associated histone acetylation. *Proc. Natl. Acad. Sci. USA* **2000**, *97*, 10014–10019. [CrossRef] [PubMed]
123. Xu, W.S.; Parmigiani, R.B.; Marks, P.A. Histone deacetylase inhibitors: molecular mechanisms of action. *Oncogene* **2007**, *26*, 5541–5552. [CrossRef] [PubMed]
124. Singh, A.K.; Kumar, R.; Pandey, A.K. Hepatocellular carcinoma: Causes, mechanism of progression and biomarkers. *Curr. Chem. Genom. Transl. Med.* **2018**, Accepted-in press.
125. Hitomi, T.; Matsuzaki, Y.; Yokota, T.; Takaoka, Y.; Sakai, T. p15 (INK4b) in HDAC inhibitor-induced growth arrest. *FEBS Lett* **2003**, *554*, 347–350. [CrossRef]
126. Suzuki, T.; Yokozaki, H.; Kuniyasu, H.; Hayashi, K.; Naka, K.; Ono, S.; Ishikawa, T.; Tahara, E.; Yasui, W. Effect of trichostatin A on cell growth and expression of cell cycle- and apoptosis-related molecules in humangastric and oral carcinoma cell lines. *Int. J. Cancer* **2000**, *88*, 992–997. [CrossRef]
127. Nakata, S.; Yoshida, T.; Horinaka, M.; Shiraishi, T.; Wakada, M.; Sakai, T. Histone deacetylase inhibitors upregulate death receptor 5/TRAIL-R2 and sensitize apoptosis induced by TRAIL/APO2-L in human malignant tumor cells. *Oncogene* **2004**, *23*, 6261–6271. [CrossRef] [PubMed]
128. Glick, R.D.; Swendeman, S.L.; Coffey, D.C.; Rifkind, R.A.; Marks, P.A.; Richon, V.M.; Michael, P.; La-Quaglia, M.P. Hybrid polar histone deacetylase inhibitor induces apoptosis and CD95/ CD95 ligand expression in human neuroblastoma. *Cancer Res.* **1999**, *59*, 4392–4399. [PubMed]
129. Insinga, A.; Monestiroli, S.; Ronzoni, S.; Gelmetti, V.; Marchesi, F.; Viale, A.; Altucci, L.; Nervi, C.; Minucci, S.; Pelicci, P.G. Inhibitors of histone deacetylases induce tumor-selective apoptosis through activation of the death receptor pathway. *Nat. Med.* **2005**, *11*, 71–76. [CrossRef] [PubMed]
130. Zhao, Y.; Tan, J.; Zhuang, L.; Jiang, X.; Liu, E.T.; Yu, Q. Inhibitors of histone deacetylases target the Rb-E2F1 pathway for apoptosis induction through activation of proapoptotic protein Bim. *Proc. Natl. Acad. Sci. USA* **2005**, *102*, 16090–16095. [CrossRef] [PubMed]
131. Ruefli, A.A.; Bernhard, D.; Tainton, K.M.; Kofler, R.; Smyth, M.J.; Johnstone, R.W. Suberoylanilide hydroxamic acid (SAHA) overcomes multidrug resistance and induces cell death in P-glycoprotein-expressing cells. *Int. J. Cancer* **2002**, *99*, 292–298. [CrossRef] [PubMed]
132. Sharma, A.K.; Kumar, S.; Chashoo, G.; Saxena, A.K.; Pandey, A.K. Cell cycle inhibitory activity of Piper longum against A549 cell line and its protective effect against metal-induced toxicity in rats. *Ind. J. Biochem. Biophys.* **2014**, *51*, 358–364.
133. Rosato, R.R.; Maggio, S.C.; Almenara, J.A.; Payne, S.G.; Atadja, P.; Spiegel, S.; Dent, P.; Grant, S. The histone deacetylase inhibitor LAQ824 induces human leukemia cell death through a process involving XIAP down-regulation, oxidative injury, and the acid sphingomyelinase-dependent generation of ceramide. *Mol. Pharmacol.* **2006**, *69*, 216–225. [CrossRef] [PubMed]
134. Shao, Y.; Gao, Z.; Marks, P.A.; Jiang, X. Apoptotic and autophagic cell death induced by histone deacetylase inhibitors. *Proc. Natl. Acad. Sci. USA* **2004**, *101*, 18030–18035. [CrossRef] [PubMed]
135. Zhang, J.; Ng, S.; Wang, J.; Zhou, J.; Tan, S.H.; Yang, N.; Lin, Q.; Xia, D.; Shen, H.M. Histone deacetylase inhibitors induce autophagy through FOXO1-dependent pathways. *Autophagy* **2015**, *11*, 629–642. [CrossRef] [PubMed]

136. Hrzenjak, A.; Kremser, M.L.; Strohmeier, B.; Moinfar, F.; Zatloukal, K.; Denk, H. SAHA induces caspase-independent, autophagic cell death of endometrial stromal sarcoma cells by influencing the mTOR pathway. *J. Pathol.* **2008**, *216*, 495–504. [CrossRef] [PubMed]
137. Liu, Y.L.; Yang, P.M.; Shun, C.T.; Wu, M.S.; Weng, J.R.; Chen, C.C. Autophagy potentiates the anti-cancer effects of the histone deacetylase inhibitors in hepatocellular carcinoma. *Autophagy* **2010**, *6*, 1057–1065. [CrossRef] [PubMed]
138. Shulak, L.; Beljanski, V.; Chiang, C.; Dutta, M.; Van Grevenynghe, J.; Belgnaoui, S.M.; Nguyen, L.; Di Lenardo, T.; Semmes, O.J.; Lin, R.; et al. Histone deacetylase inhibitors potentiate vesicular stomatitis virus oncolysis in prostate cancer cells by modulating NF-κB-dependent autophagy. *J. Virol.* **2014**, *88*, 2927–2940. [CrossRef] [PubMed]
139. Oh, M.; Choi, I.K.; Kwon, H.J. Inhibition of histone deacetylase1 induces autophagy. *Biochem. Biophys. Res. Commun.* **2008**, *369*, 1179–1183. [CrossRef] [PubMed]
140. Chiao, M.T.; Cheng, W.Y.; Yang, Y.C.; Shen, C.C.; Ko, J.L. Suberoylanilide hydroxamic acid (SAHA) causes tumor growth slowdown and triggers autophagy in glioblastoma stem cells. *Autophagy* **2013**, *9*, 1509–1526. [CrossRef] [PubMed]
141. Zupkovitz, G.; Tischler, J.; Posch, M.; Sadzak, I.; Ramsauer, K.; Egger, G.; Grausenburger, R.; Schweifer, N.; Chiocca, S.; Decker, T.; et al. Negative and positive regulation of gene expression by mouse histone deacetylase 1. *Mol. Cell Biol.* **2006**, *26*, 7913–7928. [CrossRef] [PubMed]
142. Liang, D.; Kong, X.; Sang, N. Effects of histone deacetylase inhibitors on HIF-1. *Cell Cycle* **2006**, *5*, 2430–2435. [CrossRef] [PubMed]
143. Jeong, J.W.; Bae, M.K.; Ahn, M.Y.; Kim, S.H.; Sohn, T.K.; Bae, M.H.; Yoo, M.A.; Song, E.J.; Lee, K.J.; Kim, K.W. Regulation and destabilization of HIF-1alpha by ARD1-mediated acetylation. *Cell* **2002**, *111*, 709–720. [CrossRef]
144. Qian, D.Z.; Kachhap, S.K.; Collis, S.J.; Verheul, H.M.; Carducci, M.A.; Atadja, P.; Pili, R. Class II histone deacetylases arenassociated with VHL-independent regulation of hypoxiainducible factor 1{alpha}. *Cancer Res.* **2006**, *66*, 8814–8821. [CrossRef] [PubMed]
145. Fath, D.M.; Kong, X.; Liang, D.; Lin, Z.; Chou, A.; Jiang, Y.; Fang, J.; Caro, J.; Sang, N. Histone deacetylase inhibitors repress the transactivation potential of hypoxia-inducible factors independently of direct acetylation of HIF-alpha. *J. Biol. Chem.* **2006**, *281*, 13612–13619. [CrossRef] [PubMed]
146. Deroanne, C.F.; Bonjean, K.; Servotte, S.; Devy, L.; Colige, A.; Clausse, N.; Blacher, S.; Verdin, E.; Foidart, J.M.; Nusgens, B.V.; et al. Histone deacetylases inhibitors as anti-angiogenic agents altering vascular endothelial growth factor signalling. *Oncogene* **2002**, *21*, 427–436. [CrossRef] [PubMed]
147. Cinatl, J.; Kotchetkov, R.; Blaheta, R.; Driever, P.H.; Vogel, J.U.; Cinatl, J. Induction of differentiation and suppression of malignant phenotype of human neuroblastoma BE(2)-C cells by valproic acid: Enhancement by combination with interferon α. *Int. J. Oncol.* **2002**, *20*, 97–106. [CrossRef] [PubMed]
148. Sharma, U.K.; Kumar, R.; Gupta, A.; Ganguly, R.; Pandey, A.K. Renoprotective effect of cinnamaldehyde in food color induced toxicity. *3 Biotech* **2018**, *8*, 212. [CrossRef] [PubMed]
149. Sharma, U.K.; Sharma, A.K.; Gupta, A.; Kumar, R.; Pandey, A.; Pandey, A.K. Pharmacological activities of cinnamaldehyde and eugenol: antioxidant, cytotoxic and anti-leishmanial studies. *Cell. Mol. Biol. (Noisy-le-grand)* **2017**, *63*, 73–78. [CrossRef] [PubMed]
150. Kumar, S.; Pandey, S.; Pandey, A.K. In vitro antibacterial, antioxidant, cytotoxic activities of Parthenium hysterophorus and characterization of extracts by LC MS analysis. *BioMed Res. Int.* **2014**, *2014*, 495154. [CrossRef] [PubMed]
151. Sharma, A.K.; Sharma, U.K.; Pandey, A.K. Protective effect of *Bauhinia variegata* leaf extracts against oxidative damage, cell proliferation and bacterial growth. *Proc. Natl. Acad. Sci. India, Sect. B Biol. Sci.* **2017**, *87*, 47–51. [CrossRef]
152. Rosato, R.R.; Almenara, J.A.; Grant, S. The histone deacetylase inhibitor MS-275 promotes differentiation or apoptosis in human leukemia cells through a process regulated by generation of reactive oxygen species and induction of p21CIP1/WAF1 1. *Cancer Res.* **2003**, *63*, 3637–3645. [PubMed]
153. Ruefli, A.A.; Ausserlechner, M.J.; Bernhard, D.; Sutton, V.R.; Tainton, K.M.; Kofler, R.; Smyth, M.J.; Johnstone, R.W. The histone deacetylase inhibitor and chemotherapeutic agent suberoylanilide hydroximic

acid (SAHA) induces a cell-death pathway characterized by cleavage of Bid and production of reactive oxygen species. *Proc. Natl. Acad. Sci. USA* **2001**, *98*, 10833–10838. [CrossRef] [PubMed]

154. Kumar, S.; Pandey, A.K. Free radicals: Health implications and their mitigation by herbals. *Br. J. Med. Med. Res.* **2015**, *7*, 438–457. [CrossRef]
155. Xu, W.; Ngo, L.; Perez, G.; Dokmanovic, M.; Marks, P.A. Intrinsic apoptotic and thioredoxin pathways in human prostate cancer cell response to histone deacetylase inhibitor. *Proc. Natl. Acad. Sci. USA* **2006**, *103*, 15540–15545. [CrossRef] [PubMed]
156. Saitoh, M.; Nishitoh, H.; Fujii, M.; Takeda, K.; Tobiume, K.; Sawada, Y.; Kawabata, M.; Miyazono, K.; Ichijo, H. Mammalian thioredoxin is a direct inhibitor of apoptosis signal-regulating kinase (ASK) 1. *EMBO J.* **1998**, *17*, 2596–2606. [CrossRef] [PubMed]
157. Cimini, D.; Mattiuzzo, M.; Torosantucci, L.; Degrassi, F. Histone hyperacetylation in mitosis prevents sister chromatid separation and produces chromosome segregation defects. *Mol. Biol. Cell* **2003**, *14*, 3821–3833. [CrossRef] [PubMed]
158. Kumar, S.; Chashoo, G.; Saxena, A.K.; Pandey, A.K. *Parthenium hysterophorus*: A Probable Source of Anticancer, Antioxidant and Anti-HIV Agents. *BioMed Res. Int.* **2013**, *2013*, 810734. [CrossRef] [PubMed]
159. Khabele, D. The Therapeutic Potential of Class I Selective Histone Deacetylase Inhibitors in Ovarian Cancer. *Front. Oncol.* **2014**, *4*, 111. [CrossRef] [PubMed]
160. Santoro, F.; Botrugno, O.A.; Dal, Z.R.; Pallavicini, I.; Matthews, G.M.; Cluse, L.; Barozzi, I.; Senese, S.; Fornasari, L.; Moretti, S.; et al. dual role for Hdac1: oncosuppressor in tumorigenesis, oncogene in tumor maintenance. *Blood* **2013**, 3459–3468. [CrossRef] [PubMed]

8

The Multitarget Activity of Natural Extracts on Cancer: Synergy and Xenohormesis

María Herranz-López, María Losada-Echeberría and Enrique Barrajón-Catalán *

Instituto de Biología Molecular y Celular (IBMC) and Instituto de Investigación, Desarrollo e Innovación en Biotecnología Sanitaria de Elche (IDiBE), Universitas Miguel Hernández 03202 Elche, Spain; mherranz@umh.es (M.H.-L.); mlosada@umh.es (M.L.-E.)

* Correspondence: e.barrajon@umh.es;

Abstract: It is estimated that over 60% of the approved drugs and new drug developments for cancer and infectious diseases are from natural origin. The use of natural compounds as a potential source of antitumor agents has been deeply studied in many cancer models, both in vitro and in vivo. Most of the Western medicine studies are based on the use of highly selective pure compounds with strong specificity for their targets such as colchicine or taxol. Nevertheless, approximately 60% of fairly specific drugs in their initial research fail because of toxicity or ineffectiveness in late-stage preclinical studies. Moreover, cancer is a multifaceted disease that in most cases deserves a polypharmacological therapeutic approach. Complex plant-derived mixtures such as natural extracts are difficult to characterize and hardly exhibit high pharmacological potency. However, in some cases, these may provide an advantage due to their multitargeted mode of action and potential synergistic behavior. The polypharmacology approach appears to be a plausible explanation for the multigargeted mechanism of complex natural extracts on different proteins within the same signalling pathway and in several biochemical pathways at once. This review focuses on the different aspects of natural extracts in the context of anticancer activity drug development, with special attention to synergy studies and xenohormesis.

Keywords: cancer; natural compound; synergy; xenohormesis; polypharmacology

1. Introduction

Cancer is not a single disease, but a complex clinical situation in which multiple molecular pathways and cellular processes are compromised. Each cancer type has its own molecular fingerprint and, at least one of the cancer hallmarks described in [1], is altered. However, in spite of this heterogeneous situation, all cancers have a common behavior based on uncontrolled proliferation and invasion. This invasive phenotype is the real clinical problem and, in most cases, still remains unresolved, causing morbidity and mortality.

Anticancer research and drug discovery are continuously increasing the therapeutic arsenal, and relevant advances have been made towards individualized treatments [2–5]. New antibody-based drugs, called biological treatments [6,7], have improved treatments and prognosis in some cancer types such as breast, lung, liver cancers and lymphoma. New specific inhibitor families have also been developed, especially against proliferation related kinases. These drugs are called "inibs" [8,9]. In this sense, there is a tendency to look for highly specific drugs within the low micromolar range to solve very specific, almost individual cases. In vitro and in silico approaches have propelled the development of these specific drugs, and our bibliography is full of these examples [10–13]. These specific drugs follow the classic pharmacological dogma "one drug-one target", but in spite of their undeniable value, they lack some relevant aspects that will be discussed in the following sections.

On the contrary, the molecular promiscuity of some molecules, especially those from natural origin [14,15], allow them to exert a potential multitarget mechanism of action. These compounds are able to interact with different targets, modifying different pathways or different steps of the same signaling cascade. In addition, promiscuity is not always due to a single compound but a mixture of compounds, as occurs in some complex natural extracts. In these cases, each compound is able to interact with one or multiple targets, increasing the pharmacological promiscuity of the whole drug. In addition, natural extracts or their main components can be combined with conventional chemotherapy, reducing the development of resistance to antitumor drugs and toxic effects [16].

This review will be focused on discussing the advantages and drawbacks of the use of natural extracts when compared with classical individual targeting strategy. Xenohormesis, multitargeting, synergy and drug resistance will be the main points that will be addressed.

2. Natural Compounds, Hormesis and Xenohormesis

Chemistry and analytical advances have allowed the synthesis and characterization of millions of new molecules for drug discovery. In some cases, synthesis was structurally guided using in silico or structural approaches, in others, combinatorial libraries were built based on a molecular scaffold or leads. This approach has allowed the development of new drugs not only for cancer treatment but also for other diseases. However, all these drugs have been human-designed and lack natural origin. On the contrary, natural extracts and their compounds have been selected for by millions of years of evolution as complex sources of medicinal agents. This is the basis of xenohormesis hypothesis [17,18]. They present very diverse chemical structures, from the simplest phenolic acids in plants to the most complex marine compounds [19–21]. Glycosylation, methylation and other esterifications and the presence of other moieties, increase the number and diversity of natural compounds. This constitutes a countless and invaluable source of new drugs. From a biomedical point of view, hormesis is an adaptive response in which the exposure to a low dose of an environmental factor or chemical compound, that is harmful at high concentrations, has a beneficial and/or adaptive effect on a cell or organism. Sometimes this response is mediated by some compounds that, when incorporated in the heterotroph diet, induce biological responses leading to pharmacological effects. This final effect is called xenohormesis, as the final benefit is obtained by the heterotroph organism, not for the plant that originally adapted to the stressful condition [17,18]. Xenohormesis is a way of cross-species interaction and communication.

Although hormesis is an essential concept in evolution, xenohormesis has also allowed the expansion and fixation of evolutionary advances in non-autotrophs organisms. Nowadays, xenohormesis gives us a chance to obtain benefits from natural compounds and obtain new drugs selected by nature all through the evolution process. These compounds can be used directly for anticancer drug discovery, and also as new leads in novel developments using the classical structurally guided or in silico approaches. This is one of the main advantages of natural extracts and their compounds. They can be used as any other drugs, but with the benefit of being selected by natural evolution.

3. Combined Therapies, Multitargeting and Synergy

Based on the classic pharmacological dogma "one drug-one target", monotherapy has been the traditional approach, not only to treat diseases, but also to find new active drugs against a chosen target. However, presently there is evidence pointing out that combined therapies are much more efficient than single-drug-based treatments. In this sense, combinational therapy is extended to treat not only cancer but also other diseases, such as AIDS, bacterial infections, hypertension, metabolic or rheumatic disorders [22].

Combined drug therapy design is a hard and challenging task. Individual and combined actions must be characterized and it sometimes requires new preclinical and clinical trials. In addition, these multiple comparisons are sometimes difficult to incorporate into those studies.

Combined therapies are normally based on co-administration of two or more drugs. These combined drugs can be based on the combination of pure compounds, or can be achieved by using drugs based on mixtures of natural extracts.

Combined therapies are based on targeting different molecular signatures of the disease. On the one hand, multitargeting makes drug screening more complicated as complex assays must be developed to test all possibilities. On the other hand, multitargeting creates the opportunity to obtain synergic interactions between the combined therapy elements and drug resistance development, as detailed in further sections. There is a plethora of combined chemotherapy treatments covering most of the different cancer phenotypes. In fact, most of the recommended treatment regimens include two or more drugs, but as mentioned above, combined therapy use is not exclusive to cancer treatments, it is also extended to other disciplines such as antimicrobial and antihypertensive diseases.

Synergy is therefore the most relevant characteristic of combined therapies, including natural extracts. The first impetus for synergy research came from pharmaceutical legislation which demands the verification that every compound of a combined pharmaceutical preparation contributes to the claimed complete efficacy [22]. In terms of pharmacology, synergy is the ability of some mixtures to be more potent than the sum of their individual components. This definition is exportable to other disciplines and is based on the complementary as well as additive mechanism of action. Accordingly, synergy is not an absolute factor and the pharmacological interaction between the components of a mixture can be more or less synergic. This aspect is the main difference between additive and synergic behavior and is sometimes forgotten by researchers and clinicians.

Another aspect to be analyzed is that a single mixture is able to perform in a different way depending on the proportion of its components. According to this, different proportions of the same compounds could provide different results in terms of synergy, not only in an absolute way, but also in terms of being more or less synergic [23]. In this sense, an ideal proportion which provides the highest synergy results is always mathematically possible.

There are several ways to develop synergy studies, but in all cases, a previous and detailed design is required to obtain conclusive results. Most synergy studies fail because of a deficient design, both in qualitative and quantitative ways. There are several exhaustive and relevant reviews on synergy [22,24–26], so this review will not go deeper into how to study it. However, some aspects about study design deserve a comment:

- Drug selection: The right selection of the drugs for synergy studies is the first step to succeed. There are multiple available drugs for a single disease, but not all are suitable for a synergy study. Drugs must be selected considering different molecular targets. If not, antagonism or other undesired pharmacological interactions can be obtained. These different molecular targets can be located in different molecules, in distinguished epitopes of the same molecule or even in molecules of different pathways.
- Synergy study method: As mentioned above, there are several methods to study synergy between drugs. Quantitative methods such as Combination Index (CI) [27] or Fractional Inhibitory Concentration Index (FICI) [14] calculation are preferred as they obtain better conclusions.
- Biological assay: According to the selected method for synergy studies, a robust and reliable biological assay must be selected that allows testing a high number of samples with a large variability in composition. Survival or viability tests are diverse and allow high throughput screening approaches [28]. They are commonly used for anticancer compound research, but also for most of the other areas of drug discovery in which synergy is topical, such as antimicrobial drug discovery.
- Sample testing: Once the test is selected, an adequate design of the plates is also crucial. Checkboard plate design is probably the best approach for pairwise combinations using multi-wells plates. This strategy can be used not only for pairwise combinations but also for 3-drug combinations as shown in Figure 1.

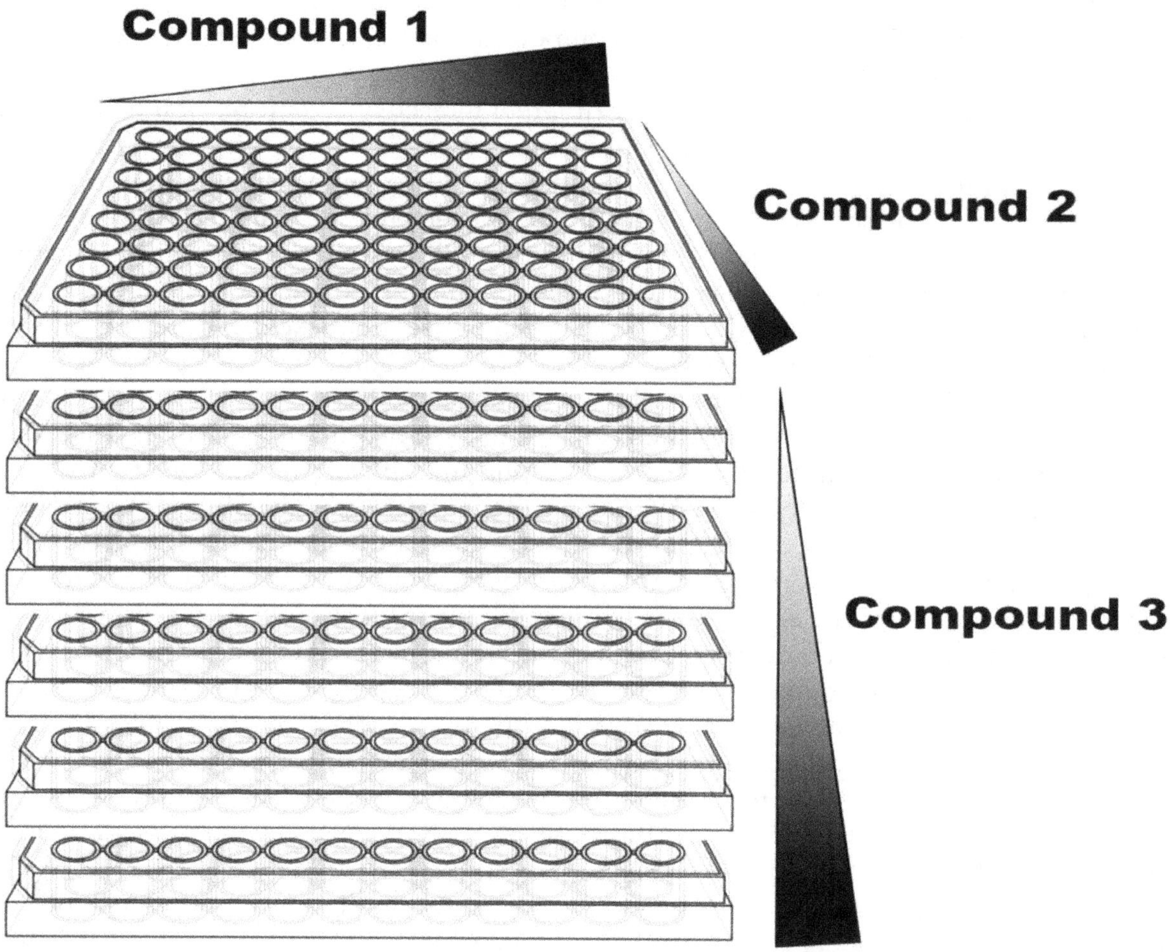

Figure 1. Checkboard plate design can be used not only for single plate experiments but also for more complex studies using three different compounds. In these cases, the concentration of each compound increases in one of the three dimensions (*x*, *y* and *z* axis) as indicated in the figure.

Following these recommendations, the final results will not only be scientifically relevant, but also comparable to other single drug or combined therapies. This will allow researchers and clinicians to obtain better conclusions and contribute to the development of new therapeutic approaches.

4. Examples of Synergy Studies

References to synergic interactions between drugs in cancer research are abundant in the bibliography. However, focusing on natural extract synergy studies, three main groups of examples can be classified. The first group includes studies covering complex extracts whose components present synergistic interactions among them. The second group includes examples of synergy between different extracts and natural compounds of different origin. Finally, the third group comprises examples of anticancer approved drugs combined with natural compounds or extracts. Some of the most relevant examples of each category are listed below and shown in Table 1.

Table 1. Examples of synergic interactions among compounds or compounds and approved drugs in cancer research. Main examples included in this manuscript are shown in this table, organized in rows. First and second columns indicate the name of the components among which synergy is obtained. Third and fourth and fifth columns show the cellular models in which synergy studies were performed (including their origin), the main effect and the bibliographic reference.

Extract/Compound	Synergy	Experimental Model (Cell Line)	Effect	References
Pomegranate extract	Among their compounds	Oral cancer (KB, CAL27), colon cancer (HT-29, HCT116, SW480, SW620) and prostate cancer (RWPE-1, 22Rv1)	Antiproliferative, apoptotic and antioxidant	[29]
Pomegranate extract	Among their compounds	Prostate cancer (DU 145)	Antiproliferative, antimetastatic and phospholipase A2 (PLA2) inhibition	[30]
Grape extract	Among their compounds and with Ara-C and tazofurin	Leukemia (HL-60)	Antiproliferative and apoptotic	[31]
Grape extract	Among their compounds	Colon cancer (HCT116)	Antiproliferative and apoptotic	[32]
Rosemary extract	Among their compounds	Colon cancer (HT-29)	Antiproliferative	[33]
Ginger extract	Among their compounds	Prostate cancer (PC-3)	Antiproliferative	[34]
Graviola flavonoids	Among their compounds	Prostate cancer (PC-3)	Antiproliferative	[35]
Turmeric extract	With rosemary compounds	Breast cancer (MDA-MB-453, MDA-MB-468, and MCF7)	Antiproliferative, G1 cell cycle arrest	[36]
Tea extract	With capsicum compounds	Cervical cancer (HeLa) and breast cancer (4T1)	Antiproliferative	[37]
Tea extract	With soy compounds	Mice *in vivo* model	Metabolic effect	[38]
Tea extract	With soy compounds	Prostate cancer (LnCAP) xenotrasplants	Antiproliferative	[39]
Tea extract	With others tea extracts	Review	Antioxidant, antimicrobial and antitumoral	[40]
Resveratrol	With quercetin and ellagic acid	Leukemia (MOLT-4)	Antiproliferative, apoptosis and cel cycle arrest	[41,42]
Carothenoids	With other phytochemicals	Prostate cancer LNCaP , PC-3 and DU-145) and breast cancer (MCF-7)	Antiproliferative	[43]
Genistein	With cisplatin, 5-fluorouracil, arsenic trioxide, doxorubicin, gemcitabine camptothecine and hidroxi-camptothecine	Pancreatic cancer (BxPC-3 xenograft, COL-357 and L3.6pl) colon cancer (HT29), hepatic cancer (HepG2, Hep3B, SK-Hep-1, HEpG2 xenograft), cervical cancer (HeLa) ovarian cancer (OAW-42), bladder cancer (TCC-SUP) and lung cancer (ME-180pt, UMSCC-5)	Antiproliferative	[44]
Curcumin	With 5-fluorouracil, oxaliplatin, cisplatin, etoposide, camptothecine and doxorubicine	Colon cancer (HT-29), ovarian cancer (2008 and C13) and human and rat glioblastoma cell lines	Antiproliferative	[44]
(-)-epìgallocatechin-3-gallate	With doxorubicin, gemcitabine and cisplatin	Carcinoma doxorubicin resistant (KB-A-1 xenograft) cholangiocarcinoma (Mz-ChA-1 cell line and xenograft) and ovarian cancer (SKOC3, CAOV3 and C200)	Antiproliferative	[44]
Quercetin	With doxorubicin, cisplatin, arsenic trioxide and temozolomide	Neuroblastoma and Edwing's sarcoma cell lines, laryngeal cancer (Hep2), leukemia (U937 and HL-60) and astrocytoma	Antiproliferative	[44]
Resveratrol	With Cisplatin and doxorubicin	Acute leukemia (ML-2/DX30, AML-2/DX100 and AML-2/DX300)	Antiproliferative	[44]

Pomegranate polyphenolic extracts have demonstrated numerous biological activities such as antioxidant, cardiovascular preventive and antitumoral activities [45–48]. These extracts are enriched in ellagitannins such as ellagic acid, punicalagin and punicalin. Synergy studies between pomegranate polyphenols have been performed in colon cancer cells [29], prostate [30] and other cellular models [49]. Grape fruit is also a well-known source of active compounds, including resveratrol as the most representative one. As with pomegranate, grape extracts present abundant biological activities [31,50]. In regards to cancer and synergy studies, grape polyphenols have shown synergy between them, especially on colon cancer cell models [32]. Rosemary terpenes have also shown antitumoral synergic activity on colon cancer cells [33]. Ginger compounds [34], graviola flavonoids and acetogenin's action on prostate cancer [35] are examples of synergic interactions between different compounds included those that are present in the same extract.

In addition to single complex natural extracts, some studies have tested the synergic interactions between different extracts and/or different natural compounds, even mixing a complex natural extract with an individual natural compound. On the one hand, turmeric extracts have showed synergic activity with rosemary extracts as well as their representative compounds, carnosic acid and curcumin [36]. Tea natural compounds, mainly catechins, synergistically interact with capsicum compounds [37], soy phytochemicals [38,39] and between different tea extracts [40]. On the other hand, individual compounds such as resveratrol, quercetin and ellagic acid also interact synergistically in human leukemia cells [41,42]. Carotenoids and other phytochemicals also presented similar behavior [43]. Finally, natural compounds and extracts synergistically interact with clinically used anticancer drugs as occurs between many polyphenols and anticancer drugs such as cisplatin, doxorubicin, 5-fluoracil and others as reviewed in Reference [44].

5. Drawbacks of Using Natural Compounds

Pure natural compounds have demonstrated the same validity as synthetic or semisynthetic drugs in drug discovery. They are single compounds with a well-known chemical structure. They can be obtained from natural resources, in most cases using synthetic or semisynthetic approaches [51,52]. However, natural extracts, regardless of vegetal, microorganism or animal origin, are usually complex mixtures. Two main consequences are derived from natural extract's complexity. First, these mixtures must be chemically characterized as much as possible. The improvement of analytical techniques such as liquid and gas chromatography coupled to mass detection, magnetic resonance and other approaches have permitted the characterization of very complex extracts [23,53–55]. The second consequence is that natural extract reproducibility is sometimes difficult due to the biological diversity of samples. This depends on origin, climate conditions, storage and extraction procedures. However, as occurred in other disciplines, this drawback can be avoided by controlling crop conditions, origin and extract production.

Natural compound bioavailability is also a drawback that deserves attention. Natural compounds have very different structures and, therefore, their bioavailability depend on the individual compound [56–58]. On the one hand, some natural compounds are quickly and fully absorbed, reaching the plasma in their native form so providing significant plasmatic concentrations. On the other hand, other natural compounds have scarce absorption, high metabolized rates and a fast excretion process. In all these cases, plasmatic concentration are low and biological activities are difficult to infer. Some strategies have been developed to improve natural compound bioavailability. Such as the use of different forms of encapsulation [59]; as nanoparticles [60,61], emulsion [62] or liposomes [63]. These approaches have been used especially to increase the solubility of highly hydrophobic compounds and extracts, and to improve the bioavailability of hydrophilic compounds with low stability or poor absorption [64,65]. However, in the end, natural compounds are not quite as different to other drugs that also present bioavailability limitations, and each case must be studied independently taking in account its solubility and the ADME processes.

Drug resistance is probably the most important problem of cancer treatments. There are many drug resistance mechanisms [66,67] and no drug is free to develop a resistant phenotype. Once again, natural compounds and extracts are not different to other drugs, and resistance phenomena may also take place. Combined therapies minimize the risk of drug resistance, as tumor cells that develops resistance against one of the drugs may be affected by other drugs or compounds present in the same mixture. In this sense, natural pure compounds perform as any other drug and can be used in combination to reduce resistance, but natural extracts are mixtures that may act as a combined therapy itself, contributing to a decrease in drug-resistant phenotypes.

6. Concluding Remarks

The current state of the art shows that combined therapies using natural extracts or combination of natural compounds and polypharmacology are quite promising. This is due to both the synergic interactions between their components and the reduction of drug resistant phenotype risk. Natural extracts are naturally occurring mixtures that have been selected by hormesis processes that can be beneficial to humans according to xenohormesis theory. They are indeed real combined therapies that, if well selected and characterized, can be used for new anticancer drugs development. In this sense, the design of high-quality synergy studies is crucial and a supplementary effort in this sense is worthy.

But not everything may be considered an advantage when using natural extracts, they share some drawbacks with conventional anticancer drugs. Poor bioavailability and drug resistance mechanisms are as common among natural extracts as with conventional drugs. However, the polypharmacological properties of natural extracts makes resistance more difficult and, as occurred with other conventional drugs, bioavailability problems can be addressed using different approaches such as encapsulation. The most important disadvantage of natural extracts is their complexity and reproducibility, but as mentioned above, technical advances and quality controls during processing can overcome this problem.

In conclusion, natural extracts are a promising source of new anticancer drugs, but also suppose a challenging issue. As in the past, natural extracts will continue to be used as sources to develop new anticancer agents. These compounds have been selected on an evolutionary basis that may suppose an advantage for their performance.

Nevertheless, the same criteria for safety, efficacy and quality that are required for their synthetic counterparts must be expected. Strong efforts must be applied in extract characterization and in synergy studies. Despite these challenges, natural extracts are an irreplaceable source of new anticancer compounds that undoubtedly will allow the development of new anticancer therapies in the future.

Acknowledgments: Authors want to thank their lab supervisor, Vicente Micol, for his invaluable support.

References

1. Hanahan, D.; Weinberg, R.A. Hallmarks of cancer: The next generation. *Cell* **2011**, *144*, 646–674. [CrossRef] [PubMed]
2. Diamandis, M.; White, N.M.A.; Yousef, G.M. Personalized medicine: Marking a new epoch in cancer patient management. *Mol. Cancer Res.* **2010**, *8*, 1175–1187. [CrossRef] [PubMed]
3. Jain, K.K. Personalized medicine. *Curr. Opin. Mol. Ther.* **2002**, *4*, 548–558. [PubMed]
4. Olopade, O.I.; Grushko, T.A.; Nanda, R.; Huo, D. Advances in breast cancer: Pathways to personalized medicine. *Clin. Cancer Res.* **2008**, *14*, 7988–7999. [CrossRef] [PubMed]
5. Wang, E.; Zaman, N.; McGee, S.; Milanese, J.S.; Masoudi-Nejad, A.; O'Connor-McCourt, M. Predictive genomics: A cancer hallmark network framework for predicting tumor clinical phenotypes using genome sequencing data. *Semin. Cancer Biol.* **2015**, *30*, 4–12. [CrossRef] [PubMed]
6. Scott, A.M.; Wolchok, J.D.; Old, L.J. Antibody therapy of cancer. *Nat. Rev. Cancer* **2012**, *12*, 278–287. [CrossRef] [PubMed]
7. Weiner, L.M.; Surana, R.; Wang, S. Monoclonal antibodies: Versatile platforms for cancer immunotherapy. *Nat. Rev. Immunol.* **2010**, *10*, 317–327. [CrossRef]
8. Lee, Y.T.; Tan, Y.J.; Oon, C.E. Molecular targeted therapy: Treating cancer with specificity. *Eur. J. Pharmacol.* **2018**, *834*, 188–196. [CrossRef]
9. Arora, A.; Scholar, E.M. Role of tyrosine kinase inhibitors in cancer therapy. *J. Pharmacol. Exp. Ther.* **2005**, *315*, 971–979. [CrossRef]
10. Edelman, L.B.; Eddy, J.A.; Price, N.D. In silico models of cancer. *Wiley Interdiscip. Rev. Syst. Biol. Med.* **2010**, *2*, 438–459. [CrossRef]
11. Ruiz-Torres, V.; Losada-Echeberría, M.; Herranz-López, M.; Barrajón-Catalán, E.; Galiano, V.; Micol, V.; Encinar, A.J. New Mammalian Target of Rapamycin (mTOR) Modulators Derived from Natural Product Databases and Marine Extracts by Using Molecular Docking Techniques. *Mar. Drugs* **2018**, *16*, 385. [CrossRef] [PubMed]

12. Bellamy, W.T. Prediction of Response to Drug Therapy of Cancer: A Review of In Vitro Assays. *Drugs* **1992**, *44*, 690–708. [CrossRef] [PubMed]
13. Nyga, A.; Cheema, U.; Loizidou, M. 3D tumour models: Novel in vitro approaches to cancer studies. *J. Cell Commun. Signal.* **2011**, *5*, 239–248. [CrossRef] [PubMed]
14. Barrajon-Catalan, E.; Herranz-Lopez, M.; Joven, J.; Segura-Carretero, A.; Alonso-Villaverde, C.; Menendez, J.A.; Micol, V. Molecular promiscuity of plant polyphenols in the management of age-related diseases: Far beyond their antioxidant properties. *Adv. Exp. Med. Biol.* **2014**, *824*, 141–159. [PubMed]
15. Joven, J.; Rull, A.; Rodriguez-Gallego, E.; Camps, J.; Riera-Borrull, M.; Hernández-Aguilera, A.; Martin-Paredero, V.; Segura-Carretero, A.; Micol, V.; Alonso-Villaverde, C.; et al. Multifunctional targets of dietary polyphenols in disease: A case for the chemokine network and energy metabolism. *Food Chem. Toxicol.* **2013**, *51*, 267–279. [CrossRef] [PubMed]
16. Rejhová, A.; Opattová, A.; Čumová, A.; Slíva, D.; Vodička, P. Natural compounds and combination therapy in colorectal cancer treatment. *Eur. J. Med. Chem.* **2018**, *144*, 582–594. [CrossRef] [PubMed]
17. Howitz, K.T.; Sinclair, D.A. Xenohormesis: Sensing the chemical cues of other species. *Cell* **2008**, *133*, 387–391. [CrossRef]
18. Menendez, J.A.; Joven, J.; Aragones, G.; Barrajon-Catalan, E.; Beltran-Debon, R.; Borras-Linares, I.; Camps, J.; Corominas-Faja, B.; Cufi, S.; Fernandez-Arroyo, S.; et al. Xenohormetic and anti-aging activity of secoiridoid polyphenols present in extra virgin olive oil: A new family of gerosuppressant agents. *Cell Cycle* **2013**, *12*, 555–578. [CrossRef]
19. Ruiz-Torres, V.; Encinar, J.; Herranz-López, M.; Pérez-Sánchez, A.; Galiano, V.; Barrajón-Catalán, E.; Micol, V. An Updated Review on Marine Anticancer Compounds: The Use of Virtual Screening for the Discovery of Small-Molecule Cancer Drugs. *Molecules* **2017**, *22*, 1037. [CrossRef]
20. Grochowski, D.M.; Skalicka-Wozniak, K.; Orhan, I.E.; Xiao, J.; Locatelli, M.; Piwowarski, J.P.; Granica, S.; Tomczyk, M. A comprehensive review of agrimoniin. *Ann. N. Y. Acad. Sci.* **2017**, *1401*, 166–180. [CrossRef]
21. Grochowski, D.M.; Locatelli, M.; Granica, S.; Cacciagrano, F.; Tomczyk, M. A Review on the Dietary Flavonoid Tiliroside. *Compr. Rev. Food Sci. Food Saf.* **2018**, *17*, 1395–1421. [CrossRef]
22. Wagner, H.; Ulrich-Merzenich, G. Synergy research: Approaching a new generation of phytopharmaceuticals. *Phytomedicine* **2009**, *16*, 97–110. [CrossRef] [PubMed]
23. Tomas-Menor, L.; Barrajon-Catalan, E.; Segura-Carretero, A.; Marti, N.; Saura, D.; Menendez, J.A.; Joven, J.; Micol, V. The promiscuous and synergic molecular interaction of polyphenols in bactericidal activity: An opportunity to improve the performance of antibiotics? *Phytother. Res.* **2015**, *29*, 466–473. [CrossRef] [PubMed]
24. Roell, K.R.; Reif, D.M.; Motsinger-Reif, A.A. An Introduction to Terminology and Methodology of Chemical Synergy-Perspectives from Across Disciplines. *Front. Pharmacol.* **2017**, *8*, 158. [CrossRef] [PubMed]
25. Chou, T.C. Drug combination studies and their synergy quantification using the chou-talalay method. *Cancer Res.* **2010**, *70*, 440–446. [CrossRef] [PubMed]
26. Greco, W.R.; Bravo, G.; Parsons, J.C. The search for synergy: A critical review from a response surface perspective. *Pharmacol. Rev.* **1995**, *47*, 331–385. [PubMed]
27. Chou, T.C. Theoretical basis, experimental design, and computerized simulation of synergism and antagonism in drug combination studies. *Pharmacol. Rev.* **2006**, *58*, 621–681. [CrossRef]
28. Stoddart, M.J. Cell viability assays: Introduction. *Methods Mol. Biol. (Clifton, N.J.)* **2011**, *740*, 1–6.
29. Seeram, N.P.; Adams, L.S.; Henning, S.M.; Niu, Y.; Zhang, Y.; Nair, M.G.; Heber, D. In vitro antiproliferative, apoptotic and antioxidant activities of punicalagin, ellagic acid and a total pomegranate tannin extract are enhanced in combination with other polyphenols as found in pomegranate juice. *J. Nutr. Biochem.* **2005**, *16*, 360–367. [CrossRef]
30. Lansky, E.P.; Jiang, W.; Mo, H.; Bravo, L.; Froom, P.; Yu, W.; Harris, N.M.; Neeman, I.; Campbell, M.J. Possible synergistic prostate cancer suppression by anatomically discrete pomegranate fractions. *Invest. New Drugs* **2005**, *23*, 11–20. [CrossRef]
31. Athar, M.; Back, J.H.; Tang, X.; Kim, K.H.; Kopelovich, L.; Bickers, D.R.; Kim, A.L. Resveratrol: A review of preclinical studies for human cancer prevention. *Toxicol. Appl. Pharmacol.* **2007**, *224*, 274–283. [CrossRef] [PubMed]
32. Radhakrishnan, S.; Reddivari, L.; Sclafani, R.; Das, U.N.; Vanamala, J. Resveratrol potentiates grape seed extract induced human colon cancer cell apoptosis. *Front. Biosci. Elite* **2011** *3E*, 1509–1523. [CrossRef]

33. Pérez-Sánchez, A.; Barrajón-Catalán, E.; Ruiz-Torres, V.; Agulló-Chazarra, L.; Herranz-López, M.; Valdés, A.; Cifuentes, A.; Micol, V. Rosemary (Rosmarinus officinalis) extract causes ROS-induced necrotic cell death and inhibits tumor growth in vivo. *Sci. Rep.* **2018**. [CrossRef]
34. Brahmbhatt, M.; Gundala, S.R.; Asif, G.; Shamsi, S.A.; Aneja, R. Ginger phytochemicals exhibit synergy to inhibit prostate cancer cell proliferation. *Nutr. Cancer* **2013**, *65*, 263–272. [CrossRef] [PubMed]
35. Yang, C.; Gundala, S.R.; Mukkavilli, R.; Vangala, S.; Reid, M.D.; Aneja, R. Synergistic interactions among flavonoids and acetogenins in Graviola (Annona muricata) leaves confer protection against prostate cancer. *Carcinogenesis* **2015**, *36*, 656–665. [CrossRef] [PubMed]
36. Einbond, L.S.; Wu, H.A.; Kashiwazaki, R.; He, K.; Roller, M.; Su, T.; Wang, X.; Goldsberry, S. Carnosic acid inhibits the growth of ER-negative human breast cancer cells and synergizes with curcumin. *Fitoterapia* **2012**, *83*, 1160–1168. [CrossRef] [PubMed]
37. Morré, D.J.; Morré, D.M. Synergistic Capsicum-tea mixtures with anticancer activity. *J. Pharm. Pharmacol.* **2003**, *55*, 987–994. [CrossRef]
38. Zhou, J.R.; Li, L.; Pan, W. Dietary soy and tea combinations for prevention of breast and prostate cancers by targeting metabolic syndrome elements in mice. *Am. J. Clin. Nutr.* **2007**, *86*, 882S–888S. [CrossRef]
39. Zhou, J.R.; Yu, L.; Zhong, Y.; Blackburn, G.L. Soy phytochemicals and tea bioactive components synergistically inhibit androgen-sensitive human prostate tumors in mice. *J. Nutr.* **2003**, *133*, 516–521. [CrossRef]
40. Malongane, F.; McGaw, L.J.; Mudau, F.N. The synergistic potential of various teas, herbs and therapeutic drugs in health improvement: A review. *J. Sci. Food Agric.* **2017**, *97*, 4679–4689. [CrossRef]
41. Mertens-Talcott, S.U.; Percival, S.S. Ellagic acid and quercetin interact synergistically with resveratrol in the induction of apoptosis and cause transient cell cycle arrest in human leukemia cells. *Cancer Lett.* **2005**, *218*, 141–151. [CrossRef] [PubMed]
42. Mertens-Talcott, S.U.; Bomser, J.A.; Romero, C.; Talcott, S.T.; Percival, S.S. Ellagic acid potentiates the effect of quercetin on p21 waf1/cip1, p53, and MAP-kinases without affecting intracellular generation of reactive oxygen species in vitro. *J. Nutr.* **2005**, *135*, 609–614. [CrossRef] [PubMed]
43. Linnewiel-Hermoni, K.; Khanin, M.; Danilenko, M.; Zango, G.; Amosi, Y.; Levy, J.; Sharoni, Y. The anti-cancer effects of carotenoids and other phytonutrients resides in their combined activity. *Arch. Biochem. Biophys.* **2015**, *572*, 28–35. [CrossRef] [PubMed]
44. Lewandowska, U.; Gorlach, S.; Owczarek, K.; Hrabec, E.; Szewczyk, K. Synergistic interactions between anticancer chemotherapeutics and phenolic compounds and anticancer synergy between polyphenols. *Postepy Hig. Med. Dosw.* **2014**, *68*, 520–540. [CrossRef] [PubMed]
45. Basu, A.; Penugonda, K. Pomegranate juice: A heart-healthy fruit juice. *Nutr. Rev.* **2009**, *67*, 49–56. [CrossRef] [PubMed]
46. Bell, C.; Hawthorne, S. Ellagic acid, pomegranate and prostate cancer—A mini review. *J. Pharm. Pharmacol.* **2008**, *60*, 139–144. [CrossRef] [PubMed]
47. Landete, J.M. Ellagitannins, ellagic acid and their derived metabolites: A review about source, metabolism, functions and health. *Food Res. Int.* **2011**, *44*, 1150–1160. [CrossRef]
48. Larrosa, M.; García-Conesa, M.T.; Espín, J.C.; Tomás-Barberán, F.A. Ellagitannins, ellagic acid and vascular health. *Mol. Aspects Med.* **2010**, *31*, 513–539. [CrossRef]
49. Bishayee, A.; Bishayee, A. Pomegranate-derived constituents as inducers of cell death: Implications in cancer prevention and therapy. In *Natural Compounds as Inducers of Cell Death*; Springer: Dordrecht, The Netherlands, 2012; Volume 1, pp. 33–47.
50. Xia, E.Q.; Deng, G.F.; Guo, Y.J.; Li, H.B. Biological activities of polyphenols from grapes. *Int. J. Mol. Sci.* **2010**, *11*, 622–646. [CrossRef]
51. Herzon, S.B.; Vanderwal, C.D. Introduction: Natural Product Synthesis. *Chem. Rev.* **2017**, *117*, 11649–11650. [CrossRef]
52. Hale, K.J. (Ed.) *The Chemical Synthesis of Natural Products*; Willey: Hobolen, NJ, USA, 2000.
53. Barrajon-Catalan, E.; Fernandez-Arroyo, S.; Roldan, C.; Guillen, E.; Saura, D.; Segura-Carretero, A.; Micol, V. A systematic study of the polyphenolic composition of aqueous extracts deriving from several Cistus genus species: Evolutionary relationship. *Phytochem. Anal.* **2011**, *22*, 303–312. [CrossRef] [PubMed]
54. Borrás-Linares, I.; Herranz-López, M.; Barrajón-Catalán, E.; Arráez-Román, D.; González-Álvarez, I.; Bermejo, M.;

Gutiérrez, A.F.; Micol, V.; Segura-Carretero, A. Permeability study of polyphenols derived from a phenolic-enriched hibiscus sabdariffa extract by UHPLC-ESI-UHR-Qq-TOF-MS. *Int. J. Mol. Sci.* **2015**, *16*, 18396–18411. [CrossRef] [PubMed]

55. Borrás-Linares, I.; Pérez-Sánchez, A.; Lozano-Sánchez, J.; Barrajón-Catalán, E.; Arráez-Román, D.; Cifuentes, A.; Micol, V.; Carretero, A.S. A bioguided identification of the active compounds that contribute to the antiproliferative/cytotoxic effects of rosemary extract on colon cancer cells. *Food Chem. Toxicol.* **2015**, *80*, 215–222. [CrossRef] [PubMed]
56. Olivares-Vicente, M.; Barrajón-Catalán, E.; Herranz-López, M.; Segura-Carretero, A.; Joven, J.; Encinar, J.A.; Micol, V. Plant-derived polyphenols in human health: Biological activity, metabolites and putative molecular targets. *Curr. Drug Metab.* **2018**, *19*, 351–369. [CrossRef] [PubMed]
57. D'Archivio, M.; Filesi, C.; Varì, R.; Scazzocchio, B.; Masella, R. Bioavailability of the polyphenols: Status and controversies. *Int. J. Mol. Sci.* **2010**, *11*, 1321–1342. [CrossRef] [PubMed]
58. Manach, C.; Scalbert, A.; Morand, C.; Rémésy, C.; Jiménez, L. Polyphenols: Food sources and bioavailability. *Am. J. Clin. Nutr.* **2004**, *79*, 727–747. [CrossRef] [PubMed]
59. Munin, A.; Edwards-Lévy, F. Encapsulation of natural polyphenolic compounds: A review. *Pharmaceutics* **2011**, *3*, 793–829. [CrossRef] [PubMed]
60. Khushnud, T.; Mousa, S.A. Potential role of naturally derived polyphenols and their nanotechnology delivery in cancer. *Mol. Biotechnol.* **2013**, *55*, 78–86. [CrossRef] [PubMed]
61. Liang, J.; Yan, H.; Puligundla, P.; Gao, X.; Zhou, Y.; Wan, X. Applications of chitosan nanoparticles to enhance absorption and bioavailability of tea polyphenols: A review. *Food Hydrocoll.* **2017**, *69*, 286–292. [CrossRef]
62. Lu, W.; Kelly, A.L.; Miao, S. Emulsion-based encapsulation and delivery systems for polyphenols. *Trends Food Sci. Technol.* **2016**, *47*, 1–9. [CrossRef]
63. Mignet, N.; Seguin, J.; Chabot, G.G. Bioavailability of polyphenol liposomes: A challenge ahead. *Pharmaceutics* **2013**, *5*, 457–471. [CrossRef] [PubMed]
64. Aditya, N.P.; Espinosa, Y.G.; Norton, I.T. Encapsulation systems for the delivery of hydrophilic nutraceuticals: Food application. *Biotechnol. Adv.* **2017**, *35*, 450–457. [CrossRef] [PubMed]
65. Barrajón-Catalán, E.; Funes, L.; Herranz-López, M.; González-Álvarez, I.; Bermejo, M.V.M. Differential absorption of curcuminoids between free and liposomed curcumin formulations. In *Curcumin: Clinical Uses, Health Effects and Potential Complications*; Martin, V., Ed.; Nova Publishers: Hauppauge, NY, USA, 2016; pp. 99–110.
66. Gottesman, M.M. Mechanisms of cancer drug resistance. *Annu. Rev. Med.* **2002**, *53*, 615–627. [CrossRef] [PubMed]
67. Mimeault, M.; Hauke, R.; Batra, S.K. Recent advances on the molecular mechanisms involved in the drug resistance of cancer cells and novel targeting therapies. *Clin. Pharmacol. Ther.* **2008**, *83*, 673–691. [CrossRef] [PubMed]

9

Pro-Apoptotic and Anti-Cancer Properties of Diosgenin

Gautam Sethi [1,2,3,*,†], Muthu K. Shanmugam [3,†], Sudha Warrier [4], Myriam Merarchi [3], Frank Arfuso [5], Alan Prem Kumar [3] and Anupam Bishayee [6,*]

1 Department for Management of Science and Technology Development, Ton Duc Thang University, Ho Chi Minh City 700000, Vietnam
2 Faculty of Pharmacy, Ton Duc Thang University, Ho Chi Minh City 700000, Vietnam
3 Department of Pharmacology, Yong Loo Lin School of Medicine, National University of Singapore, Singapore 117600, Singapore; phcsmk@nus.edu.sg (M.K.S.); myriammerarchi@hotmail.fr (M.M.); phcapk@nus.edu.sg (A.P.K.)
4 Division of Cancer Stem Cells and Cardiovascular Regeneration, Manipal Institute of Regenerative Medicine, Manipal University, Bangalore 560065, India; sudha.warrier@manipal.edu
5 Stem Cell and Cancer Biology Laboratory, School of Biomedical Sciences, Curtin Health Innovation Research Institute, Curtin University, Perth, WA 6102, Australia; frank.arfuso@curtin.edu.au
6 Department of Pharmaceutical Sciences, College of Pharmacy, Larkin University, 18301 N. Miami Avenue, Miami, FL 33169, USA
* Correspondence: gautam.sethi@tdt.edu.vn or phcgs@nus.edu.sg (G.S.); abishayee@ULarkin.org or abishayee@gmail.com (A.B.)
† These authors contributed equally to this work.

Abstract: Novel and alternative options are being adopted to combat the initiation and progression of human cancers. One of the approaches is the use of molecules isolated from traditional medicinal herbs, edible dietary plants and seeds that play a pivotal role in the prevention/treatment of cancer, either alone or in combination with existing chemotherapeutic agents. Compounds that modulate these oncogenic processes are potential candidates for cancer therapy and may eventually make it to clinical applications. Diosgenin is a naturally occurring steroidal sapogenin and is one of the major bioactive compounds found in dietary fenugreek (*Trigonella foenum-graecum*) seeds. In addition to being a lactation aid, diosgenin has been shown to be hypocholesterolemic, gastro- and hepato-protective, anti-oxidant, anti-inflammatory, anti-diabetic, and anti-cancer. Diosgenin has a unique structural similarity to estrogen. Several preclinical studies have reported on the pro-apoptotic and anti-cancer properties of diosgenin against a variety of cancers, both in in vitro and in vivo. Diosgenin has also been reported to reverse multi-drug resistance in cancer cells and sensitize cancer cells to standard chemotherapy. Remarkably, diosgenin has also been reported to be used by pharmaceutical companies to synthesize steroidal drugs. Several novel diosgenin analogs and nano-formulations have been synthesized with improved anti-cancer efficacy and pharmacokinetic profile. In this review we discuss in detail the multifaceted anti-cancer properties of diosgenin that have found application in pharmaceutical, functional food, and cosmetic industries; and the various intracellular molecular targets modulated by diosgenin that abrogate the oncogenic process.

Keywords: diosgenin; steroidal sapogenins; anti-cancer; apoptosis; oncogenic; metastasis

---

1. Introduction

Cancer is a complex and heterogeneous disease that afflicts men and women worldwide; it is expected to increase due to human lifestyle changes and a rapidly aging population [1]. Hanahan and Weinberg's proposed hallmarks of cancer are widely accepted towards understanding the biology of cancer cells, through a multi-stage and progressive process [2–6]. These hallmarks include sustained proliferation of cells, constitutive activation of pro-survival transcription factors, deregulated cellular functions, evading cell death signals and growth suppressors, an increased pro-inflammatory tumor microenvironment, camouflaging against immune cell destruction, promoting angiogenesis, activating cell movement from the primary site and metastasis, enabling replicative immortality, and finally, severe genome instability [2,3,5–10]. In addition, several deregulated cellular signaling networks underlying the above hallmarks have been extensively investigated in pre-clinical and clinical drug development [3,4,11–18]. In spite of detailed information of these semi-synthetic and synthetic anti-cancer agents, they only provide limited therapeutic advantages to patients due to highly toxic unwanted side effects and the development of chemoresistance [19–21]. Emerging approaches should include the identification of novel drug targets that are very effective in inhibiting the growth of cancer cells, while exhibiting fewer adverse effects. Natural products are a good source of compounds with novel chemical structures that are effective and less toxic [18,22–27]. High throughput technologies should be exploited for the screening of a large library of compounds for their anti-cancer activities [28–30]. The mainstream of United States Food and Drug Administration (US FDA)-approved compounds divulge that natural products and their derivatives occupy one-third of all novel drugs [22–24,31]. These natural compounds, in general, show multi-targeted effects and can modulate several oncogenic transcription factors that block the tumor microenvironment targets that usually sustain tumor growth [22,27,32]. These compounds can also be classified as cytotoxic or cytostatic compounds [30]. Therefore, many secondary metabolites and pure molecules isolated from herbs, spices, dietary fruits and vegetables, and even marine sources have been explored [33–35].

Several novel bioactive molecules have been found in various edible cereals, pulses, roots, and in several parts of medicinal plants. Fenugreek (*Trigonella foenum-graecum*) belongs to the family Leguminosae and is considered a traditional medicinal herb that is commonly used in India, China, Thailand, and South-East Asian countries; it is also cultivated in the Mediterranean region and Northern Africa [36–41]. Fenugreek seeds, shoots and leaves are used in Indian curry preparation as a condiment. Bibliometric data indicates that fenugreek extract has several pharmacological properties, such as being hypocholesterolemic, a lactation aid, antibacterial, a gastric stimulant, anti-anorexic, antidiabetic, galactogogic, hepatoprotective, and anti-cancer both in in vitro and in vivo studies [40–43]. Fenugreek seed extract contains several bioactive molecules in various classes of compounds, such as saponins, flavonoids, coumarins, and alkaloids that target several molecules involved in inflammation and cancer cell proliferation, invasion, migration, angiogenesis, and metastasis [40]. Sapogenins are a class of compounds that widely occur in natural products in their glycoside form and promote general healthy living. Among these compounds, steroidal sapogenins (otherwise known as spirostans) are the most potent bioactive compounds isolated from natural product sources [44,45]. Steroidal sapogenins exhibit ubiquitous pharmacological properties and the majority of them demonstrate anti-cancer activity in vitro and in pre-clinical animal models. Several clinical trials have been conducted with fenugreek seed extract, they are either completed or ongoing; however, diosgenin anti-cancer trials are yet to start [36,41]. Diosgenin is the most abundant steroidal sapogenin in fenugreek seeds. Fujii and Matsukawa isolated and identified diosgenin from *Dioscorea tokoro* Makino in 1935 [41,46] (Figure 1). Diosgenin is a phytosteroidal saponin and a major bioactive compound found in the seeds of *T. foenum-graecum*, commonly known as fenugreek, and in the roots of wild yam (*Dioscorea villosa*) [36,40, 41,47,48]. Interestingly, diosgenin is also found in high levels in numerous plant species including *Costus speciosus*, *Smilax menispermoidea*, species of *Paris*, *Aletris* and *Trillum*, and in species of *Dioscorea* [41,49,50]. The steroidal saponin, diosgenin, is biosynthesized from cholesterol. Cholesterol is formed from lanosterol and catalysed by the cytochrome P450 system. Several other routes of synthesis have been identified, such as from squalene-2,3-oxide in two ways: From cycloartenol through the formation of sitosterol [51] and from lanosterol via cholesterol [52]. Several studies have demonstrated the diverse biological activities of diosgenin, such as hypolipidemic, anti-inflammatory, anti-proliferative, hypoglycemic activity, and as a potent anti-oxidant [44]. In addition, diosgenin inhibited cancer cell proliferation and induced apoptosis in a variety of cancer cell lines including colorectal, hepatocellular, breast, osteosarcoma, and leukemia [53–55]. The primary mechanism of action of diosgenin is through the modulation of multiple cell signaling pathways that play prominent roles in cell-cycle regulation, differentiation, and apoptosis [56]. Remarkably, pharmaceutical companies use diosgenin as a principal precursor compound for the manufacturing of several steroidal drugs [48]. Diosgenin is also an attractive molecule with multifaceted properties that has found application in pharmaceutical, functional food, and cosmetic industries. In this review we provide an in-depth evaluation of literature on diosgenin and its pharmacodynamics and pharmacokinetics, and discuss several of its novel derivatives and nanoformulations that increase its bioavailability and therapeutic efficacy. Diosgenin, over the years, has provided abundant data on the prevention and treatment of various inflammation-driven diseases, including cancers [36] (Figure 2).

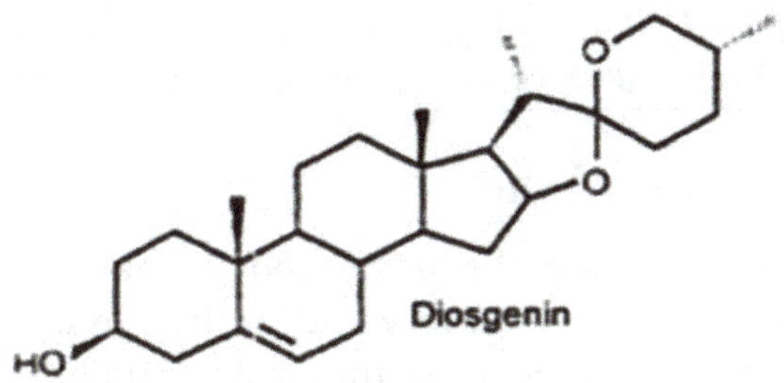

Figure 1. Chemical structure of diosgenin.

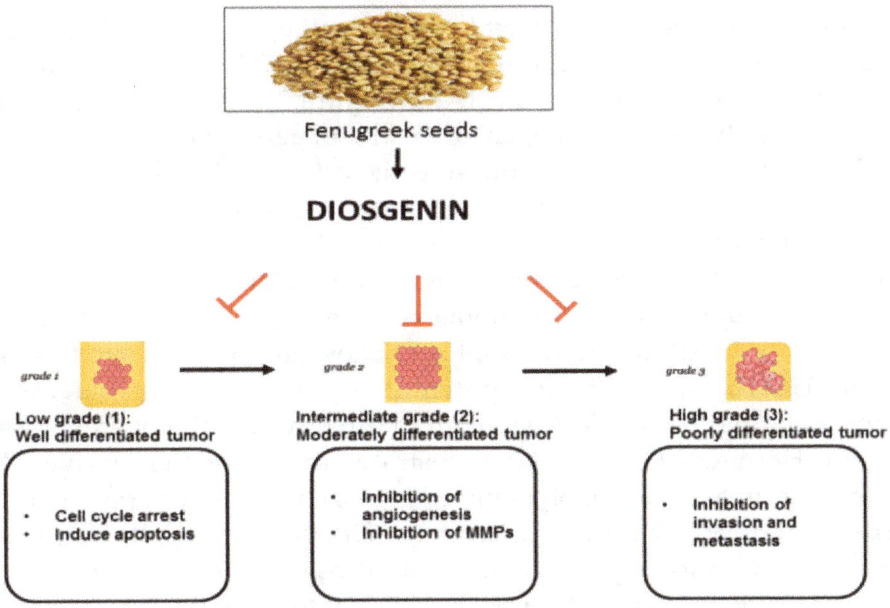

Figure 2. Tumor stage-specific inhibition of molecular targets by diosgenin.

2. Fenugreek Seed Bioactive Compounds

Fenugreek contains several chemical constituents, such as alkaloids, steroidal sapogenins, saponins, flavonoids, lipids, amino acids, and carbohydrates. Diosgenin is a major bioactive steroidal sapogenin in the fenugreek seed, which is reported to have chemopreventive and therapeutic effects against inflammation and chronic inflammation-driven cancers in preclinical in vitro and in vivo models of cancer [36,57]. Table 1 illustrates the major constituents of fenugreek seeds and leaves.

Table 1. Main phytochemical constituents of fenugreek (*T. foenum-graecum*).

Class of Compounds	Phytochemical Constituents	Reference
Steroidal sapogenins	Diosgenin, Yamogenin, Smilagenin, Sarsasapogenin, Tigogenin, Neotigogenin, Gitogenin, Yuccagenin, Saponaretin	[40]
Flavonoids	Quercetin, Rutin, Vitexin, Isovitexin	[40]
Saponins	Graecunins, Fenugrin B, Fenugreekine, Trigofoenosides A–G	[40]
Alkaloids	Trimethylamine, Neurin, Trigonelline, Choline, Gentianine, Carpaine, and Betain	[40]
Fibers	Gum, Neutral detergent fiber	[40]
Lipids	Lipids, Triacylglycerols, Diacylglycerols, Monoacylglycerols, Phosphatidylcholine, Phosphatidylethanolamine, Phosphatidylinositol, Free fatty acids	[40]
Others	Coumarin, Amino acids, Vitamins, Minerals. 28% Mucilage; 22% Proteins; 5% of a stronger swelling, Bitter fixed oil	[40]

3. In Vitro Anti-Cancer Effects of Diosgenin

Diosgenin, the major steroidal sapogenin in the fenugreek seed, has been shown to potently suppress constitutively-activated pro-inflammatory and pro-survival signaling pathways in a variety of cancer cells, and induced apoptosis [58]. Some of the earlier studies by Shishodia and Aggarwal [58] reported that diosgenin abrogated TNF-α-induced NF-κB activation and suppressed osteoclastogenesis in RAW 264.7 macrophage cells [58]. In Her-2 positive breast cancer cells, diosgenin inhibited the expression of AKT, mTOR, JNK and their associated pro-survival signaling pathways, and induced apoptosis in these cells [53]. In another study by Li et al., they reported that diosgenin could inactivate the STAT3 signaling pathway in hepatocellular carcinoma (HCC) cells, by inhibiting intracellular signaling molecules such as c-SRC, JAK1, and JAK2 (Figure 3). Diosgenin also suppressed STAT3 transcriptional activity and the expression of its downstream gene products involved in proliferation, invasion and metastasis. In addition, diosgenin sensitized HCC cells to doxorubicin and paclitaxel, and synergistically augmented apoptosis, thereby suggesting that diosgenin is a potential bioactive compound for the treatment of HCC and other cancers [54]. Diosgenin inhibited proliferation, AKT and JNK in a dose- and time-dependent manner and induced caspase-dependent apoptosis in A431 and Hep2 skin squamous cell carcinoma cells [59]. HT-29 colon cancer cells have been reported to be resistant to TRAIL-induced apoptosis. Diosgenin was shown to sensitize the HT-29 colon cancer cell to TRAIL. In addition, it potently suppressed cell proliferation and induced apoptosis by suppressing the p38/MAPK signaling pathway and the overexpression of DR5 [60]. Furthermore, Romero-Hernandez et al. [61] demonstrated that diosgenin-derived thio(seleno)ureas and glycomimetics, bearing a 1,2,3-triazolyl tether on C-3, showed more potent anti-cancer activity against MDA-MB-231 and MCF-7 breast cancer cells, HepG2 hepatocellular carcinoma cells, and induced apoptosis, compared to its parent compound diosgenin [61]. In another study, diosgenin conjugated to methotrexate was found to be more potent in inhibiting the growth of transport-resistant breast cancer cells and dihydrofolate reductase (enzyme involved in DNA synthesis), compared to the parent diosgenin [62]. In chronic myeloid leukemia cells, diosgenin-induced autophagy inhibited the mTOR signaling pathway and induced apoptotic cell death [63]. Diosgenin induced cytotoxicity and significantly inhibited the growth and proliferation of MCF-7 breast cancer cells in a dose- and time-dependent manner. Diosgenin was also shown to inhibit *N*-nitroso-*N*-methylurea-induced breast cancer in rats [64].

Of several factors that contribute to the sustained growth and proliferation of tumors, one important factor is the abundant neovascularization or formation of new micro blood vessels at the tumor site, or within the tumor. This process is also known as tumor angiogenesis. Thus, the formation of new blood vessels in tumors actively supplies the essential nutrients and growth factors that allow tumors to acquire the ability to reject chemotherapeutic drugs and develop chemoresistance [27,65–68]. Diosgenin is also a potent inhibitor of cancer cell invasion, migration, and tumor-associated angiogenesis [27,69]. He et al., reported that diosgenin inhibited the invasion and migration of triple-negative breast cancer cells and was associated with the concomitant suppression of actin polymerization, phosphorylation of Vav2, and activation of Cdc42 oncoprotein expression. These proteins have been shown to be involved in the initiation of cancer cells' invasive and migratory potential [70]. Similarly, diosgenin was found to inhibit PC3 androgen-independent prostate cancer cell invasion and migration. The inhibitory effect was mediated by the downregulation of matrix metalloproteinase (MMP)-2 and MMP-9, the key enzymes in matrix degradation and stroma invasion. Furthermore, diosgenin also downregulated the tissue inhibitors of metalloproteinase (TIMP)-2, vascular endothelial growth factor (VEGF), extracellular regulated kinase (ERK), Janus kinase (JNK), phosphotidyl-inositol-3 kinase/protein kinase B (PI3K/AKT), and NF-κB transcriptional activity [56]. In addition, diosgenin was reported to inhibit the expression of E-cadherin, integrin 5a and 6b, invasion, migration, and angiogenesis in hypoxia-sensitive BGC-823 gastric cancer cells [71]. Diosgenin was reported to inhibit proliferation of ER-positive MCF-7 breast cancer cells by the upregulation of the p53 tumor suppressor gene and activation of caspase 3, while it downregulated BCL2 in ER negative MDA-MB-231 triple-negative breast cancer cells [72]. Diosgenin, either alone, or in combination with thymoquinone, inhibited A431 and Hep2 squamous cell carcinoma cell proliferation, increased the Bax/Bcl2 ratio, and induced caspase 3-mediated apoptosis [59] (Table 2). The potential effect of diosgenin on NF-κB and STAT3 signaling pathways in tumor cells, is shown in Figure 3.

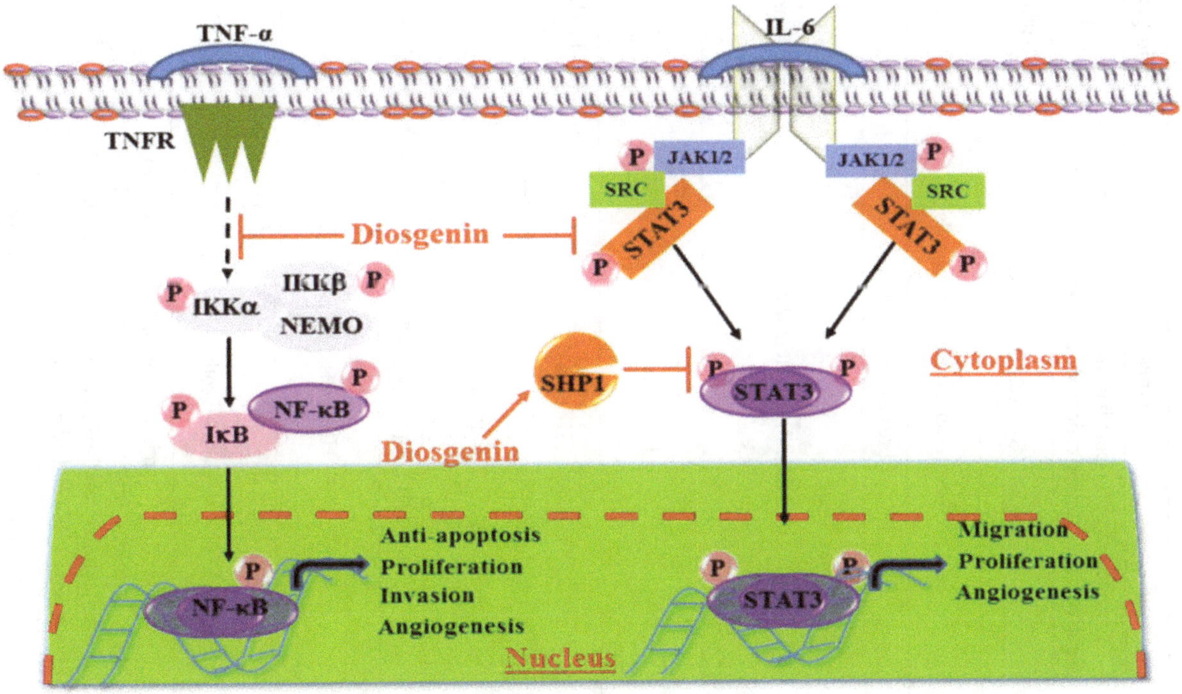

Figure 3. Role of diosgenin in NF-κB and STAT3 signaling pathways. Diosgenin abrogates TNF-α -induced activation of NF-κB and IL6-induced STAT3 signaling pathways in tumor cells. Diosgenin can hence prevent proliferation, invasion and angiogenesis; and induce apoptosis, a characteristic vastly looked for in cancer therapy.

Table 2. In vitro anti-cancer effects of diosgenin.

Cancer model	Cell Lines	Diosgenin Dose	Molecular Target	References
Breast carcinoma	Estrogen receptor positive and estrogen receptor negative human breast cancer MCF-7 and MDA 231 cells	20 µM and 30 µM	Inhibition of cell proliferation Induces apoptosis	[72]
	MDA-MB-231 breast cancer cells	20 µM, 40 µM, and 60 µM	Downregulation of Bcl2	[57]
	Her2 over-expressing breast cancer cells	5–20 µM	Modulation of Akt, mTOR, and JNK phosphorylation	[53]
	MCF-7 breast cancer cells	20 µM and 40 µM	Upregulation of p53 tumor suppressor gene	[73]
Hepatocellular carcinoma	C3A, HUH-7, and HepG2 cells	50 µM and 100 µM	Downregulation of STAT3 signaling pathway Upregulates SH-PTP2 expression Induces apoptosis Potentiates the apoptotic effects of doxorubicin and paclitaxel	[54]
Prostate carcinoma	PC3 cells	5 µM, 10 µM, and 20 µM	Downregulates NF-κB signaling pathway Inhibits matrix metalloproteinases Inhibits invasion and migration of cells	[56]
Osteosarcoma	1547 cells	40 µM, 80 µM, and 100 µM	Inhibits cell proliferation Induces apoptosis	[55]
	1547 cells	40 µM	Inhibits cell proliferation Induces apoptosis Upregulation of p53 tumor suppressor gene	[74]
Human erythroleukemia	HEL cells, K562 cells	40 µM	Inhibits NF-κB signaling pathway	[75]
	HEL cells	40 µM	Inhibits proliferation Induces apoptosis Upregulation of p21	[76]
Human Laryngocarcinoma Human Melanoma	HEp-2 cells M4Beu cells	40 µM	Inhibits cell proliferation Induces caspase-3 dependent apoptosis Upregulates p53 tumor suppressor gene	[77]
Human cancer cells	Human epithelial carcinoma cell line (A431), human NSCLC cell line (A549), human ovarian cancer cell line (A2780), Human erythroleukemia (K562) and Dukes' type C, colorectal adenocarcinoma (HCT-15)	10 mmol/L	Induces apoptosis via mitochondrial dependent pathway	[78]
	Multiple myeloma (U266), leukemia (U937), and breast cancer (MCF-7)	50 µM and 100 µM	Inhibits NF-κB signaling pathway	[58]

4. In Vivo Anti-Cancer Effects of Diosgenin

In addition to in vitro inhibition of cancer cell proliferation by dietary fenugreek seeds and its bioactive constituent diosgenin, several studies have provided evidence that diosgenin is a potent inhibitor of tumor growth in vivo in rodent models of cancer. In a rat colorectal tumor model, administration of diosgenin, given during the promotional stage, reduced azoxymethane (AOM)-induced colonic aberrant crypt foci formation [79]. Similarly, Malisetty et al., showed that diosgenin, at a dose of 15 mg/kg, significantly suppressed both the incidence and invasive potential of AOM-induced rat colon adenocarcinoma mass by 60% and colon tumor multiplicity (adenocarcinomas/rat) by 68% [80]. However, in the murine model of AOM/dextran sodium sulfate-induced colon aberrant crypt foci, diosgenin at doses of 20, 100 and 200 mg/kg b.w. in the diet did not reduce adenocarcinoma mass; nonetheless, a significant reduction in tumor multiplicity was observed with all three doses tested [81]. In another study, diosgenin (at a dose of 10 mg/kg b.w. administered intra-tumorally) significantly inhibited the growth of MCF-7 and MDA-MB-231 human breast cancer xenografts in mice [72]. In another study using inbred T739 mice, diosgenin was shown to significantly inhibit the growth of mouse LA795 lung adenocarcinoma tumors by 33.94% [82]. Diosgenin, at a dose of 80 mg/kg administered by oral gavage, was reported to inhibit the growth of oral tumors in a DMBA-induced hamster buccal pouch model [64]. Diosgenin, in combination with thymoquinone, exhibited significant tumor growth inhibition in a mice xenograft model [59]. Therefore, diosgenin modulates multiple targets and suppresses tumor growth in preclinical models of cancer. However, diosgenin's poor solubility in organic solvents and its lack of bioavailability greatly hinder its translational process as a therapeutic compound. Further clinical trials are required to evaluate its potential either as a preventive or therapeutic anti-cancer agent.

5. Semisynthetic Derivatives of Diosgenin That Exhibit Anti-Cancer Activity

Diosgenin is used in the pharmaceutical industry as the main precursor in the synthesis of steroids [83]. It has the ability to penetrate cell membranes and bind to specific receptors [84]. Steroidal sapogenins are bioactive molecules that have shown exceptional antiproliferative activity against several human cancer cells. By making specific changes in the steroidal structure of diosgenin, it can affect its biological activity. In a recent report, using diosgenin as the parent molecule, the authors synthesized two novel steroidal oxime compounds that showed significant antiproliferative activity on cervical cancer cells and human lymphocytes. These compounds induced apoptosis and activated caspase 3 [85]. In another study Mohammad et al., reported on the anti-proliferative activity of diosgenin and its semi-synthetic derivatives against breast (HBL-100), colon (HCT-116 and HT-19) and lung (A549) cancer cells. A structure-activity relationship study revealed that the potent anti-proliferative activity was mainly attributed to the analogs with the simple phenyl R moiety or electron-withdrawing ortho-substituted R moieties attached to the parent diosgenin [86]. In another study, diosgenin was used as a parent compound to synthesize 1α-hydroxysolasodine; it showed significant anti-cancer activity against prostate cancer (PC3), cervical carcinoma (HeLa), and hepatocellular carcinoma (HepG2) cells [87]. Twelve different analogs of diosgenin containing a long chain fatty acid/ester of diosgenin-7-ketoxime exhibited anti-cancer activity when tested against a panel of cancer cell lines. Compound 16 in this series exhibited potent anti-proliferative activity against DU145 prostate cancer cells, which was associated to the suppression of lipopolysaccharide-induced activation of TNF-α and IL6. The compound was also identified as safe, with a maximum tolerated dose of 300 mg/kg in Swiss albino mice [88]. In a recent article by Ghosh et al., they reported the synthesis of diosgenin functionalized iron oxide nanoparticles that exhibited anti-breast cancer activity by inhibiting proliferation and migration, and by inducing apoptosis [89].

6. Conclusions and Future Perspectives

Compounds derived either from medicinal or dietary plant sources embrace distinct advantages, such as novel bioactive structures, low toxicity, and being multi-targeted in abrogating oncogenic processes; thereby, they may form the source of improved therapeutic options. A vast body of pre-clinical experimental evidence suggests that diosgenin has great potential as an anti-cancer agent. In this review we have compiled and analyzed the role of diosgenin in modulating various oncogenic transcription factors and intracellular molecular targets that drive tumor initiation, progression and metastasis. It is well known that the majority of cancers are a consequence of chronic inflammation, infection, dysfunctional cell death mechanisms, and deregulation of cell cycle molecules. The ability of diosgenin to prevent carcinogenesis by acting as an anti-oxidant and anti-inflammatory agent, and its ability to induce apoptosis of cancer cells, suggests that it can be useful as an anti-carcinogenic agent. Due to the complexities in the cellular processes involved, several new studies need to be conducted to decipher the exact molecular targets that can be exploited to prevent cancer progression. Interestingly, there are 12 reported clinical trials on fenugreek seed extract on a variety of human ailments, as reported in www.clinicaltrials.gov. However, to date, there are no cancer-related clinical trials reported either on diosgenin or on fenugreek seed extract. Several novel synthetic diosgenin derivatives have been shown to improve its anti-cancer efficacy. Several nano-formulations and delivery systems of diosgenin are also shown to improve its bioavailability. In conclusion, several challenges such as developing novel delivery systems, pharmaceutical formulations, and semi-synthetic derivatives that are water soluble, need to be overcome to uncover diosgenin's benefits either as a chemopreventive or therapeutic agent.

Author Contributions: G.S. and M.K.S. wrote the paper, F.A., A.P.K., S.W., M.M. and A.B. critically analyzed and revised the manuscript.

Acknowledgments: A.P.K. was supported by grants from National Medical Research Council of Singapore, Medical Science Cluster, Yong Loo Lin School of Medicine, National University of Singapore and by the National Research Foundation Singapore and the Singapore Ministry of Education under its Research Centers of Excellence initiative to Cancer Science Institute of Singapore, National University of Singapore.

References

1. Siegel, R.L.; Miller, K.D.; Jemal, A. Cancer statistics, 2017. *CA Cancer J. Clin.* **2017**, *67*, 7–30. [CrossRef] [PubMed]
2. Hanahan, D.; Weinberg, R.A. The hallmarks of cancer. *Cell* **2000**, *100*, 57–70. [CrossRef]
3. Hanahan, D.; Weinberg, R.A. Hallmarks of cancer: The next generation. *Cell* **2011**, *144*, 646–674. [CrossRef] [PubMed]
4. Hanahan, D. Rethinking the war on cancer. *Lancet* **2014**, *383*, 558–563. [CrossRef]
5. Floor, S.L.; Dumont, J.E.; Maenhaut, C.; Raspe, E. Hallmarks of cancer: Of all cancer cells, all the time? *Trends Mol. Med.* **2012**, *18*, 509–515. [CrossRef] [PubMed]
6. Pietras, K.; Ostman, A. Hallmarks of cancer: Interactions with the tumor stroma. *Exp. Cell Res.* **2010**, *316*, 1324–1331. [CrossRef] [PubMed]
7. Massague, J.; Obenauf, A.C. Metastatic colonization by circulating tumour cells. *Nature* **2016**, *529*, 298–306. [CrossRef] [PubMed]
8. Chaffer, C.L.; Weinberg, R.A. How does multistep tumorigenesis really proceed? *Cancer Discov.* **2015**, *5*, 22–24. [CrossRef] [PubMed]
9. Iwatsuki, M.; Mimori, K.; Yokobori, T.; Ishi, H.; Beppu, T.; Nakamori, S.; Baba, H.; Mori, M. Epithelial-mesenchymal transition in cancer development and its clinical significance. *Cancer Sci.* **2010**, *101*, 293–299. [CrossRef] [PubMed]
10. Almendro, V.; Marusyk, A.; Polyak, K. Cellular heterogeneity and molecular evolution in cancer. *Annu. Rev. Pathol.* **2013**, *8*, 277–302. [CrossRef] [PubMed]
11. Steeg, P.S. Targeting metastasis. *Nat. Rev. Cancer* **2016**, *16*, 201–218. [CrossRef] [PubMed]

12. Wang, Z.; Dabrosin, C.; Yin, X.; Fuster, M.M.; Arreola, A.; Rathmell, W.K.; Generali, D.; Nagaraju, G.P.; El-Rayes, B.; Ribatti, D.; et al. Broad targeting of angiogenesis for cancer prevention and therapy. *Semin. Cancer Biol.* **2015**, *35*, S224–S243. [CrossRef] [PubMed]
13. Sethi, G.; Ahn, K.S.; Aggarwal, B.B. Targeting nuclear factor-kappa B activation pathway by thymoquinone: Role in suppression of antiapoptotic gene products and enhancement of apoptosis. *Mol. Cancer Res.* **2008**, *6*, 1059–1070. [CrossRef] [PubMed]
14. Tang, C.H.; Sethi, G.; Kuo, P.L. Novel medicines and strategies in cancer treatment and prevention. *BioMed Res. Int.* **2014**, *2014*, 474078. [CrossRef] [PubMed]
15. Ahn, K.S.; Sethi, G.; Aggarwal, B.B. Nuclear factor-kappa B: From clone to clinic. *Curr. Mol. Med.* **2007**, *7*, 619–637. [CrossRef] [PubMed]
16. Chai, E.Z.; Shanmugam, M.K.; Arfuso, F.; Dharmarajan, A.; Wang, C.; Kumar, A.P.; Samy, R.P.; Lim, L.H.; Wang, L.; Goh, B.C.; et al. Targeting transcription factor stat3 for cancer prevention and therapy. *Pharmacol. Ther.* **2016**, *162*, 86–97. [CrossRef] [PubMed]
17. Li, F.; Zhang, J.; Arfuso, F.; Chinnathambi, A.; Zayed, M.E.; Alharbi, S.A.; Kumar, A.P.; Ahn, K.S.; Sethi, G. NF-kappaB in cancer therapy. *Arch. Toxicol.* **2015**, *89*, 711–731. [CrossRef] [PubMed]
18. Shanmugam, M.K.; Kannaiyan, R.; Sethi, G. Targeting cell signaling and apoptotic pathways by dietary agents: Role in the prevention and treatment of cancer. *Nutr. Cancer* **2011**, *63*, 161–173. [CrossRef] [PubMed]
19. Deorukhkar, A.; Krishnan, S.; Sethi, G.; Aggarwal, B.B. Back to basics: How natural products can provide the basis for new therapeutics. *Expert Opin. Investig. Drugs* **2007**, *16*, 1753–1773. [CrossRef] [PubMed]
20. Kneller, R. The importance of new companies for drug discovery: Origins of a decade of new drugs. *Nat. Rev. Drug Discov.* **2010**, *9*, 867–882. [CrossRef] [PubMed]
21. Bishayee, A.; Sethi, G. Bioactive natural products in cancer prevention and therapy: Progress and promise. *Semin. Cancer Biol.* **2016**, *40–41*, 1–3. [CrossRef] [PubMed]
22. Newman, D.J.; Cragg, G.M. Natural products as sources of new drugs from 1981 to 2014. *J. Nat. Prod.* **2016**, *79*, 629–661. [CrossRef] [PubMed]
23. Newman, D.J. Developing natural product drugs: Supply problems and how they have been overcome. *Pharmacol. Ther.* **2016**, *162*, 1–9. [CrossRef] [PubMed]
24. Newman, D.J. Bioactive cyclic molecules and drug design. *Expert Opin. Drug Discov.* **2018**, *13*, 379–385. [CrossRef] [PubMed]
25. Shanmugam, M.K.; Lee, J.H.; Chai, E.Z.; Kanchi, M.M.; Kar, S.; Arfuso, F.; Dharmarajan, A.; Kumar, A.P.; Ramar, P.S.; Looi, C.Y.; et al. Cancer prevention and therapy through the modulation of transcription factors by bioactive natural compounds. *Semin. Cancer Biol.* **2016**, *40–41*, 35–47. [CrossRef] [PubMed]
26. Shanmugam, M.K.; Nguyen, A.H.; Kumar, A.P.; Tan, B.K.; Sethi, G. Targeted inhibition of tumor proliferation, survival, and metastasis by pentacyclic triterpenoids: Potential role in prevention and therapy of cancer. *Cancer Lett.* **2012**, *320*, 158–170. [CrossRef] [PubMed]
27. Shanmugam, M.K.; Warrier, S.; Kumar, A.P.; Sethi, G.; Arfuso, F. Potential role of natural compounds as anti-angiogenic agents in cancer. *Curr. Vasc. Pharmacol.* **2017**, *15*, 503–519. [CrossRef] [PubMed]
28. Mishra, K.P.; Ganju, L.; Sairam, M.; Banerjee, P.K.; Sawhney, R.C. A review of high throughput technology for the screening of natural products. *Biomed. Pharmacother.* **2008**, *62*, 94–98. [CrossRef] [PubMed]
29. Cragg, G.M.; Grothaus, P.G.; Newman, D.J. Impact of natural products on developing new anti-cancer agents. *Chem. Rev.* **2009**, *109*, 3012–3043. [CrossRef] [PubMed]
30. Harvey, A.L.; Edrada-Ebel, R.; Quinn, R.J. The re-emergence of natural products for drug discovery in the genomics era. *Nat. Rev. Drug Discov.* **2015**, *14*, 111–129. [CrossRef] [PubMed]
31. Newman, D.J. Natural products as leads to potential drugs: An old process or the new hope for drug discovery? *J. Med. Chem.* **2008**, *51*, 2589–2599. [CrossRef] [PubMed]
32. Chai, E.Z.; Siveen, K.S.; Shanmugam, M.K.; Arfuso, F.; Sethi, G. Analysis of the intricate relationship between chronic inflammation and cancer. *Biochem. J.* **2015**, *468*, 1–15. [CrossRef] [PubMed]
33. Sung, B.; Prasad, S.; Yadav, V.R.; Aggarwal, B.B. Cancer cell signaling pathways targeted by spice-derived nutraceuticals. *Nutr. Cancer* **2012**, *64*, 173–197. [CrossRef] [PubMed]
34. Newman, D.J.; Cragg, G.M. Current status of marine-derived compounds as warheads in anti-tumor drug candidates. *Mar. Drugs* **2017**, *15*, 99. [CrossRef] [PubMed]
35. Newman, D.J.; Cragg, G.M. Drugs and drug candidates from marine sources: An assessment of the current "state of play". *Planta Med.* **2016**, *82*, 775–789. [CrossRef] [PubMed]

36. El Bairi, K.; Ouzir, M.; Agnieszka, N.; Khalki, L. Anticancer potential of trigonella foenum graecum: Cellular and molecular targets. *Biomed. Pharmacother.* **2017**, *90*, 479–491. [CrossRef] [PubMed]
37. Shabbeer, S.; Sobolewski, M.; Anchoori, R.K.; Kachhap, S.; Hidalgo, M.; Jimeno, A.; Davidson, N.; Carducci, M.A.; Khan, S.R. Fenugreek: A naturally occurring edible spice as an anticancer agent. *Cancer Biol. Ther.* **2009**, *8*, 272–278. [CrossRef] [PubMed]
38. Aggarwal, B.B.; Kunnumakkara, A.B.; Harikumar, K.B.; Tharakan, S.T.; Sung, B.; Anand, P. Potential of spice-derived phytochemicals for cancer prevention. *Planta Med.* **2008**, *74*, 1560–1569. [CrossRef] [PubMed]
39. Kenny, O.; Smyth, T.J.; Hewage, C.M.; Brunton, N.P. Antioxidant properties and quantitative UPLC-MS analysis of phenolic compounds from extracts of Fenugreek (*Trigonella foenum-graecum*) seeds and bitter melon (*Momordica charantia*) fruit. *Food Chem.* **2013**, *141*, 4295–4302. [CrossRef] [PubMed]
40. Wani, S.A.; Kumar, P. Fenugreek: A review on its nutraceutical properties and utilization in various food products. *J. Saudi Soc. Agric. Sci.* **2018**, *17*, 97–106. [CrossRef]
41. Kim, J.K.; Park, S.U. An update on the biological and pharmacological activities of diosgenin. *EXCLI J.* **2018**, *17*, 24–28. [PubMed]
42. Bahmani, M.; Shirzad, H.; Mirhosseini, M.; Mesripour, A.; Rafieian-Kopaei, M. A review on ethnobotanical and therapeutic uses of Fenugreek (*Trigonella foenum-graceum* L.). *J. Evid. Based Complement. Altern. Med.* **2016**, *21*, 53–62. [CrossRef] [PubMed]
43. Srinivasan, K. Fenugreek (*Trigonella foenum-graecum*): A review of health beneficial physiological effects. *Food Rev. Int.* **2006**, *22*, 203–224. [CrossRef]
44. Jesus, M.; Martins, A.P.; Gallardo, E.; Silvestre, S. Diosgenin: Recent highlights on pharmacology and analytical methodology. *J. Anal. Methods Chem.* **2016**, *2016*, 4156293. [CrossRef] [PubMed]
45. Yang, S.F.; Weng, C.J.; Sethi, G.; Hu, D.N. Natural bioactives and phytochemicals serve in cancer treatment and prevention. *Evid. Based Complement. Altern. Med.* **2013**, *2013*, 698190. [CrossRef] [PubMed]
46. Djerassi, C.; Rosenkranz, G.; Pataki, J.; Kaufmann, S. Steroids, xxvii. Synthesis of allopregnane-3beta, 11beta, 17alpha-, 20beta, 21-pentol from cortisone and diosgenin. *J. Biol. Chem.* **1952**, *194*, 115–118. [PubMed]
47. Patel, K.; Gadewar, M.; Tahilyani, V.; Patel, D.K. A review on pharmacological and analytical aspects of diosmetin: A concise report. *Chin. J. Integr. Med.* **2013**, *19*, 792–800. [CrossRef] [PubMed]
48. Chen, Y.; Tang, Y.M.; Yu, S.L.; Han, Y.W.; Kou, J.P.; Liu, B.L.; Yu, B.Y. Advances in the pharmacological activities and mechanisms of diosgenin. *Chin. J. Nat. Med.* **2015**, *13*, 578–587. [CrossRef]
49. Tang, Y.; Yi, T.; Chen, H.; Zhao, Z.; Liang, Z.; Chen, H. Quantitative comparison of multiple components in dioscorea nipponica and d. Panthaica by ultra-high performance liquid chromatography coupled with quadrupole time-of-flight mass spectrometry. *Phytochem. Anal.* **2013**, *24*, 413–422. [CrossRef] [PubMed]
50. Tang, Y.N.; Pang, Y.X.; He, X.C.; Zhang, Y.Z.; Zhang, J.Y.; Zhao, Z.Z.; Yi, T.; Chen, H.B. UPLC-QTOF-MS identification of metabolites in rat biosamples after oral administration of dioscorea saponins: A comparative study. *J. Ethnopharmacol.* **2015**, *165*, 127–140. [CrossRef] [PubMed]
51. Ciura, J.; Szeliga, M.; Grzesik, M.; Tyrka, M. Next-generation sequencing of representational difference analysis products for identification of genes involved in diosgenin biosynthesis in Fenugreek (*Trigonella foenum-graecum*). *Planta* **2017**, *245*, 977–991. [CrossRef] [PubMed]
52. Vaidya, K.; Ghosh, A.; Kumar, V.; Chaudhary, S.; Srivastava, N.; Katudia, K.; Tiwari, T.; Chikara, S.K. De novo transcriptome sequencing in *Trigonella foenum-graecum* L. to identify genes involved in the biosynthesis of diosgenin. *Plant. Genome* **2013**, *6*, 1–11. [CrossRef]
53. Chiang, C.T.; Way, T.D.; Tsai, S.J.; Lin, J.K. Diosgenin, a naturally occurring steroid, suppresses fatty acid synthase expression in HER2-overexpressing breast cancer cells through modulating Akt, mTOR and JNK phosphorylation. *FEBS Lett.* **2007**, *581*, 5735–5742. [CrossRef] [PubMed]
54. Li, F.; Fernandez, P.P.; Rajendran, P.; Hui, K.M.; Sethi, G. Diosgenin, a steroidal saponin, inhibits STAT3 signaling pathway leading to suppression of proliferation and chemosensitization of human hepatocellular carcinoma cells. *Cancer Lett.* **2010**, *292*, 197–207. [CrossRef] [PubMed]
55. Moalic, S.; Liagre, B.; Corbiere, C.; Bianchi, A.; Dauca, M.; Bordji, K.; Beneytout, J.L. A plant steroid, diosgenin, induces apoptosis, cell cycle arrest and cox activity in osteosarcoma cells. *FEBS Lett.* **2001**, *506*, 225–230. [CrossRef]
56. Chen, P.S.; Shih, Y.W.; Huang, H.C.; Cheng, H.W. Diosgenin, a steroidal saponin, inhibits migration and invasion of human prostate cancer pc-3 cells by reducing matrix metalloproteinases expression. *PLoS ONE* **2011**, *6*, e20164. [CrossRef] [PubMed]

57. Raju, J.; Rao, C.V. Diosgenin, a steroid saponin constituent of yams and fenugreek: Emerging evidence for applications. In *Bioactive Compounds Medicine in Phytomedicine*; Rasooli, I., Ed.; InTech.: London, UK, 2012; pp. 125–142.
58. Shishodia, S.; Aggarwal, B.B. Diosgenin inhibits osteoclastogenesis, invasion, and proliferation through the downregulation of Akt, I kappa B kinase activation and NF-kappa B-regulated gene expression. *Oncogene* **2006**, *25*, 1463–1473. [CrossRef] [PubMed]
59. Das, S.; Dey, K.K.; Dey, G.; Pal, I.; Majumder, A.; MaitiChoudhury, S.; kundu, S.C.; Mandal, M. Antineoplastic and apoptotic potential of traditional medicines thymoquinone and diosgenin in squamous cell carcinoma. *PLoS ONE* **2012**, *7*, e46641. [CrossRef] [PubMed]
60. Lepage, C.; Leger, D.Y.; Bertrand, J.; Martin, F.; Beneytout, J.L.; Liagre, B. Diosgenin induces death receptor-5 through activation of p38 pathway and promotes trail-induced apoptosis in colon cancer cells. *Cancer Lett.* **2011**, *301*, 193–202. [CrossRef] [PubMed]
61. Romero-Hernandez, L.L.; Merino-Montiel, P.; Montiel-Smith, S.; Meza-Reyes, S.; Vega-Baez, J.L.; Abasolo, I.; Schwartz, S., Jr.; Lopez, O.; Fernandez-Bolanos, J.G. Diosgenin-based thio(seleno)ureas and triazolyl glycoconjugates as hybrid drugs. Antioxidant and antiproliferative profile. *Eur. J. Med. Chem.* **2015**, *99*, 67–81. [CrossRef] [PubMed]
62. Cai, B.; Liao, A.; Lee, K.K.; Ban, J.S.; Yang, H.S.; Im, Y.J.; Chun, C. Design, synthesis of methotrexate-diosgenin conjugates and biological evaluation of their effect on methotrexate transport-resistant cells. *Steroids* **2016**, *116*, 45–51. [CrossRef] [PubMed]
63. Jiang, S.; Fan, J.; Wang, Q.; Ju, D.; Feng, M.; Li, J.; Guan, Z.B.; An, D.; Wang, X.; Ye, L. Diosgenin induces ros-dependent autophagy and cytotoxicity via mtor signaling pathway in chronic myeloid leukemia cells. *Phytomedicine* **2016**, *23*, 243–252. [CrossRef] [PubMed]
64. Jagadeesan, J.; Langeswaran, K.; Gowthamkumar, S.; Balasubramanian, M.P. Diosgenin exhibits beneficial efficiency on human mammary carcinoma cell line MCF-7 and against N-nitroso-N-methylurea (NMU) induced experimental mammary carcinoma. *Biomed. Prev. Nutr.* **2013**, *3*, 381–388. [CrossRef]
65. Albini, A.; Tosetti, F.; Li, V.W.; Noonan, D.M.; Li, W.W. Cancer prevention by targeting angiogenesis. *Nat. Rev. Clin. Oncol.* **2012**, *9*, 498–509. [CrossRef] [PubMed]
66. Folkman, J. Tumor angiogenesis: Therapeutic implications. *N. Engl. J. Med.* **1971**, *285*, 1182–1186. [PubMed]
67. Folkman, J. Role of angiogenesis in tumor growth and metastasis. *Semin. Oncol.* **2002**, *29*, 15–18. [CrossRef] [PubMed]
68. Folkman, J. Angiogenesis: An organizing principle for drug discovery? *Nat. Rev. Drug Discov.* **2007**, *6*, 273–286. [CrossRef] [PubMed]
69. Selim, S.; Al Jaouni, S. Anti-inflammatory, antioxidant and antiangiogenic activities of diosgenin isolated from traditional medicinal plant, costus speciosus (Koen ex.Retz.) Sm. *Nat. Prod. Res.* **2016**, *30*, 1830–1833. [CrossRef] [PubMed]
70. He, Z.; Chen, H.; Li, G.; Zhu, H.; Gao, Y.; Zhang, L.; Sun, J. Diosgenin inhibits the migration of human breast cancer MDA-MB-231 cells by suppressing VAV2 activity. *Phytomedicine* **2014**, *21*, 871–876. [CrossRef] [PubMed]
71. Mao, Z.J.; Tang, Q.J.; Zhang, C.A.; Qin, Z.F.; Pang, B.; Wei, P.K.; Liu, B.; Chou, Y.N. Anti-proliferation and anti-invasion effects of diosgenin on gastric cancer BGC-823 cells with HIF-1alpha shrnas. *Int. J. Mol. Sci.* **2012**, *13*, 6521–6533. [CrossRef] [PubMed]
72. Srinivasan, S.; Koduru, S.; Kumar, R.; Venguswamy, G.; Kyprianou, N.; Damodaran, C. Diosgenin targets AKT-mediated prosurvival signaling in human breast cancer cells. *Int. J. Cancer* **2009**, *125*, 961–967. [CrossRef] [PubMed]
73. Sowmyalakshmi, S.; Ranga, R.; Gairola, C.G.; Chendil, D. Effect of diosgenin (Fenugreek) on breast cancer cells. *Proc. Am. Assoc. Cancer Res.* **2005**, *46*, 1382.
74. Corbiere, C.; Liagre, B.; Bianchi, A.; Bordji, K.; Dauca, M.; Netter, P.; Beneytout, J.L. Different contribution of apoptosis to the antiproliferative effects of diosgenin and other plant steroids, hecogenin and tigogenin, on human 1547 osteosarcoma cells. *Int. J. Oncol.* **2003**, *22*, 899–905. [CrossRef] [PubMed]
75. Liagre, B.; Bertrand, J.; Leger, D.Y.; Beneytout, J.L. Diosgenin, a plant steroid, induces apoptosis in COX-2 deficient K562 cells with activation of the p38 map kinase signalling and inhibition of NF-kappaB binding. *Int. J. Mol. Med.* **2005**, *16*, 1095–1101. [CrossRef] [PubMed]

76. Leger, D.Y.; Liagre, B.; Corbiere, C.; Cook-Moreau, J.; Beneytout, J.L. Diosgenin induces cell cycle arrest and apoptosis in hel cells with increase in intracellular calcium level, activation of CPLA2 and COX-2 overexpression. *Int. J. Oncol.* **2004**, *25*, 555–562. [CrossRef] [PubMed]
77. Corbiere, C.; Liagre, B.; Terro, F.; Beneytout, J.L. Induction of antiproliferative effect by diosgenin through activation of p53, release of apoptosis-inducing factor (AIF) and modulation of caspase-3 activity in different human cancer cells. *Cell. Res.* **2004**, *14*, 188–196. [CrossRef] [PubMed]
78. Wang, S.L.; Cai, B.; Cui, C.B.; Liu, H.W.; Wu, C.F.; Yao, X.S. Diosgenin-3-O-alpha-L-rhamnopyranosyl-(1→4)-beta-d-glucopyranoside obtained as a new anticancer agent from dioscorea futschauensis induces apoptosis on human colon carcinoma HCT-15 cells via mitochondria-controlled apoptotic pathway. *J. Asian Nat. Prod. Res.* **2004**, *6*, 115–125. [CrossRef] [PubMed]
79. Raju, J.; Patlolla, J.M.; Swamy, M.V.; Rao, C.V. Diosgenin, a steroid saponin of *Trigonella foenum graecum* (Fenugreek), inhibits azoxymethane-induced aberrant crypt foci formation in F344 rats and induces apoptosis in HT-29 human colon cancer cells. *Cancer Epidemiol. Biomarkers Prev.* **2004**, *13*, 1392–1398. [PubMed]
80. Malisetty, V.S.; Patlolla, J.M.R.; Raju, J.; Marcus, L.A.; Choi, C.L.; Rao, C.V. Chemoprevention of colon cancer by diosgenin, a steroidal saponin constituent of fenugreek. *Proc. Am. Assoc. Cancer Res.* **2005**, *46*, 2473.
81. Miyoshi, N.; Nagasawa, T.; Mabuchi, R.; Yasui, Y.; Wakabayashi, K.; Tanaka, T.; Ohshima, H. Chemoprevention of azoxymethane/dextran sodium sulfate-induced mouse colon carcinogenesis by freeze-dried yam sanyaku and its constituent diosgenin. *Cancer Prev. Res. (Phila.)* **2011**, *4*, 924–934. [CrossRef] [PubMed]
82. Yan, L.L.; Zhang, Y.J.; Gao, W.Y.; Man, S.L.; Wang, Y. In vitro and in vivo anticancer activity of steroid saponins of paris polyphylla var. Yunnanensis. *Exp. Oncol.* **2009**, *31*, 27–32. [PubMed]
83. Marker, R.E.; Sterols, C.V. The preparation of testosterone and related compounds from sarsasapogenin and diosgenin. *J. Am. Chem. Soc.* **1940**, *62*, 2543–2547. [CrossRef]
84. Tietze, L.F.; Bell, H.P.; Chandrasekhar, S. Natural product hybrids as new leads for drug discovery. *Angew. Chem. Int. Ed.* **2003**, *42*, 3996–4028. [CrossRef] [PubMed]
85. Sanchez-Sanchez, L.; Hernandez-Linares, M.G.; Escobar, M.L.; Lopez-Munoz, H.; Zenteno, E.; Fernandez-Herrera, M.A.; Guerrero-Luna, G.; Carrasco-Carballo, A.; Sandoval-Ramirez, J. Antiproliferative, cytotoxic, and apoptotic activity of steroidal oximes in cervicouterine cell lines. *Molecules* **2016**, *21*, 1533. [CrossRef] [PubMed]
86. Masood Ur, R.; Mohammad, Y.; Fazili, K.M.; Bhat, K.A.; Ara, T. Synthesis and biological evaluation of novel 3-O-tethered triazoles of diosgenin as potent antiproliferative agents. *Steroids* **2017**, *118*, 1–8. [CrossRef] [PubMed]
87. Liu, C.; Xie, F.; Zhao, G.D.; Wang, D.F.; Lou, H.X.; Liu, Z.P. Synthetic studies towards 1alpha-hydroxysolasodine from diosgenin and the unexpected tetrahydrofuran ring opening in the birch reduction process. *Steroids* **2015**, *104*, 214–219. [CrossRef] [PubMed]
88. Hamid, A.A.; Kaushal, T.; Ashraf, R.; Singh, A.; Chand Gupta, A.; Prakash, O.; Sarkar, J.; Chanda, D.; Bawankule, D.U.; Khan, F.; et al. (22beta,25R)-3beta-hydroxy-spirost-5-en-7-iminoxy-heptanoic acid exhibits anti-prostate cancer activity through caspase pathway. *Steroids* **2017**, *119*, 43–52. [CrossRef] [PubMed]
89. Ghosh, S.; More, P.; Derle, A.; Kitture, R.; Kale, T.; Gorain, M.; Avasthi, A.; Markad, P.; Kundu, G.C.; Kale, S.; et al. Diosgenin functionalized iron oxide nanoparticles as novel nanomaterial against breast cancer. *J. Nanosci. Nanotechnol.* **2015**, *15*, 9464–9472. [CrossRef] [PubMed]

10

Potential Anticancer Properties of Osthol: A Comprehensive Mechanistic Review

Yalda Shokoohinia [1,2], Fataneh Jafari [1], Zeynab Mohammadi [3], Leili Bazvandi [3], Leila Hosseinzadeh [1], Nicholas Chow [4], Piyali Bhattacharyya [5], Mohammad Hosein Farzaei [1,*], Ammad Ahmad Farooqi [6], Seyed Mohammad Nabavi [7], Mükerrem Betül Yerer [8] and Anupam Bishayee [9,*]

1 Pharmaceutical Sciences Research Center, School of Pharmacy, Kermanshah University of Medical Sciences, Kermanshah 67146, Iran; yshokoohinia@kums.ac.ir (Y.S.); fataneh.jafari@yahoo.com (F.J.); lhosseinzadeh90@yahoo.com (L.H.)
2 Department of Pharmacognosy and Biotechnology, School of Pharmacy, Kermanshah University of Medical Sciences, Kermanshah 67146, Iran
3 Students Research Committee, School of Pharmacy, Kermanshah University of Medical Sciences, Kermanshah 67146, Iran; zeynabmohamadi47@yahoo.com (Z.M.); leilibazvandi@yahoo.com (L.B.)
4 Department of Clinical and Administrative Sciences, College of Pharmacy, Larkin University, Miami, FL 33169, USA; NChow@ularkin.org
5 School of Health Sciences, University of Turabo, Gurabo, PR 00778, USA; pbhattacharyya@suagm.edu
6 Laboratory for Translational Oncology and Personalized Medicine, Rashid Latif Medical College, Lahore 54000, Pakistan; ammadfarooqi@rlmclahore.com
7 Applied Biotechnology Research Center, Baqiyatallah University of Medical Sciences, Tehran 1435916471, Iran; Nabavi208@gmail.com
8 Department of Pharmacology, Faculty of Pharmacy, University of Erciyes, 38039 Kayseri, Turkey; eczbetul@yahoo.com
9 Department of Pharmaceutical Sciences, College of Pharmacy, Larkin University, Miami, FL 33169, USA
* Correspondence: mh.farzaei@gmail.com (M.H.F.); abishayee@ularkin.org or abishayee@gmail.com (A.B.)

Abstract: Cancer is caused by uncontrolled cell proliferation which has the potential to occur in different tissues and spread into surrounding and distant tissues. Despite the current advances in the field of anticancer agents, rapidly developing resistance against different chemotherapeutic drugs and significantly higher off-target effects cause millions of deaths every year. Osthol is a natural coumarin isolated from Apiaceaous plants which has demonstrated several pharmacological effects, such as antineoplastic, anti-inflammatory and antioxidant properties. We have attempted to summarize up-to-date information related to pharmacological effects and molecular mechanisms of osthol as a lead compound in managing malignancies. Electronic databases, including PubMed, Cochrane library, ScienceDirect and Scopus were searched for in vitro, in vivo and clinical studies on anticancer effects of osthol. Osthol exerts remarkable anticancer properties by suppressing cancer cell growth and induction of apoptosis. Osthol's protective and therapeutic effects have been observed in different cancers, including ovarian, cervical, colon and prostate cancers as well as chronic myeloid leukemia, lung adenocarcinoma, glioma, hepatocellular, glioblastoma, renal and invasive mammary carcinoma. A large body of evidence demonstrates that osthol regulates apoptosis, proliferation and invasion in different types of malignant cells which are mediated by multiple signal transduction cascades. In this review, we set spotlights on various pathways which are targeted by osthol in different cancers to inhibit cancer development and progression.

Keywords: osthol; cancer; phytochemicals; natural product; malignancies; apoptosis

1. Introduction

Cancer is a multifaceted and therapeutically challenging disease and rapidly emerging pre-clinical and clinical studies have started to shed light on the molecular mechanisms which underlie cancer development and progression [1]. Based on the United States National Cancer Institute's categorization, diverse types of cancer include myeloma, carcinoma, leukemia, lymphoma and central nervous system cancer depending on cell type involved [2].

In the next couple of decades, the prevalence of cancer is predicted to rise to 70%, amounting to 22 million cases. The most common sites of cancer diagnosed in 2012 were lung, breast, prostate, colon, stomach, cervix and liver carcinomas. One-third of cancer deaths can be attributed to five life style and nutritive factors, such as overweight, low fresh and fiber food intake, absence of physical activity as well as tobacco and alcohol use [1]. Moreover, malignancies affect the psychological well-being (e.g., depression, anxiety, distress and somatization) of patients and their caregivers [3].

The goals of cancer treatment are to destroy tumors or to markedly prolong survival and improve a patient's quality of life [1]. Deregulations in spatio-temporally controlled signaling mechanisms, including nuclear factor kappa-light-chain-enhancer of activated B cells (NF-κB) [4], activator protein-1 (Ap-1) [4,5] and mitogen-activated protein kinase (MAPK) signaling pathways, played contributory role in carcinogenesis and drug resistance [6–8]. Additionally, microtubules have been targeted to disrupt the normal function of the mitotic spindle [9]. Although chemotherapy and radiotherapy are greatly efficient approaches in the treatment of cancer, malignant cells continue to develop resistance to these treatments [4].

Natural products, containing bioactive secondary metabolites, have beneficial effects on human health [10,11] and the active ingredients are strong candidates to be lead compounds for the development of new drugs [12]. From 1930 to 2012, 183 drugs were approved as antitumor agents; 30% of these were obtained from natural sources, 57% were natural agents with semisynthetic modifications and 34% had natural product mimetic pharmacophores [13]. Although targeted therapies, such as monoclonal antibodies, have greatly improved, the perfect treatment of several cancers, such as leukemia, gastrointestinal and breast cancers, remain to be achieved through new therapies [10]. Natural products exert anticancer effects through various mechanisms such as alteration of cell cycle [4,14] interference with microtubules [15], topoisomerase inhibitory activities [16], immunomodulatory effects [17] and chemopreventive effects [18] achieved by modulation of various oncogenic signaling molecules and pathways [19–21].

Coumarins are derivatives of 2H-1-benzopyran-2-one which can be obtained mainly from cyclization of a C-2 oxygenated *cis*-cinnamic acid. These compounds are widely found in plants in the form of free coumarins or their glycosides [22]. Coumarins naturally occurr with several molecular structures, especially in the Apiaceae [23,24] and Rutaceae families, as well as many other plant families, including Asteraceae, Poaceae and Rubiaceae [22]. Coumarins have various biological properties related to their chemical structure [25–27]. Some coumarins have vasorelaxant activity in coronary vessels and some other showed hypotensive [22], antiviral [28], antileishmanial [29] anti-inflammatory [30] and antispasmodic [31] effects. Furanocoumarins are also widely used in the treatment of leucoderma and psoriasis due to their photosensitivity properties [32,33]. Some hydroxy- and methoxy-coumarins are able to absorb ultraviolet radiation and are commonly used in sunblock creams [22].

Coumarins have prominent anticancer properties with low adverse effects based on the functional groups in the original structure [34,35]. They can affect different cellular pathways, including suppression of angiogenesis, several types of heat shock proteins (HSPs) and cell proliferation as well as inhibition of the enzymes chiefly involved in the pathophysiology of cancer, such as telomerase, monocarboxylate transporters, carbonic anhydrase, aromatase and sulfatase [35,36].

Osthol (osthole), 7-methoxy-8-(3-methyl-2-butenyl)-2*H*-1-benzopyran-2-one, a natural coumarin obtained from *Cnidium* spp. and other Apiaceous plants [37], has been found to exert health-promoting effects [38]. *Cnidium monnieri* fruits rich in osthol are popularly used in traditional Chinese medicine [39].

Osthol is a prenylated coumarin with a wide range of pharmacological effects, such as neuroprotective [40], spasmolytic [41] immunomodulatory [42], osteogenic [43], hepatoprotective [44], vasorelaxant [45], antimicrobial [45], antiviral [46] and antileishmanial properties [47], many of which could be implicated in the primary or secondary prevention of cancer. In this review, we aim to provide a critical and mechanistic insight into the biological and pharmacological properties of osthol that are useful in the treatment of cancer.

2. Literature Search Methodology

Electronically available databases, including PubMed, Science Direct, Cochrane library and Scopus, were searched for cellular, animal or human studies which assessed the anticancer effects of osthol. We have followed the preferred reporting items for systematic review and meta-analysis (PRISMA) criteria which are preferred for reporting systematic reviews. Relevant and high-quality publications were collected for the years 1966–2017 (up to January). Unpublished results were not included. Only English language papers were included in this review. The search terms were "osthol" or "osthole" in title and abstract. Results from primary search were screened by two independent investigators. Included articles were checked for verification of scientific name of source plant, the dose of administration, type of cancer as well as type of cell line for cellular studies and the animal model for animal studies. Results were reviewed for significant effects on proliferation, apoptosis, pro-inflammatory cytokines, oxidative markers, antioxidant enzymes and tissue damage biomarkers.

From total 1354 results, 676 reports were excluded because of duplication and 17 were omitted as they were review papers. Additionally, two were ruled out since they were not in English and 31 were excluded because the subject was on other compounds rather than osthol. Among 628 retrieved studies, 355 were excluded out as they were analytical and phytochemical aspects of osthol rather than pharmacological effects; 273 reports on pharmacological effects of osthol were retrieved amongst which 248 were omitted since they assessed pharmacological effects of osthol other than anticancer properties. Twenty five reports including one in vivo and 24 in vitro studies were finally included. Figure 1 shows a flow diagram of the selective procedure for literature included in this review.

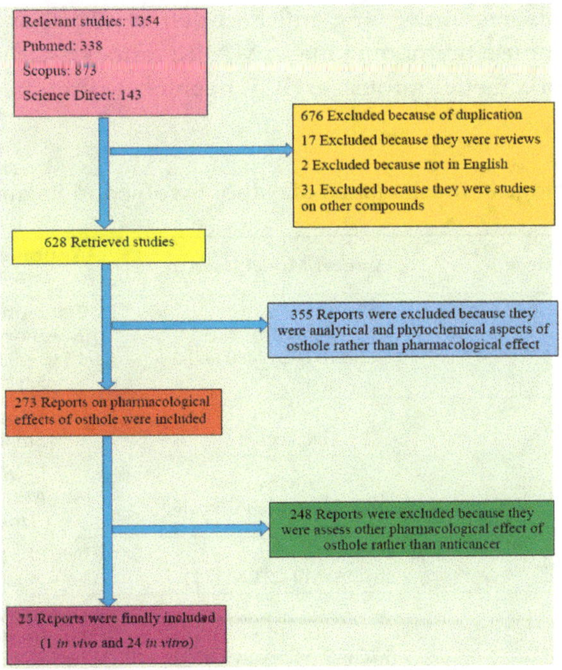

Figure 1. Study selection diagram.

3. Cellular and Molecular Mechanisms of Anticancer Effects of Osthol

A comprehensive review of the reported literature on anticancer activity of osthol indicated that this therapeutic agent could potentially exert anticancer and antitumor activity via several mechanisms, including cell cycle inhibition, apoptosis induction, anti-angiogenesis, inhibition of metastasis, and suppression of cell proliferation and cell migration (Figure 2). Based on the type of cancer, the effective dose and the mechanism of action could be different. A detailed data on the anticancer mechanism of osthol is presented below and Table 1.

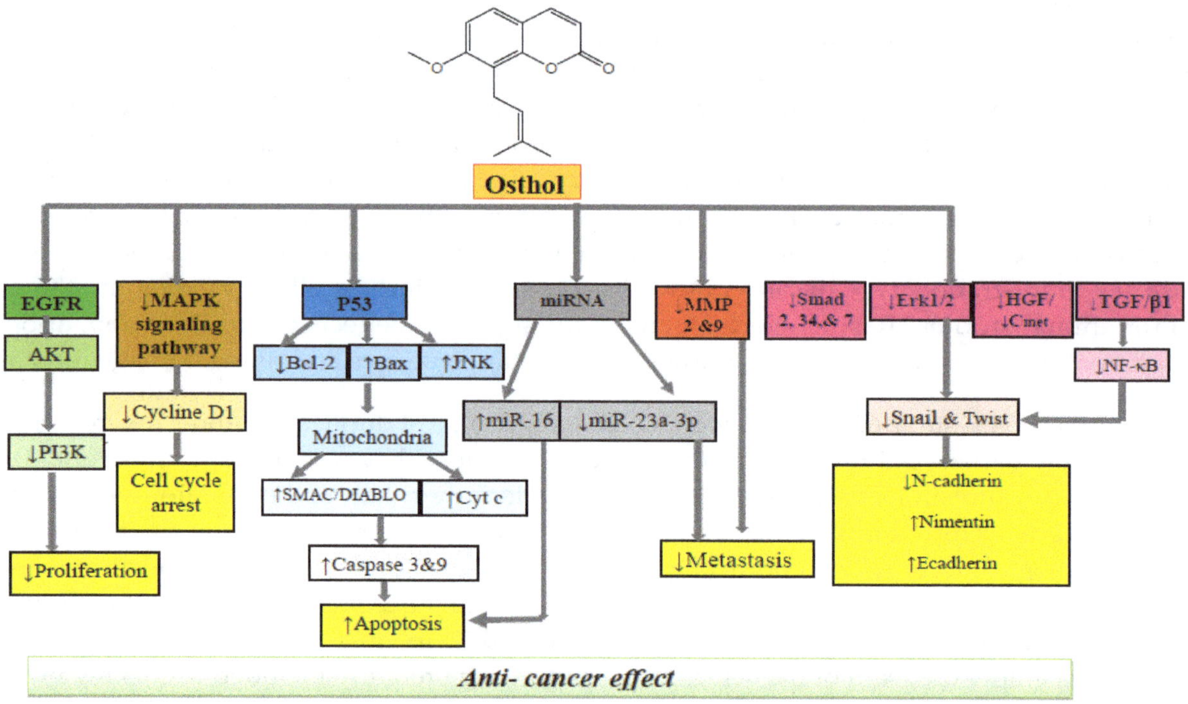

Figure 2. Molecular mechanisms underlying anticancer effect of osthol. EGFR, epidermal growth factor receptor; Akt, AKR mouse thymoma kinase; MAPK, mitogen-activated protein kinase; RNA, ribonucleic acid; MMP, matrix metalloprotease; HGF, hepatocyte growth factor; TGF, tumor growth factor; NF-κB, nuclear factor-κB.

Table 1. Pharmacological mechanisms of osthol involved in its anticancer activities.

Type of Cancer	Conc. or Dose	Cancer Model Used	Anticancer Effects and Mechanisms	Reference
Colon	1, 3 & 10 mM	In vitro (HCT116 & SW480 cells)	↓Cell motility; ↑apoptosis; ↑phosphorylation of p53 on Ser15 (p-p53); ↑acetylation of p53; ↑ROS; ↑JNK	[48]
Prostate	100 mM	In vitro (PC3 cells)	↑Apoptosis; ↓Bcl-; ↑Bax; ↑Smac/DIABLO	[49]
Prostate	20~80 μM	In vitro (AIPC, DU145 & PC3 cells)	↓TGF-β, ↓Akt, JNK& ERK ↓miR-23a-3p	[50]
Breast	15 mM	In vitro (MDA-MB-231 & 4T1)	↓TbetaRII; ↓Smad2; ↓Smad3; ↓Smad4	[51]
Breast	20 mM	In vitro (MCF-7, MDA-MB-453, MDA-MB-231 & BT-20 cells)	↓c-Met signaling; ↓FASN; ↓HGF- induced EMT; ↓c-Met protein levels; ↓cell migration; ↓invasion; ↓c-Met/Akt/mTOR	[52]

Table 1. *Cont.*

Type of Cancer	Conc. or Dose	Cancer Model Used	Anticancer Effects and Mechanisms	Reference
Breast	5, 10, 24, 40 & 80 mM	In vitro (MDA-MB-231, MCF-7, HBL-100 & HER2-overexpressing human cancer cell lines)	↓proliferation; ↑apoptosis; ↓FASN; ↓Akt; ↓mTOR; ↑paclitaxel-induced cytotoxicity	[53]
Breast	5.25 mg/kg	In vivo (Mice treated orally twice weekly)	↑IL-8; ↑M-CSF; ↑PTHrP; ↓OPG/RANKL	[54]
Breast	20–90 mM	In vitro (MDA-231BO cells)	↓Cell viability; ↓proliferation; ↑apoptosis; ↓TGF-β/Smads	[54]
Brain	50, 100 & 200 mM	In vitro (U87 cells)	↓proliferation; ↑apoptosis; ↑miR16; ↓MMP9	[55]
Brain	25, 50 & 100 mM	In vitro (Rat glioma cells)	↓Proliferation; ↓PI3K/Akt/MAPK	[56]
Brain	10–100 mM	In vitro (GBM8401 cells)	↓EMT; ↓Akt and GSK3β; ↓Snail; ↓Twist; ↓I3K/Akt	[57]
Brain	100 mM	In vitro (SKNMC cells)	↑Apoptosis by ↑Bcl; ↑Bax; ↑Smac/DIABLO	[49]
Lung	50, 100 & 150 mM	In vitro (A549 cells)	↑G2/M arrest; ↑apoptosis; ↓Cyclin B1; ↓p-Cdc2; ↓Bcl-2; ↑Bax, ↓PI3K/Akt signaling pathway	[58]
Lung	20, 40, 60 mM 80 mM	In vitro (A549 cells)	↓MMP-2; ↓MMP-9	[58]
Lung	5–20 mM	In vitro (A549 cells)	↓NF-κB mediated snail activation; ↓invasion; ↓migration; ↓adhesion	[59]
Lung	100 mM	In vitro (H1299 cells)	↑Apoptosis; ↓Bcl; ↑Bax; ↑Smac/DIABLO	[49]
Leukemia	5 mM 15 mM	In vitro (K562/ADM cells)	↓MDR in myelogenous leukemia	[60]
Leukemia	30 mg/kg for 8 days	In vivo (CDF1 female mice transplanted with P-388 D1 cells)	↑Apoptosis; ↓P-388 D1 cells	[61]
Cervix	77.96 mM 64.94 mM	In vitro (HeLa cells)	↑Apoptosis	[61]
Ovary	20, 40, 80, 120, 160 and 200	In vitro (A2780 & OV2008 cells)	↓Cells proliferation; ↑apoptosis	[62]
Ovary	5, 10, 24, 40 mM 80 mM	In vitro (SKOV3 human cancer cells)	↓FASN; ↓proliferation; ↑apoptosis; ↓Akt; ↓mTOR; ↑paclitaxel-induced cytotoxicity	[53]
Renal	20–30 mM	In vitro (Caki & U251MG cells)	↑Apoptosis; ↓MMP level; ↑cytochrome *c*; ↓c-FLIP	[63]
Liver	20, 40, 80, 120, 160 or 200 mM	In vitro (SMCC-7721, MHCC-97H, HCC-LM3 & BEL-7402 cells)	↓Proliferation; ↑DNA damage; ↓migration; ↓Cdc2; ↓cyclin B1; ↑ERCC1	[64]

Arrows (↑ and ↓) show increase and decrease in the obtained variables, respectively. H1299, human non-small cell lung carcinoma; GSK3β, glycogen synthase kinase 3-β; EMT, epithelial-mesenchymal transition; Akt, AKR mouse thymoma kinase; PI3K, phosphatidylinositol-3-kinase; IGF, insulin-like growth factor; EGFR, epidermal growth factor receptor; COX-2, cyclooxygenase 2; TPK, tyrosine protein kinase; VEGF, vascular endothelial growth factor; NF-κB, nuclear factor kappa-light-chain-enhancer of activated B cells; MAPK, mitogen-activated protein kinase; ROS, reactive oxygen species; JNK, c-Jun N-terminal kinase; c-MET, cellular mesenchymal to epithelial transition factor; mTOR, mammalian target of rapamycin; MDR, multiple drug resistance; Bax: BCL2-Associated X Protein; TGFβRII, transforming growth factor-β receptor, type II; GMP, guanosine monophosphate.

3.1. Colon Cancer

Epidemiological and scientific studies have considerably enhanced our understanding of the evolutionary process underpinning colon cancer development and progression. Metastasis of primary tumors affects the survival of patients [65]. In a study conducted by Huang et al. [48] using HCT116 and SW480 human colon cancer cell lines, osthol demonstrated specific antitumor effect with concentrations of 1, 3 and 10 μM (Table 1). Osthol significantly decreased cell motility in both cell lines through activation of pro-apoptotic signaling pathways and up-regulation of p53 expression; p53 protein has a main role in the regulation of several genes involved in growth inhibition process, apoptosis, cell cycle arrest as well as DNA repair [66]. Apoptosis-induction capacity has been accepted as a mechanism of action for the antitumor drugs [12]; therefore, considerable effort is being directed towards the development of potential medicines that induce apoptosis in tumor cells.

Apoptosis can occur in two main pathways: the mitochondrial (intrinsic) pathway and the death receptor (extrinsic) pathway [67]. In the intrinsic pathway, the mitochondria have a principle role. It is characterized by cytochrome c release from the mitochondrial which activates a family of cysteine protease enzymes, caspases. This process is controlled by the Bcl-2 family of proteins. This family is an essential member of the programmed cell death process, acting to either inhibit (Bcl-2 and Bcl-xl) or promote (Bax and Bcl-xS) cell death [68]. The elevation of the Bax/Bcl-2 ratio, which has a pivotal contribution in apoptosis, is considered as one of the important mechanisms of osthol in the induction of apoptosis and disturbance in permeability of mitochondrial membranes in cancer cells. Osthol exerted apoptotic effect on colon cancer cell line via several mechanisms, including enhancement of the p53 phosphorylation on Ser15 (p-p53) and p53 acetylation on Lys379 (acetylp53). The p53 protein, acting as a tumor suppressor, plays key roles in activating apoptosis through sensing both intrinsic and extrinsic stresses [69]. Moreover, p53 protein has a significant participation in the regulation of cell cycle arrest, and DNA repair, activating c-Jun N-terminal kinase (JNK) pathway, generation of ROS, modulating PI3K/Akt signaling pathway as well as promoting G2/M arrest. Another mechanism which is involved in pro-apoptotic activity of osthol is p53-independent apoptosis process via stimulating JNK and reactive oxygen species (ROS) formation as summarized in Figure 2 [48].

3.2. Prostate Cancer

Genome sequencing and gene expression analyses have highlighted essential roles of epigenetic and genetic changes in prostate carcinogenesis. Almost all prostate cancers are adenocarcinomas. Mounting evidences have suggested that prostate cancer is found more often in African-American men in comparison to white men [70]. In a cellular study performed by Shokoohinia et al. [18], potential anticancer effect of osthol was assessed on PC3 human prostate cancer cell line. Results of this investigation suggested that osthol acts as a powerful cytotoxic agent against PC3 cells. Caspase activation through intrinsic or extrinsic pathway was significantly involved in the induction of apoptotic cell death. Osthol could remarkably boost the expression of caspase-9 and caspase-3 in PC3 cells. This natural coumarin also activated apoptosis by down-regulation of the antiapoptotic agent, Bcl-2, and up-regulation of the proapoptotic gene Bax (BCL2-Associated X Protein) as well as Smac/DIABLO, a mitochondrial protein released in response to apoptosis stimuli and suppresses the activity apoptosis inhibitors; thus, can facilitate apoptosis [67].

It has previously been convincingly revealed that ectopic expression of miR-23a-3p in DU145 cells induced considerable reversal of osthol-mediated reduction in invasive potential of prostate cancer cells. Detailed mechanistic insights suggested that osthol markedly downregulated miR-23a-3p in DU145 cells [50].

3.3. Breast Cancer

Breast cancer is a common malignancy responsible for cancer-related deaths in females around the world, and accordingly, exploring therapeutic approaches in order to suppressing this disease is immediately vital [71]. In an in vitro study reported by Ye et al. [51] on MDA-MB-231 and 4T1, two invasive mammary carcinoma cell lines, osthol at 15 μM showed inhibitory effect on cell proliferation and invasion. Results showed that osthol in combination with platycodin D, a triterpene saponin, could dramatically reduce tumor growth factor-β receptor II (TGFβRII), Smad2, Smad3 and Smad4 gene or protein expressions and efficiently suppressed TGF-β-induced Smad2 and Smad3 phosphorylation. The latter is the main mechanism of osthol in the reduction of proliferation and invasion of breast cancer cells. Hepatocyte growth factor (HGF) is able to induce epithelial–mesenchymal passage in cancerous cells which can result in cancer cell migration. In an in vitro study performed by Hung et al. [48], a series of human breast cancer cells, such as MDA-MB-453, MDA-MB-23, BT-20 and MCF-7, were treated with osthol. It has been observed that osthol significantly suppressed HGF-induced cell distribution, invasion and migration in MCF-7 cell cultures. Abnormal stimulation of the HGF/c-Met (cellular mesenchymal to epithelial transition factor) pathway has a remarkable role in the progression of various models of cancers as well as advancement of tumor invasion and metastatic system. Osthol inhibited HGF-induced c-Met phosphorylation along with a reduction in the total c-Met protein expression in MCF-7 cells which is intervened by C75 (pharmacological inhibitor) of fatty acid synthase (FASN).

In addition to the effects of osthol in breast cancer, this compound reduces the metastasis of this cancer to the bone marrow. In an in vivo study [54], the researchers used a mouse model to investigate the preventive effect of osthol against the metastasis of human breast cancer cells to the bone. Results showed that osthol blocked breast cancer cell growth, migration and invasion, along with enhancement of apoptosis of breast cancer cells.

Osteoprotegerin (OPG) is a soluble decoy receptor which lacks a trans-membrane domain. It protects the skeleton from excessive bone resorption. Mechanistically, it was shown that OPG interacted with receptor activator of nuclear factor-κB ligand (RANKL) and prevented its structural binding with RANK. The role of osthol in prevention of bone marrow metastasis is mediated by the regulation of OPG/RANKL cascade in the interactions between osteoblasts and breast cancer cells and also suppressing TGF-β/Smads pathway which has a pivotal role in breast cancer bone metastasis. However, many researchers are trying to find strategies to suppress tumor growth as well as tumor metastasis [72].

3.4. Brain Cancer

Glioma, a highly relapsing type of tumor, represents 44.6% of central nervous system tumors and has a high rate of morbidity [73]. In vitro investigation by Lin et al. [55] on glioma cell line U87 showed a significant inhibition of proliferation and augmentation of apoptosis at concentrations of 50, 100 and 200 μM of osthol. Mechanistically, it has been shown that osthol upregulated miR-16 in the U87 cells. These effects were mediated through up-regulation of expression miR-16 and down-regulation of matrix metalloprotease (MMP)-9 expression [74]. MicroRNAs (miRNAs) are a class of non-coding, small molecule RNAs and act as regulators of gene expression [55]. Ding et al. [56] investigated the anticancer effect of osthol on C6 rat glioma cell. Results showed that osthol apparently prevented glioma cell proliferation. This natural compound was also able to induce apoptosis by up-regulating the expression of pro-apoptotic proteins as well as reduction of anti-apoptotic factors expression. Furthermore, the compound could inhibit C6 cell migration and invasion. Results showed that inhibition occurred through phosphatidylinositol-3-kinase (PI3K)/AKR mouse thymoma kinase (Akt) and MAPK signaling pathway [75]. MAPK pathway was significantly involved in regulation of the phospho-proteome of brain tumors. MAPK activation can also induce cell-cycle arrest via cyclin D1 activation and reduction of apoptosis through modulation of the BCL-2-family [76]. Several proteins control cell proliferation processes, amongst which cyclin-dependent kinases (CDKs) are the most important ones. A CDK binds a regulatory protein called cyclin. This complex (CDK-cyclin) has a modulatory role in cell cycle progression and drive cells to enter the next phase at the appropriate time. Increased cyclin D1 expression has been involved in several types of cancer. Osthol is demonstrated to reduce D1 expression. The PI3K/Akt signaling pathway is involved in regulation of cancer development and progression mainly through triggering an increase in phosphorylated levels of Akt [77].

Glioblastoma multiform (GBM) is a progressive type of brain tumor in adults. Recent treatment approaches for GBM include surgical resection, radiotherapy and chemotherapy [78,79]. An in vitro study on insulin-like growth factor (IGF)-1-induced GBM8401 cells exposed to different concentration of osthol showed that this natural agent can reverse IGF-1-induced morphological changes, mediated by increasing epithelial marker expression and reducing mesenchymal marker expression. It has been found that IGF-1 can result in the conversion of GBM8401 cells to fibroblastic phenotype and in this condition the intercellular space becomes expanded. In addition, a wound-healing experiment indicated that osthol could suppress IGF-1-induced migration of GBM8401 cells. Suppression of MMP-2 and MMP-9 plays a significant role in the inhibition of IGF-1-induced cell migration in GBM8401 cells. Osthol reduced the phosphorylation of Akt and glycogen synthase kinase 3β (GSK3β) and regained the GSK3β activity [57]. Pretreatment with IGF-1 can lead to phosphorylation of Akt and Erk1/2 involved in expression of Snail and Twist. Osthol can remarkably suppress the IGF-1-induced down-regulation of ZO-1 and β-catenin as well as up regulation of vimentin, N-cadherin, Snail and Twist in a dose- and time-dependent manner. Suppressing Snail and Twist expression which is characteristic of mesenchymal tumor areas, is one of the main mechanism of osthol in inhibiting the induction of EMT in epithelial neoplasms [80]. One of the mechanisms by which the growth suppressive effect of osthol suppresses the growth of the malignant cells is mediated via the effects of osthol on the PI3K/Akt mTOR pathway. EMT is the critical step for metastatically competent brain cancer cells to spread and invade distant sites. This process is mediated through growth factors. It is interesting that osthol is able to inhibit IGF-1-induced EMT through PI3K/Akt pathway inhibition in human brain cancer cells [81].

3.5. Lung Cancer

Lung cancer is the leading cause of cancer-related deaths all over the world, and non-small cell lung cancer (NSCLC) is responsible for about 80% of all cases [82,83]. In an in vitro study by Xu et al. [84], A549 human lung cancer cells were exposed to osthol at various concentrations. Osthol significantly reduced cell growth and arrested the cells in G_2/M phase. It has been revealed that the osthol cellular mechanism of action includes down-regulation of cyclin B1, p-Cdc2 and Bcl-2 expressions and up-regulation of Bax expression in A549 cells. Osthol could also suppress the PI3K/Akt signaling pathway which might be one of the molecular mechanisms by which the compound exerts anticancer effects. In another study by Xu et al. [58], the effects of various concentration of osthol on the migratory and invasive potential of A549 cells were evaluated. Osthol dose-dependently exerted inhibitory effects on lung cancer cells and effectively suppressed proliferation, migration and invasion of cancerous cells. Cellular mechanisms which are essential for these effects were associated with the inhibition of MMP-2 and MMP-9 expression in the human lung cancer cells which have a significant role in cell invasion and migration. Moreover, Feng et al. [59] investigated the effect of osthol on adenocarcinomic human alveolar basal epithelial cells (A549). The cancerous cells were treated with osthol in 5–20 mM for 48 h. Results showed that osthol extremely suppressed TGF-β1-induced epithelial-to-mesenchymal transition (EMT), adhesion, invasion and migration in A549 which is mediated by adjusting NF-κB and Snail signaling pathways. This molecule can interact with cell adhesion molecules which are involved in angiogenesis. The process of angiogenesis is under regulation of several pro-angiogenic genes as well as growth factors including epidermal growth factor (EGF), vascular endothelial growth factor (VEGF), basic fibroblast growth factor (bFGF), platelet derived growth factors (PDGF), angiopoetin-1 and 2 and MMPs [81].

3.6. Leukemia

Chronic myeloid leukemia (CML) is a type of hematologic malignancy [85]. Multidrug resistance (MDR) has an important role in CML chemotherapy failure through drug resistance [86]. Wang et al. [60] showed that osthol has a remarkable effect on CML. In this research, K562/ADM cells were treated with osthol for 24 h. The potential of osthol to overcome MDR caused by P-glycoprotein (P-gp) was measured by the CCK-8 assay in the K562/ADM cell line. Results demonstrated that osthol remarkably reduced P-gp expression through suppression of the PI3K/Akt signaling pathway which is associated with modulation of MDR mediated by P-gp in different types of leukemia. The authors concluded that the PI3K/Akt signaling pathway is a key mechanism triggered in the reversal effect of osthol in the MDR.

Chou et al. [61] evaluated pharmacological properties of osthol against human leukemia via in vivo and in vitro assessments. P-388 D1 murine leukemia cells were intraperitoneally administered into CDF1 female mice (BALB/c female × DBA/2 male). CDF1 mice with leukemia received osthol (30 mg/kg, orally) once a day for a period of nine days. Data clearly suggested that osthol significantly prolonged lifespan of P-388 D1 tumor-bearing mice by more than 37.5% in comparison to solvent-treated animals. Importantly, survival of one mouse of the osthol-treated group was noted to be more than 60 days.

3.7. Cervical Cancer

A common type of malignancy in women all over the world is cervical cancer [87]. In an in vitro study that utilized HeLa human cervical cancer cells, osthol concentration- and time-dependently suppressed cell growth. Furthermore, cytotoxic effects were non-significant in coumarin-treated primary cultured normal cervical fibroblasts which indicates its specific pharmacological effects on cancer cells. It has been revealed that osthol performs its anticancer potential on cervical cancer cells by elevating DNA fragmentation as well as activation of poly (ADP-ribose) polymerase (PARP) which has an essential contribution in programmed cell death resulting in induction of apoptosis in HeLa cells [61].

3.8. Ovarian Cancer

Ovarian cancer is considered as the most lethal gynecologic cancer [88] in women. Epidemiological studies demonstrated that the proportion of ovarian cancer patients who experienced a five-year survival rate is less than 50% post-diagnosis. The main therapeutic approach for ovarian cancer patients is cytoreductive surgery along with paclitaxel-based chemical agents [88,89]. Clinical evidence reported good primary response in many cases; however, there are still remarkable challenges such as multi-chemotherapy drug resistance. In an in vitro study reported by Jiang et al. [62] uncontrolled proliferation and migration of ovarian cancer cells, including OV2008 and A2780, were assessed. Osthol remarkably reduced cell viability of ovarian cancer cells; whereas no toxicity was detected in normal ovarian cells. Subsequent to treatment with osthol, migratory potential, expression levels and functionalities of MMP-9 and MMP-2 were noted to be significantly suppressed in wound healing and trans-well assays. This natural coumarin repressed cells proliferation via promoting G_2/M phase cell cycle arrest and activation of apoptosis process in malignant cells. It has been suggested that other underlying mechanisms of its anticancer action were the enhancement of the apoptotic protein caspase-3, caspase-9 and Bax/Bcl-2.

3.9. Renal Cancer

In an in vitro study, Min et al. [63] showed that osthol increased TNF-related apoptosis-inducing ligand (TRAIL)-mediated cell death in Caki cell line. Induction of apoptotic cell death by osthol (20–30 μM for 24 h) is mediated by regulation of the FLICE like inhibitory protein (c-FLIP) expression in human renal carcinoma cells. c-FLIP overexpression markedly inhibited apoptosis; however, osthol significantly reduced c-FILP levels and sensitized resistant cells to TRAIL. Also, osthol significantly decreased MMP levels and synergistic treatment with TRAIL induced an increase in cytosolic accumulation of cytochrome c. These findings provided evidence that osthol worked synergistically with TRAIL and induced apoptosis in TRAIL-resistant cell lines. Moreover, osthol blocks the growth and invasion of bladder cancer cells by inhibiting the expression of the angiogenesis-related proteins COX-2, VEGF, MMP-2 and NF-κB. Future studies must converge on detailed investigation of osthol-mediated regulation of the TRAIL pathway in resistant cancer cells. We still have insufficient information about regulation of death receptors (DR4 and DR5) by osthol in cancer cells.

3.10. Liver Cancer

In an in vitro study, Lin et al. [64] reported that osthol reduced hepatocellular carcinoma (HCC) cell proliferation. The chemotherapeutic potential of osthol on HCC cell proliferation was mediated through induction of DNA damage and cell cycle arrest as well as inhibition of migration of HCC cells. It remarkably suppressed the cell cycle in the G_2/M phase by blocking the expression of Cdc2. Cyclin-dependent kinase 1 (CDK1)-cyclin B, also known as cell division control protein kinase 2 (Cdc2)-cyclin B is a member of cyclin-dependent kinases with a significant role in regulation of the cell cycle. It has been found that down-regulation of MMP-2 and MMP-9 is involved in suppression of migration of HCC cells by this natural agent. Finally, the authors demonstrated that osthole inhibited EMT by increasing epithelial biomarkers E-cadherin and β-catenin and simultaneously repressing the levels of N-cadherin and vimentin. This phytoconstituents also damaged DNA by induction of DNA excision repair protein (ERCC) 1 expression enhancing epithelial biomarkers E-cadherin and β-catenin, and reducing mesenchymal N-cadherin are among the main cellular factors which have a key role in suppression of EMT by osthol [90]. These cellular pathways suggest an interesting chemotherapeutic effect of osthol on HCC. The interaction of DNA and other coumarins have been reported previously [91].

3.11. Protectice Effect against Toxicity of Chemotherpy

The positive effects of osthol in modulating cancer include direct anticarcinogenic activity along with protective effects against side effects of conventional chemotherapeutic agents. One of the chemotherapeutic drugs that are used for treatment of several types of cancers is doxorubicin [55] which shows several adverse effects due to its inherent pro-oxidant activity. Protective effects of osthol against doxorubicin-induced oxidative stress and apoptosis in the neuronal cell line (PC12) has been confirmed. The protective mechanisms of osthol include enhancement of mitochondrial membrane potential, elevation of Bax/Bcl-2 ratio, improvement in loss of cell viability, suppression of intracellular reactive oxygen species (ROS) generation as well as increases in mitochondrial membrane potential in PC12 cells [18,92]. Fatty acid synthase (FASN) is the only enzyme engaged in long-chain saturated fatty acid synthesis and is implicated in cancer progression by regulating lipid raft function. Thus, one of the molecular pathways by which osthol performs its protective action against cancer progression is its potent inhibitory effect on FASN [53].

4. Toxicity of Osthol

Reviewing current literature can help to collect information regarding the bio-efficacy and safety of the administration of significant phytochemicals in the prevention and management of different malignancies and their relevant complications. Since osthol safety has been investigated, the no-observed adverse-effect level (NOAEL) of osthol for both male and female rats is considered to be less than 5 mg/kg [93]. We suggest to perform randomized, controlled, trials with adequate sample size in order to validate the safety and efficacy of osthol in managing patients with malignancies.

5. Conclusions and Future Directions

Osthol is a natural coumarin isolated from Umbelliferae plants with a wide range of pharmacological effects. The goal of the present review was to provide a summary of current knowledge on the anticancer effects of osthol as a lead compound in malignancy therapy along with in-depth molecular mechanisms. This natural phytochemical suppresses the activation of different apoptotic proteins such as caspase-3 and caspase-9, Smac/DIABLO, poly-ADP ribose polymerase and survivin, which are associated with the intrinsic pathways of apoptosis. Osthol is demonstrated to induce apoptosis in different carcinoma cell lines through up-regulation of p53 expression. It has also been shown that osthol induces apoptosis through a mechanism independent of the tumor-suppressing properties of p53. This effect of osthol seems to be promising since the compound demonstrated antitumor effects in several types of cancers in which a p53 regulatory system is involved [94]. It also can diminish metastasis via different molecular mechanisms such as reducing the expression of Smad 2, 3 and 4, C75, and inhibition of the HGF/c-Met signaling pathway as well as HGF-induced c-Met phosphorylation. Osthol also has a stimulatory effect on the extrinsic apoptotic pathway by increasing levels of caspase-8 (unique to the extrinsic pathway). Furthermore, ability of osthol to inhibit NF-κB-mediated cell survival pathway plays an important contribution in its pro-apoptotic properties, as summarized in Figure 2.

Results obtained from studies evaluating anticancer potential of osthol have confirmed its protective and therapeutic effect on various types of malignancies including ovarian cancer, cervical cancer, chronic myeloid leukemia, lung adenocarcinoma cells, glioma as well as glioblastoma multiform cells, invasive mammary carcinoma cells, colon cancer, and prostate cancer. Recent investigations, mentioned previously, have suggested that osthol has a significant action in the brain by protecting neurons. Additionally, the ability of osthol in penetrating the blood–brain barrier indicates its potential as a future drug for chemotherapy of brain tumors.

Based on the insights gleaned from decades of research, it seems clear that a "one size fits all" approach will not be effective in clinical settings. There has been a paradigm shift in our understanding about the heterogeneous nature of cancer, and accordingly, researchers are now focusing on multi-targeted approaches. Osthol has emerged as a promising phytochemical reportedly involved in the regulation of different signaling pathways. However, we have just started to scratch the surface of information related to the potential of osthol to target multiple proteins and signaling pathways. We still need to have a better understanding of how osthol regulates specific signaling pathways, such as VEGF/VEGFR, PDGF/PDGFR and SHH/GLI pathways, and exert differential modulation of oncogenic and tumor suppressor microRNAs.

Numerous studies presented here clearly suggest that osthol possesses the potential to act in an inhibitory role in the progression of malignancies. A large body of evidence demonstrated that osthol regulates apoptosis, proliferation and invasion in different types of malignant cells which is mediated by multiple cellular signaling pathways. However, the mechanisms of function of osthol toward various cancers are not the same. As it was mentioned, osthol possesses antioxidant activity, causing inhibition of ROS overproduction in different cells. ROS can activate several pathways involved in metastasis and possess critical roles in invasion and invadopodia formation; moreover, ROS also possess prominent roles on signaling cascades relating to resistance to apoptosis, neovascularization, and proliferation. Therefore, ROS contribute in various mechanisms [95–98], and reduction of ROS using antioxidants is a promising way to inhibit different cancers. Based on the different roles of ROS in cancer cells and their contribution in different mechanistic pathways, the function of antioxidants such as osthol in excretion of anticancer activity could be probably different. Regarding the remarkable pharmacological functions of osthol in the protection and treatment of malignancies as described above, this natural compound is becoming a significant natural structure for drug discovery. Furthermore, mechanistic investigations for exploring precise intracellular mechanisms of osthol in defending and fighting against cancer are recommended. Also, well-designed randomized clinical trials are important to evaluate the safety and efficacy of osthol in patients with different types of cancers.

Acknowledgments: Authors are grateful to the deputy of Research, Kermanshah University of Medical Sciences, Kermanshah, Iran for the grant No. 93487.

Author Contributions: Y.S., M.H.F. and L.H. designed the structure of the paper and drafted the manuscript. F.J., Z.M., L.B. performed the literature search and contributed in writing the manuscript. A.B., P.B., N.C., M.B.Y., A.A.F. and S.M.N. reviewed and revised the manuscript. All authors had full access to the final version of the manuscript and gave their approval before publishing.

References

1. World-Health-Organization. Cancer: Fact Sheet No. 297. 2015. Available online: http://www.who.int (accessed on 2 October 2016).
2. Jena, J.; Ranjan, R.; Ranjan, P.; Sarangi, M.K. A Study on Natural Anticancer Plants. *Int. J. Pharm. Chem. Sci.* **2012**, *1*, 365–368.
3. Padmaja, G.; Vanlalhruaii, C.; Rana, S.; Nandinee, D.; Hariharan, M. Care givers' depression, anxiety, distress, and somatization as predictors of identical symptoms in cancer patients. *J. Cancer Res. Ther.* **2016**, *12*, 53–57. [CrossRef] [PubMed]
4. Safarzadeh, E.; Sandoghchian, S.S.; Baradaran, B. Herbal medicine as inducers of apoptosis in cancer treatment. *Adv. Pharm. Bull.* **2014**, *4*, 421–427. [PubMed]
5. HemaIswarya, S.; Doble, M. Potential synergism of natural products in the treatment of cancer. *Phytother. Res.* **2006**, *20*, 239–249. [CrossRef] [PubMed]
6. Cragg, G.M.; Newman, D.J. Plants as a source of anti-cancer agents. *J. Ethnopharmacol.* **2005**, *100*, 72–79. [CrossRef] [PubMed]
7. Guan, X.; Sun, Z.; Chen, X.; Wu, H.; Zhang, X. Inhibitory effects of Zengshengping fractions on DMBA-induced buccal pouch carcinogenesis in hamsters. *Chin. Med. J.* **2012**, *125*, 332–337. [CrossRef] [PubMed]
8. Sadeghi-Aliabadi, H.; Aliasgharluo, M.; Fattahi, A.; Mirian, M.; Ghanadian, M. In vitro cytotoxic evaluation of some synthesized COX-2 inhibitor derivatives against a panel of human cancer cell lines. *Res. Pharm. Sci.* **2013**, *8*, 298–303. [PubMed]
9. Mukhtar, E.; Adhami, V.M.; Mukhtar, H. Targeting microtubules by natural agents for cancer therapy. *Mol. Cancer Ther.* **2014**, *13*, 275–284. [CrossRef] [PubMed]
10. Basmadjian, C.; Zhao, Q.; Bentouhami, E.; Djehal, A.; Nebigil, C.G.; Johnson, R.A.; Serova, M.; De Gramont, A.; Faivre, S.; Raymond, E.; et al. Cancer wars: Natural products strike back. *Front. Chem.* **2014**, *2*, 20. [CrossRef] [PubMed]
11. Vergara, D.; De Domenico, S.; Tinelli, A.; Stanca, E.; Del Mercato, L.L.; Giudetti, A.M.; Simeone, P.; Guazzelli, N.; Lessi, M.; Manzini, C.; et al. Anticancer effects of novel resveratrol analogues on human ovarian cancer cells. *Mol. BioSyst.* **2017**, *13*, 1131–1141. [CrossRef] [PubMed]
12. Ahmadi, F.; Derakhshandeh, K.; Jalalizadeh, A.; Mostafaie, A.; Hosseinzadeh, L. Encapsulation in PLGA-PEG enhances 9-nitro-camptothecin cytotoxicity to human ovarian carcinoma cell line through apoptosis pathway. *Res. Pharm. Sci.* **2015**, *10*, 161–168. [PubMed]
13. Newman, D.J.; Giddings, L.-A. Natural products as leads to antitumor drugs. *Phytochem. Rev.* **2014**, *13*, 123–137. [CrossRef]
14. Farzaei, M.H.; Bahramsoltani, R.; Rahimi, R. Phytochemicals as adjunctive with conventional anticancer therapies. *Curr. Pharm. Des.* **2016**, *22*, 4201–4218. [CrossRef] [PubMed]
15. Nobili, S.; Lippi, D.; Witort, E.; Donnini, M.; Bausi, L.; Mini, E.; Capaccioli, S. Natural compounds for cancer treatment and prevention. *Pharmacol. Res.* **2009**, *59*, 365–378. [CrossRef] [PubMed]
16. Ashley, R.E.; Osheroff, N. Natural products as topoisomerase II poisons: Effects of thymoquinone on DNA cleavage mediated by human topoisomerase IIα. *Chem. Res. Toxicol.* **2014**, *27*, 787–793. [CrossRef] [PubMed]
17. Schafer, G.; Kaschula, C.H. The immunomodulation and anti-inflammatory effects of garlic organosulfur compounds in cancer chemoprevention. *Anti-Cancer Agents Med. Chem.* **2014**, *14*, 233–240. [CrossRef]
18. Shokoohinia, Y.; Hosseinzadeh, L.; Moieni-Arya, M.; Mostafaie, A.; Mohammadi-Motlagh, H.-R. Osthole attenuates doxorubicin-induced apoptosis in PC12 cells through inhibition of mitochondrial dysfunction and ROS production. *BioMed Res. Int.* **2014**, *2014*, 156848. [CrossRef] [PubMed]
19. Bishayee, A.; Sethi, G. Bioactive natural products in cancer prevention and therapy: Progress and promise. *Semin. Cancer Biol.* **2016**, *40–41*, 1–3. [CrossRef] [PubMed]

20. Block, K.I.; Gyllenhaal, C.; Lowe, L.; Amedei, A.; Amin, A.R.; Amin, A.; Aquilano, K.; Arbiser, J.; Arreola, A.; Arzumanyan, A. Designing a broad-spectrum integrative approach for cancer prevention and treatment. *Semin. Cancer Biol.* **2015**, *35*, S276–S304. [CrossRef] [PubMed]
21. Shanmugam, M.K.; Lee, J.H.; Chai, E.Z.P.; Kanchi, M.M.; Kar, S.; Arfuso, F.; Dharmarajan, A.; Kumar, A.P.; Ramar, P.S.; Looi, C.Y. Cancer prevention and therapy through the modulation of transcription factors by bioactive natural compounds. *Semin. Cancer Biol.* **2016**, *40–41*, 35–47. [CrossRef] [PubMed]
22. Waksmundzka-Hajnos, M.; Sherma, J.; Kowalska, T. *Thin Layer Chromatography in Phytochemistry*; CRC Press: Boca Raton, FL, USA, 2008.
23. Sajjadi, S.; Zeinvand, H.; Shokoohinia, Y. Isolation and identification of osthol from the fruits and essential oil composition of the leaves of *Prangos asperula* Boiss. *Res. Pharm. Sci.* **2009**, *4*, 19–23.
24. Sajjadi, S.E.; Shokoohinia, Y.; Hemmati, S. Isolation and identification of furanocoumarins and a phenylpropanoid from the acetone extract and identification of volatile constituents from the essential oil of *Peucedanum pastinacifolium*. *Chem. Nat. Compd.* **2012**, *48*, 668–671. [CrossRef]
25. Ahmadi, F.; Valadbeigi, S.; Sajjadi, S.; Shokoohinia, Y.; Azizian, H.; Taheripak, G. Grandivittin as a natural minor groove binder extracted from Ferulago macrocarpa to ct-DNA, experimental and in silico analysis. *Chem. Biol. Interact.* **2016**, *258*, 89–101. [CrossRef] [PubMed]
26. Venugopala, K.-N.; Rashmi, V.; Odhav, B. Review on natural coumarin lead compounds for their pharmacological activity. *BioMed Res Int.* **2013**, *2013*, 963248. [CrossRef] [PubMed]
27. Shokoohinia, Y.; Gheibi, S.; Kiani, A.; Sadrjavadi, K.; Nowroozi, A.; Shahlaei, M. Multi-spectroscopic and molecular modeling investigation of the interactions between prantschimgin and matrix metalloproteinase 9 (MMP9). *Luminescence* **2015**, *31*, 587–593. [CrossRef] [PubMed]
28. Ghannadi, A.; Fattahian, K.; Shokoohinia, Y.; Behbahani, M.; Shahnoush, A. Anti-viral evaluation of sesquiterpene coumarins from *Ferula assa-foetida* against HSV-1. *Iran. J. Pharm. Res.* **2014**, *13*, 523–530. [PubMed]
29. Sajjadi, S.E.; Eskandarian, A.-A.; Shokoohinia, Y.; Yousefi, H.-A.; Mansourian, M.; Asgarian-Nasab, H.; Mohseni, N. Antileishmanial activity of prenylated coumarins isolated from *Ferulago angulata* and *Prangos asperula*. *Res. Pharm. Sci.* **2016**, *11*, 324–331. [CrossRef] [PubMed]
30. Kiani, A.; Almasi, K.; Shokoohinia, Y.; Sadrjavadi, K.; Nowroozi, A.; Shahlaei, M. Combined spectroscopy and molecular modeling studies on the binding of galbanic acid and MMP9. *Int. J. Biol. Macromol.* **2015**, *81*, 308–315. [CrossRef] [PubMed]
31. Sadraei, H.; Shokoohinia, Y.; Sajjadi, S.E.; Mozafari, M. Antispasmodic effects of *Prangos ferulacea* acetone extract and its main component osthole on ileum contraction. *Res. Pharm. Sci.* **2013**, *8*, 137–144. [PubMed]
32. Ceska, O.; Chaudhary, S.; Warrington, P.; Ashwood-Smith, M. Photoactive furocoumarins in fruits of some umbellifers. *Phytochemistry* **1986**, *26*, 165–169. [CrossRef]
33. Ranjbar, S.; Shokoohinia, Y.; Ghobadi, S.; Bijari, N.; Gholamzadeh, S.; Moradi, N.; Ashrafi-Kooshk, M.R.; Aghaei, A.; Khodarahmi, R. Studies of the interaction between isoimperatorin and human serum albumin by multispectroscopic method: Identification of possible binding site of the compound using esterase activity of the protein. *Sci. World J.* **2013**, *2013*, 305081. [CrossRef] [PubMed]
34. Bijari, N.; Shokoohinia, Y.; Ashrafi-Kooshk, M.R.; Ranjbar, S.; Parvaneh, S.; Moieni-Arya, M.; Khodarahmi, R. Spectroscopic study of interaction between osthole and human serum albumin: Identification of possible binding site of the compound. *J. Lumin.* **2013**, *143*, 328–336. [CrossRef]
35. Thakur, A.; Singla, R.; Jaitak, V. Coumarins as anticancer agents: A review on synthetic strategies, mechanism of action and SAR studies. *Eur. J. Med. Chem.* **2015**, *101*, 476–495. [CrossRef] [PubMed]
36. Geisler, J.; Sasano, H.; Chen, S.; Purohit, A. Steroid sulfatase inhibitors: Promising new tools for breast cancer therapy? *J. Steroid Biochem. Mol. Biol.* **2011**, *125*, 39–45. [CrossRef] [PubMed]
37. Jelodarian, Z.; Shokoohinia, Y.; Rashidi, M.; Ghiasvand, N.; Hosseinzadeh, L.; Iranshahi, M. New polyacetylenes from *Echinophora cinerea* (Boiss.) Hedge et Lamond. *Nat. Prod. Res.* **2017**, *31*, 2256–2263. [CrossRef] [PubMed]
38. You, L.; Feng, S.; An, R.; Wang, X. Osthole: A promising lead compound for drug discovery from a traditional Chinese medicine (TCM). *Nat. Prod. Commun.* **2009**, *4*, 297–302. [PubMed]
39. Zhang, Q.; Qin, L.; He, W.; Van Puyvelde, L.; Maes, D.; Adams, A.; Zheng, H.; De Kimpe, N. Coumarins from *Cnidium monnieri* and their antiosteoporotic activity. *Planta Med.* **2007**, *73*, 13–19. [CrossRef] [PubMed]

40. Wang, S.-J.; Lin, T.-Y.; Lu, C.-W.; Huang, W.-J. Osthole and imperatorin, the active constituents of *Cnidium monnieri* (L.) Cusson, facilitate glutamate release from rat hippocampal nerve terminals. *Neurochem. Int.* **2008**, *53*, 416–423. [CrossRef] [PubMed]
41. Sadraei, H.; Shokoohinia, Y.; Sajjadi, S.; Ghadirian, B. Antispasmodic effect of osthole and *Prangos ferulacea* extract on rat uterus smooth muscle motility. *Res. Pharm. Sci.* **2012**, *7*, 141–149. [PubMed]
42. Resch, M.; Steigel, A.; Chen, Z.-L.; Bauer, R. 5-Lipoxygenase and cyclooxygenase-1 inhibitory active compounds from *Atractylodes lancea*. *J. Nat. Prod.* **1998**, *61*, 347–350. [CrossRef] [PubMed]
43. Zhang, W.; Ma, D.; Zhao, Q.; Ishida, T. The effect of the major components of *Fructus Cnidii* on osteoblasts in vitro. *J. Acupunct. Meridian Stud.* **2010**, *3*, 32–37. [CrossRef]
44. Huang, R.; Chen, C.; Huang, Y.; Hsieh, D.; Hu, C.; Chang, C. Osthole increases glycosylation of hepatitis B surface antigen and suppresses the secretion of hepatitis B virus in vitro. *Hepatology* **1996**, *24*, 508–515. [CrossRef] [PubMed]
45. Guh, J.-H.; Yu, S.-M.; Ko, F.-N.; Wu, T.-S.; Teng, C.-M. Antiproliferative effect in rat vascular smooth muscle cells by osthole, isolated from *Angelica pubescens*. *Eur. J. Pharmacol.* **1996**, *298*, 191–197. [CrossRef]
46. Gholamzadeh, S.; Behbahani, M.; Fattahi, A.; Sajjadi, S.; Shokoohinia, Y. Antiviral evaluation of coumarins from *Prangos ferulacea* L. (Lindl). *Res. Pharm. Sci.* **2012**, *7*, S783.
47. Kermani, E.-K.; Sajjadi, S.-E.; Hejazi, S.-H.; Arjmand, R.; Saberi, S.; Eskandarian, A.-A. Anti-Leishmania activity of osthole. *Pharmacog. Res.* **2016**, *8* (Suppl. 1), S1. [CrossRef] [PubMed]
48. Huang, S.-M.; Tsai, C.-F.; Chen, D.-R.; Wang, M.-Y.; Yeh, W.-L. p53 is a key regulator for osthole-triggered cancer pathogenesis. *BioMed Res. Int.* **2014**, *2014*, 175247. [CrossRef] [PubMed]
49. Shokoohinia, Y.; Hosseinzadeh, L.; Alipour, M.; Mostafaie, A.; Mohammadi-Motlagh, H.-R. Comparative evaluation of cytotoxic and apoptogenic effects of several coumarins on human cancer cell lines: Osthole induces apoptosis in p53-deficient H1299 cells. *Adv. Pharmacol. Sci.* **2014**, *2014*, 847574. [CrossRef] [PubMed]
50. Wen, Y.-C.; Lee, W.-J.; Tan, P.; Yang, S.-F.; Hsiao, M.; Lee, L.-M.; Chien, M.-H. By inhibiting snail signaling and miR-23a-3p, osthole suppresses the EMT-mediated metastatic ability in prostate cancer. *Oncotarget* **2015**, *6*, 21120–21136. [CrossRef] [PubMed]
51. Ye, Y.; Han, X.; Guo, B.; Sun, Z.; Liu, S. Combination treatment with platycodin D and osthole inhibits cell proliferation and invasion in mammary carcinoma cell lines. *Environ. Toxicol. Pharmacol.* **2013**, *36*, 115–124. [CrossRef] [PubMed]
52. Hung, C.-M.; Kuo, D.-H.; Chou, C.-H.; Su, Y.-C.; Ho, C.-T.; Way, T.-D. Osthole suppresses hepatocyte growth factor (HGF)-induced epithelial-mesenchymal transition via repression of the c-Met/Akt/mTOR pathway in human breast cancer cells. *J. Agric. Food Chem.* **2011**, *59*, 9683–9690. [CrossRef] [PubMed]
53. Lin, V.C.-H.; Chou, C.-H.; Lin, Y.-C.; Lin, J.-N.; Yu, C.-C.; Tang, C.-H.; Lin, H.-Y.; Way, T.-D. Osthole suppresses fatty acid synthase expression in HER2-overexpressing breast cancer cells through modulating Akt/mTOR pathway. *J. Agric. Food Chem.* **2010**, *58*, 4786–4793. [CrossRef] [PubMed]
54. Wu, C.; Sun, Z.; Guo, B.; Ye, Y.; Han, X.; Qin, Y.; Liu, S. Osthole inhibits bone metastasis of breast cancer. *Oncotarget* **2017**, *8*, 58480–58493. [CrossRef] [PubMed]
55. Lin, K.; Gao, Z.; Shang, B.; Sui, S.; Fu, Q. Osthole suppresses the proliferation and accelerates the apoptosis of human glioma cells via the upregulation of microRNA-16 and downregulation of MMP-9. *Mol. Med. Rep.* **2015**, *12*, 4592–4597. [CrossRef] [PubMed]
56. Ding, D.; Wei, S.; Song, Y.; Li, L.; Du, G.; Zhan, H.; Cao, Y. Osthole exhibits anti-cancer property in rat glioma cells through inhibiting PI3K/Akt and MAPK signaling pathways. *Cell. Physiol. Biochem.* **2013**, *32*, 1751–1760. [CrossRef] [PubMed]
57. Lin, Y.-C.; Lin, J.-C.; Hung, C.-M.; Chen, Y.; Liu, L.-C.; Chang, T.-C.; Kao, J.-Y.; Ho, C.-T.; Way, T.-D. Osthole inhibits insulin-like growth factor-1-induced epithelial to mesenchymal transition via the inhibition of PI3K/Akt signaling pathway in human brain cancer cells. *J. Agric. Food Chem.* **2014**, *62*, 5061–5071. [CrossRef] [PubMed]
58. Xu, X.-M.; Zhang, Y.; Qu, D.; Feng, X.-W.; Chen, Y.; Zhao, L. Osthole suppresses migration and invasion of A549 human lung cancer cells through inhibition of matrix metalloproteinase-2 and matrix metallopeptidase-9 in vitro. *Mol. Med. Rep.* **2012**, *6*, 1018–1022. [CrossRef] [PubMed]
59. Feng, H.; Lu, J.-J.; Wang, Y.; Pei, L.; Chen, X. Osthole inhibited TGF β-induced epithelial–mesenchymal transition (EMT) by suppressing NF-κB mediated Snail activation in lung cancer A549 cells. *Cell Adhes. Migr.* **2017**, *11*, 464–475. [CrossRef] [PubMed]

60. Wang, H.; Jia, X.-H.; Chen, J.-R.; Wang, J.-Y.; Li, Y.-J. Osthole shows the potential to overcome P-glycoprotein-mediated multidrug resistance in human myelogenous leukemia K562/ADM cells by inhibiting the PI3K/Akt signaling pathway. *Oncol. Rep.* **2016**, *35*, 3659–3668. [CrossRef] [PubMed]
61. Chou, S.Y.; Hsu, C.S.; Wang, K.T.; Wang, M.C.; Wang, C.C. Antitumor effects of Osthol from *Cnidium monnieri*: An in vitro and in vivo study. *Phytother. Res.* **2007**, *21*, 226–230. [CrossRef] [PubMed]
62. Jiang, G.; Liu, J.; Ren, B.; Tang, Y.; Owusu, L.; Li, M.; Zhang, J.; Liu, L.; Li, W. Anti-tumor effects of osthole on ovarian cancer cells in vitro. *J. Ethnopharmacol.* **2016**, *193*, 368–376. [CrossRef] [PubMed]
63. Min, K.-J.; Han, M.; Kim, S.; Park, J.-W.; Kwon, T.K. Osthole enhances TRAIL-mediated apoptosis through downregulation of c-FLIP expression in renal carcinoma Caki cells. *Oncol. Rep.* **2017**, *37*, 2348–2354. [CrossRef] [PubMed]
64. Lin, Z.-K.; Liu, J.; Jiang, G.-Q.; Tan, G.; Gong, P.; Luo, H.-F.; Li, H.-M.; Du, J.; Ning, Z.; Xin, Y. Osthole inhibits the tumorigenesis of hepatocellular carcinoma cells. *Oncol. Rep.* **2017**, *37*, 1611–1618. [CrossRef] [PubMed]
65. Friend, S. p53: A glimpse at the puppet behind the shadow play. *Science* **1994**, *265*, 334–336. [CrossRef] [PubMed]
66. Livingstone, L.R.; White, A.; Sprouse, J.; Livanos, E.; Jacks, T.; Tlsty, T.D. Altered cell cycle arrest and gene amplification potential accompany loss of wild-type p53. *Cell* **1992**, *70*, 923–935. [CrossRef]
67. Hosseinzadeh, L.; Behravan, J.; Mosaffa, F.; Bahrami, G.; Bahrami, A.R.; Karimi, G. Effect of curcumin on doxorubicin-induced cytotoxicity in H9c2 cardiomyoblast cells. *Iran. J. Basic Med. Sci.* **2011**, *14*, 49–56.
68. Elmore, S. Apoptosis: A review of programmed cell death. *Toxicol. Pathol.* **2007**, *35*, 495–516. [CrossRef] [PubMed]
69. Amaral, J.D.; Xavier, J.M.; Steer, C.J.; Rodrigues, C.M. The role of p53 in apoptosis. *Discov. Med.* **2010**, *9*, 145–152. [PubMed]
70. Mao, H.L.; Liu, P.S.; Zheng, J.F.; hai Zhang, P.; Zhou, L.G.; Xin, G.; Liu, C. Transfection of Smac/DIABLO sensitizes drug-resistant tumor cells to TRAIL or paclitaxel-induced apoptosis in vitro. *Pharmacol. Res.* **2007**, *56*, 483–492. [CrossRef] [PubMed]
71. Jemal, A.; Bray, F.; Center, M.M.; Ferlay, J.; Ward, E.; Forman, D. Global cancer statistics. *CA Cancer J. Clin.* **2011**, *61*, 69–90. [CrossRef] [PubMed]
72. De Cicco, P.; Panza, E.; Armogida, C.; Ercolano, G.; Taglialatela-Scafati, O.; Shokoohinia, Y.; Camerlingo, R.; Pirozzi, G.; Calderone, V.; Cirino, G.; et al. The hydrogen sulfide releasing molecule acetyl deacylasadisulfide inhibits metastatic melanoma. *Front. Pharmacol.* **2017**, *8*, 65. [CrossRef] [PubMed]
73. Sun, Y.-C.; Wang, J.; Guo, C.-C.; Sai, K.; Wang, J.; Chen, F.-R.; Yang, Q.-Y.; Chen, Y.-S.; Wang, J.; To, T.S.-S.; et al. MiR-181b sensitizes glioma cells to teniposide by targeting MDM2. *BMC Cancer* **2014**, *14*, 611. [CrossRef] [PubMed]
74. Gheibi, S.; Shokohinia, Y.; Kiani, A.; Sadrjavadi, K.; Nowroozi, A.; Shahlaei, M. Molecular insight into the Grandivitin-matrix metalloproteinase 9 interactions. *J. Photochem. Photobiol. B* **2016**, *162*, 493–499. [CrossRef] [PubMed]
75. Tatevossian, R.G.; Lawson, A.R.; Forshew, T.; Hindley, G.F.; Ellison, D.W.; Sheer, D. MAPK pathway activation and the origins of pediatric low-grade astrocytomas. *J. Cell. Physiol.* **2010**, *222*, 509–514. [CrossRef] [PubMed]
76. Balmanno, K.; Cook, S. Tumour cell survival signalling by the ERK1/2 pathway. *Cell Death Differ.* **2009**, *16*, 368–377. [CrossRef] [PubMed]
77. Luo, J.; Manning, B.D.; Cantley, L.C. Targeting the PI3K-Akt pathway in human cancer: Rationale and promise. *Cancer Cell* **2003**, *4*, 257–262. [CrossRef]
78. Buckner, J.C. Factors influencing survival in high-grade gliomas. In *Seminars in Oncology*; WB Saunders: Philadelphia, PA, USA, 2003; Volume 30, pp. 10–14.
79. Chen, Y.-H.; Hung, M.-C.; Shyu, W.-C. Role of cancer stem cells in brain tumors. *Biomedicine* **2012**, *2*, 84–91. [CrossRef]
80. Zhang, X.; Chen, T.; Zhang, J.; Mao, Q.; Li, S.; Xiong, W.; Qiu, Y.; Xie, Q.; Ge, J. Notch1 promotes glioma cell migration and invasion by stimulating β-catenin and NF-κB signaling via AKT activation. *Cancer Sci.* **2012**, *103*, 181–190. [CrossRef] [PubMed]
81. Wilken, R.; Veena, M.S.; Wang, M.B.; Srivatsan, E.S. Curcumin: A review of anti-cancer properties and therapeutic activity in head and neck squamous cell carcinoma. *Mol. Cancer* **2011**, *10*, 12. [CrossRef] [PubMed]

82. Jemal, A.; Siegel, R.; Ward, E.; Hao, Y.; Xu, J.; Murray, T.; Thun, M.J. Cancer statistics, 2008. *CA Cancer J. Clin.* **2008**, *58*, 71–96. [CrossRef] [PubMed]
83. Parkin, D.M.; Bray, F.; Ferlay, J.; Pisani, P. Global cancer statistics, 2002. *CA Cancer J. Clin.* **2005**, *55*, 74–108. [CrossRef] [PubMed]
84. Xu, X.; Zhang, Y.; Qu, D.; Jiang, T.; Li, S. Osthole induces G2/M arrest and apoptosis in lung cancer A549 cells by modulating PI3K/Akt pathway. *J. Exp. Clin. Cancer Res.* **2011**, *30*, 33. [CrossRef] [PubMed]
85. Mathisen, M.S.; Kantarjian, H.M.; Cortes, J.; Jabbour, E. Mutant BCR-ABL clones in chronic myeloid leukemia. *Haematologica* **2011**, *96*, 347–349. [CrossRef] [PubMed]
86. Souza, P.S.; Vasconcelos, F.C.; De Souza Reis, F.R.; De Moraes, G.N.; Maia, R.C. P-glycoprotein and survivin simultaneously regulate vincristine-induced apoptosis in chronic myeloid leukemia cells. *Int. J. Oncol.* **2011**, *39*, 925–933. [PubMed]
87. Echelman, D.; Feldman, S. Management of cervical precancers: A global perspective. *Hematol. Oncol. Clin. N. Am.* **2012**, *26*, 31–44. [CrossRef] [PubMed]
88. Mei, L.; Chen, H.; Wei, D.M.; Fang, F.; Liu, G.J.; Xie, H.Y.; Wang, X.; Zou, J.; Han, X.; Feng, D. Maintenance chemotherapy for ovarian cancer. *Curr. Oncol. Rep.* **2013**, *5*, 454–458.
89. Park, J.T.; Chen, X.; Trope, C.G.; Davidson, B.; Shih, I.-M.; Wang, T.-L. Notch3 overexpression is related to the recurrence of ovarian cancer and confers resistance to carboplatin. *Am. J. Pathol.* **2010**, *177*, 1087–1094. [CrossRef] [PubMed]
90. Wells, A.; Grahovac, J.; Wheeler, S.; Ma, B.; Lauffenburger, D. Targeting tumor cell motility as a strategy against invasion and metastasis. *Trends Pharmacol. Sci.* **2013**, *34*, 283–289. [CrossRef] [PubMed]
91. Ahmadi, F.; Shokoohinia, Y.; Javaheri, S.; Azizian, H. Proposed binding mechanism of galbanic acid extracted from *Ferula assa-foetida* to DNA. *J. Photochem. Photobiol. B* **2017**, *166*, 63–73. [CrossRef] [PubMed]
92. Shokoohinia, Y.; Khajouei, S.; Ahmadi, F.; Ghiasvand, N.; Hosseinzadeh, L. Protective effect of bioactive compounds from *Echinophora cinerea* against cisplatin-induced oxidative stress and apoptosis in the PC12 cell line. *Iran. J. Basic Med. Sci.* **2017**, *20*, 438–445. [PubMed]
93. Shokoohinia, Y.; Bazargan, S.; Miraghaee, S.; Javadirad, E.; Hosseinzadeh, L. Safety assessment of osthole isolated from *Prangos ferulacea*: Acute and subchronic toxicities and modulation of cytochrome P450. *Jundishapur J. Nat. Pharm. Prod.* **2017**. [CrossRef]
94. Davatgaran-Taghipour, Y.; Masoomzadeh, S.; Farzaei, M.H.; Bahramsoltani, R.; Karimi-Soureh, Z.; Rahimi, R.; Abdollahi, M. Polyphenol nanoformulations for cancer therapy: Experimental evidence and clinical perspective. *Int. J. Nanomed.* **2017**, *12*, 2689–2702. [CrossRef] [PubMed]
95. Peiris-Pagès, M.; Martinez-Outschoorn, U.E.; Sotgia, F.; Lisanti, M.P. Metastasis and oxidative stress: Are antioxidants a metabolic driver of progression? *Cell Metabol.* **2015**, *22*, 956–958. [CrossRef] [PubMed]
96. Panieri, E.; Santoro, M.M. ROS homeostasis and metabolism: A dangerous liaison in cancer cells. *Cell Death Dis.* **2016**, *7*, e2253. [CrossRef] [PubMed]
97. Nelson, K.K.; Melendez, J.A. Mitochondrial redox control of matrix metallopro-teinases. *Free Radic. Biol. Med.* **2004**, *37*, 768–784. [CrossRef] [PubMed]
98. Morry, J.; Ngamcherdtrakul, W.; Yantasee, W. Oxidative stress in cancer and fibrosis: Opportunity for therapeutic intervention with antioxidant compounds, enzymes, and nanoparticles. *Redox Biol.* **2017**, *11*, 240–253. [CrossRef] [PubMed]

11

Anticancer Effects of Green Tea and the Underlying Molecular Mechanisms in Bladder Cancer

Yasuyoshi Miyata *, Tomohiro Matsuo, Kyohei Araki, Yuichiro Nakamura, Yuji Sagara, Kojiro Ohba and Hideki Sakai

Department of Urology, Nagasaki University Graduate School of Biomedical Sciences, Nagasaki 852-8501, Japan; tomozo1228@hotmail.com (T.M.); k-araki205@cameo.plala.or.jp (K.A.); yn1238056@yahoo.co.jp (Y.N.); gaasara3@gmail.com (Y.S.); ohba-k@nagasaki-u.ac.jp (K.O.); hsakai@nagasaki-u.ac.jp (H.S.)

* Correspondence: int.doc.miya@m3.dion.ne.jp;

Abstract: Green tea and green tea polyphenols (GTPs) are reported to inhibit carcinogenesis and malignant behavior in several diseases. Various in vivo and in vitro studies have shown that GTPs suppress the incidence and development of bladder cancer. However, at present, opinions concerning the anticancer effects and preventive role of green tea are conflicting. In addition, the detailed molecular mechanisms underlying the anticancer effects of green tea in bladder cancer remain unclear, as these effects are regulated by several cancer-related factors. A detailed understanding of the pathological roles and regulatory mechanisms at the molecular level is necessary for advancing treatment strategies based on green tea consumption for patients with bladder cancer. In this review, we discuss the anticancer effects of GTPs on the basis of data presented in in vitro studies in bladder cancer cell lines and in vivo studies using animal models, as well as new treatment strategies for patients with bladder cancer, based on green tea consumption. Finally, on the basis of the accumulated data and the main findings, we discuss the potential usefulness of green tea as an antibladder cancer agent and the future direction of green tea-based treatment strategies for these patients.

Keywords: animal model; treatment; bladder cancer; epidemiology; green tea

---

1. Introduction

Green tea is obtained from the leaves of the plant *Camellia sinensis*, and it is one of the most popular beverages worldwide, particularly in Asia. Green tea is recognized to have health-promoting effects that are attributed to green tea polyphenols (GTPs), such as epicatechin, epigallocatechin, epicatechin-3-gallate (ECG), and epigallocatechin-3-gallate (EGCG) [1]. In addition, its antioxidant, anti-inflammatory, and antibacterial properties have been reported to provide various benefits to its consumers [2]. Several investigators have reported that the addition of GTPs to drinking water can prevent carcinogenesis and the development of various types of malignancies [3–5]. In addition, laboratory-based evidence of the anticancer effects of GTPs has been increasing [4,6]. On the other hand, other studies have shown that green tea consumption does not decrease the risk for various types of cancers, including brain cancer and breast cancer [7,8]. In addition, a meta-analysis of published case-control and cohort studies showed that green tea consumption is not associated with risk of pancreatic cancer [9]. Furthermore, no significant association between green tea consumption and colon cancer risk was observed (summary RR: 0.99; 95% CI: 0.79, 1.24) in prospective cohort studies [10]. Additionally, it has been reported that green tea consumption might be associated with an increased risk of upper aerodigestive tract cancer [11]. Taken together, the anticancer effects of green tea consumption and GTPs remain controversial. With regard to bladder cancer, various in vivo and in vitro studies have provided inconsistent results.

Below, we first present a general discussion on the relationship between green tea consumption and cancer risk on the basis of data from epidemiological studies, the mechanisms underlying these anticancer effects, the safety and adverse effects of GTPs, and trials of treatment strategies based on green tea consumption. Then, we present a detailed review of these topics with a focus on bladder cancer. Previously, excellent reviews of studies, particularly epidemiological investigations, on the relationship between green tea consumption and bladder cancer risk have been published [12,13]. Therefore, in the present review, we paid attention to the molecular mechanisms underlying the anticancer effects, findings from studies involving animal models, and novel treatment strategies based on green tea consumption for patients with bladder cancer, as these topics have been less well addressed in previous reviews.

2. Anticancer Effects of Green Tea Polyphenols

GTPs exhibit anticancer effects via the regulation of different cancer-related processes and factors, including DNA methylation, histone modification, micro-RNA, and proteins [5,14–17]. They also play an important role via the regulation of apoptosis, growth, invasion, and angiogenesis in various types of malignancies [13,15,18,19]. A recent study showed that GTPs can influence the pathological roles of not only cancer cells, but also cancer stem cells [17]. These findings have led to a hypothesis that GTPs have strong anticancer effects in vivo and in vitro. In the next section, findings that support this hypothesis are discussed.

2.1. Anticancer Effects Shown in Epidemiological Studies

When discussing the anticancer effects of GTPs, it is necessary to focus on the different phases in the natural evolution of malignant cells. Briefly, green tea extracts are thought to be useful for primary prevention (prevention and delay of cancer onset) and tertiary prevention (prevention of recurrence and metastasis) [17]. With regard to primary prevention, several epidemiological studies have shown that the average age at cancer onset in individuals with high levels of green tea consumption was significantly higher than that in individuals with low levels of green tea consumption [17,20,21]. These studies have also shown that the consumption of more than 10 cups of green tea was associated with a reduced incidence of lung, colorectum, liver, and stomach cancer [17,20,21]. Furthermore, several reports have shown that GTPs were effective in preventing transformation from a premalignant status to frank malignancy [14,22].

With regard to tertiary cancer prevention, on the other hand, one study reported that the recurrence rate for stage I and stage II breast cancer was significantly lower for patients consuming ≥5 cups of green tea daily (16.7%) than in those consuming ≤4 cups (24.3%; $p < 0.005$) [23]. However, these preventive effects were not observed for stage III breast cancer recurrence. Another report stated that the hazard ratio for stage I breast cancer recurrence showed a statistically significant decrease (hazard ratio, 0.43; 95% confidential interval, 0.22–0.84) [24]. Similar preventive effects on cancer recurrence have also been reported for other cancers. For example, a study showed that the recurrence rate for colorectal cancer was significantly lower in an experimental group (daily consumption of green tea plus tablets of green tea extracts (GTEs) than in a control group (31.0% vs. 15.0%; $p < 0.05$) [25]. In addition, GTEs reportedly showed inhibitory effects on metastasis in various types of malignancies. For example, lung metastasis from melanoma was inhibited by GTEs in an animal experiment [26].

2.2. Mechanisms Underlying the Anticancer Effects of Green Tea

Various cancer-related molecules have been reported to be modulated by GTPs. In fact, many studies have reported that GTPs inhibited cell growth and induced apoptosis in various types of malignancies [19,27,28]. In addition, these polyphenols modulate the functions of various cancer-related signaling molecules. For example, the function and expression of vascular endothelial growth factor (VEGF), which is a strong stimulator of angiogenesis, are mediated by GTPs in oral cancer and esophageal squamous cell carcinoma [14,29]. Furthermore, in these malignancies, cyclin

D1, which is a cell cycle regulator, and caspase-3, which is an important determinant for apoptosis, are associated with GTPs [14,29].

EGCG has also been reported to affect the pathological behavior of stem cells in several cancers. For example, they inhibited the proliferation and induced the apoptosis of lung cancer stem cells [30] and suppressed tumor spheroid formation by colorectal cancer stem cells [16].

Numerous previous reports have presented detailed information on the mechanisms underlying the general anticancer effects of green tea; thus, we present the details only for bladder cancer.

2.3. Cancer Treatment Strategies Based on Green Tea Consumption

While GTPs inhibit tumor growth in human lung cancer cell lines, their inhibitory effects were approximately 250-fold less effective than those of doxorubicin (Adriamycin) [31]. Therefore, it has been suggested that GTPs are more suitable for use in cancer prevention than as cancer treatment [17]. In fact, chemoprevention by oral administration of green tea catechins was investigated in volunteers with high-grade prostate intraepithelial neoplasia, a precancerous change [22]. Furthermore, EGCG administration was reported to be useful as an adjuvant therapy after complete tumor resection [32]. Various GTPs can also increase the sensitivity of anticancer agents and prevent drug resistance [33,34]. In fact, new cancer treatment strategies using a combination of GTPs and anticancer agents, such as cisplatin, paclitaxel, and tamoxifen, have been recommended for several types of malignancies [35,36]. The molecular mechanisms underlying these synergistic effects are partially clear. For example, in osteosarcoma, SOX overlapping transcript variant 7 is known to contribute to an improvement in the clinical efficacy of combination therapy with EGCG and doxorubicin via inhibition of both autophagy and stemness [37]. In addition to anticancer agents, various natural compounds have also been shown to exhibit anticancer effects when combined with GTPs. For example, in a xenograft model of human leukemia, the oral intake of green tea and intraperitoneal injection of quercetin, which is a polyphenol present in fruits and vegetables, induced apoptosis and suppressed tumor growth [38]. Furthermore, another study reported that EGCG and quercetin enhanced the anticancer effects of doxorubicin via regulation of cell cycle arrest and apoptosis in prostate cancer [39].

As mentioned above, the anticancer effects of GTPs are relatively weak, and a higher concentration of GTPs near cancer cells is considered to improve their anticancer effects. Polymeric micelles are used as the drug-delivery systems in various treatments. In recent years, several anticancer drug-loaded micellar nanocomplexes based on GTE-derivatives have been developed [40,41]. A micellar nanocomplex based on the self-assembly of EGCG and doxorubicin inhibited tumor growth in a xenograft model of human liver cancer [41]; similar results were reported for a micellar nanocomplex prepared by complexation of oligomerized EGCG with trastuzumab (Herceptin) in a mouse model of breast cancer [40]. These findings indicate that more detailed in vivo studies and clinical trials of such combined therapies are important for development of new treatment strategies of bladder cancer.

3. Bladder Cancer and Green Tea

Bladder cancer is a common malignancy in 43 countries around the globe, although the incidence among men, women, and both sexes has decreased in 11, 10, and 12 countries, respectively [42]. Bladder cancer imposes a substantial psychological, physical, and economic burden, and its prognosis is poor, despite various multidisciplinary therapeutic approaches, particularly in cases with muscle invasion and/or metastasis [43]. Therefore, more detailed information will be useful for devising preventive and treatment strategies.

Many studies have focused on the clinical benefits of food choices in terms of chemoprevention, treatment, and survival in bladder cancer [44]. Furthermore, complementary and alternative medicine (CAM), defined as a diverse medical and healthcare system, is recognized as a strategy commonly used by patients with malignancies, including bladder cancer [45]. Green tea consumption and GTPs intake are suggested as CAM strategies [46].

3.1. Epidemiological Studies on Bladder Cancer

3.1.1. Case-Control and Cohort Studies

As mentioned above, no consensus has been derived from the findings of epidemiological studies on green tea consumption, and the effects thereof on carcinogenesis and tumor development and growth remain controversial. Similarly, with regard to bladder cancer, opinions about the relationship between green tea consumption and cancer risk are conflicting. For example, it was reported that the risk of bladder cancer in individuals with high green tea consumption (≥0.14 servings/day) was lower than that in individuals who never consumed the beverage (odds ratio, 0.60; 95% confidential interval, 0.45–0.79; $p < 0.001$) [47]. However, to our knowledge, this is the only study supporting the hypothesis that a high level of green tea consumption suppresses the risk of bladder cancer. On the other hand, surprisingly, another study reported that the risk of bladder cancer was significantly higher for individuals who consumed five to nine cups of green tea daily than in those who did not consume green tea (odds ratio, 2.67; 95% confidential interval, 0.49–2.84) [48]. However, the same study also showed that bladder cancer risk was similar for individuals who consumed ≥10 cups daily than for those who did not consume green tea (odds ratio, 1.18; 95% confidential interval, 1.44–4.94) [48]. Table 1 summarizes the findings of previous studies on the relationship between green tea consumption and bladder cancer risk.

Table 1. Previous reports on the relationship between green tea consumption and bladder cancer risk.

Case-Control Study				Cohort Study			
Author/Year /Country/Ref	**Daily Intake**	**OR/RR**	**95% CI**	**Author/Year Country/Ref**	**Daily Intake**	**OR/RR**	**95% CI**
Waikens et al.	Cases/controls = 271/522			Chyou et al.			
/1996	(Men)			/1993	Never	1.0	
/USA	Q1	1.0		/USA	Ever	1.34	0.79–2.27
/[49]	Q2	1.1	0.6−1.9	/[50]			
	Q3	1.1	0.6–2.3				
	(Women)			Nagano et al.			
	Q1	1.0		/2000	0–1 cup	1.0	
	Q2	0.8	0.3–2.1	/Japan	2–4	1.07	0.61–2.00
	Q2	0.9	0.3–2.6	/[51]	≥5	1.07	0.58–2.08
Wakai et al.		124/744		Kurahashi et al.			
/2004	<	1.0		/2009	(Men)		
/Japan	1–4	1.40	0.74–2.62	/Japan	<1 cup	1.0	
/[47]	5–9	2.67	1.44–4.94	/[52]	1–2	1.18	0.73–1.91
	≥10	1.18	0.49–2.84		3–4	0.71	0.43–1.18
					≥5	0.90	0.56–1.45
Hemelt et al.		381/371			(Women)		
/2010	0	1.00			<3	1.0	
/China	<Daily	0.83	0.54–1.27		3–4	1.22	0.49–3.00
/[53]	Daily	1.02	0.71–1.48		≥5	2.29	1.06–4.92
	<4	1.23	0.76–1.97				
	≥4	0.83	0.53–1.28				
Wang et al.		1007/1299					
/2013	Never	1.0					
/USA	0.1–0.13	0.82	0.61–1.11				
/[49]	≥0.14	0.60	0.45–0.79				

ref: reference. OR: odds ratio. RR: relative ratio. CI: confidential interval.

As shown in Table 1, four of the seven studies were performed in Asian countries. In addition, among the three studies performed in the USA, the subjects were of Japanese ancestry in one and in another were Japanese individuals living in the USA [47,49,50]. Case-control and cohort studies have not been performed in Central and South America, Europe, or Africa. This does not mean that researchers and residents in these countries are not interested in the anticancer effects of tea extracts, including catechins, in bladder cancer. In fact, to clarify the relationship between fluid intake and the risk of urothelial cancer, a multicenter cohort study was designed for 233 and 236 subjects from 23 centers in 10 European countries [54]. The findings of that study revealed that the intake of tea and herbal tea was not associated with the risk of urothelial cancer. However, the effects of green tea per se were not investigated. Moreover, information concerning the anticancer effects of green tea in white and black individuals is scarce.

With regard to epidemiological studies, we should also pay attention to the fact that various units are used to measure green tea consumption, such as frequency/day, cups/day, and mL/day. In addition, the volume per cup differs among countries and regions. For example, the volume of representative cups used for consuming green tea in Japan (120–140 mL) is less than that in Western countries. This information is important when considering the clinical usefulness of green tea. It would be useful if more detailed information about the amount of green tea consumed were included in such reports in future.

3.1.2. Meta-Analyses

There have been several reports of meta-analyses of the relationship between green tea consumption and bladder cancer risk. In this review, we have focused on meta-analyses published in English, because we could not verify the content of publications in other languages. A summary of these meta-analyses is presented in Table 2.

Table 2. Meta-analyses of the relationship between green tea consumption and bladder cancer risk.

Author/Year /Reference	Number of Case-Control Studies	Number of Cohort Studies	Odds Ratio	95% Confidence Interval
Qin et al./2012/[55]	2	3	0.97	0.73–1.21
Wang et al./2013/[13]	2	2	0.81	0.68–0.98
Wu et al./2013/[56]	3	2	1.03	0.82–1.31
Zhang et al./2015/[57]	0	3	1.02	0.95–1.11
Weng et al./2017/[58]	4	3	0.95	0.73–1.24

Only one meta-analysis showed a negative correlation between green tea consumption and bladder cancer risk [13], while the remaining four showed no association between green tea consumption and the risk. A meta-analysis of three cohort studies and three hospital-based case-control studies showed that green tea consumption was not related to a decreased risk of bladder cancer (odds ratio, 0.97; 95% confidential interval, 0.73–1.21) [55]; in addition, another meta-analysis of two cohort studies and three case-control studies showed that there was no significant relationship (relative risk, 1.03; 95% confidential interval, 0.82–1.31) between green tea consumption and bladder cancer risk [56]. Yet, another dose–response meta-analysis of 25 case-control studies and seven prospective cohort studies showed no significant association between green tea consumption and bladder cancer risk [58].

On other hand, it should be noted that the number of studies included in these meta-analyses was relatively small. Although the meta-analysis by Weng et al. assessed the relationship between the consumption of various types of tea (black tea, oolong tea, herbal tea, etc.) and bladder cancer risk in 32 studies (25 case-control studies and seven cohort studies), it included only seven studies involving green tea consumption [58]. Another limitation of these meta-analyses is that they did not include papers published in languages other than English. We found a meta-analysis of five studies showing that increased consumption of green tea may have a protective effect on bladder cancer (odds ratio, 0.76; 95% confidential interval, 0.66–0.95); however, only three of those five studies were verifiable [59]. Considering that green tea is a major beverage for Asians, the majority of whom are not native English speakers, we believe that the publication of English versions of studies published in Asian languages is important.

3.2. Mechanisms Underlying the Anticancer Effects of Green Tea in Bladder Cancer

Although it remains unclear how GTPs regulate malignant aggressiveness, various cancer-related mechanisms and molecules are known to play important roles in the anticancer effects of green tea. In addition, green tea and its extracts have been suggested to affect multiple pathological activities and signaling pathways [60]. Therefore, we evaluated the relationships between GTP and cancer-related functions, including cell survival, cell death, migration, and the cell cycle, in bladder cancer cell lines (Table 3).

Table 3. Relationships between green tea polyphenol treatment and various cancer-related functions in in vitro studies of bladder cancer cell lines.

Cell Line	Type	Dosage/Concentration	Author/Year/Reference
Growth inhibition			
AY-27	EGCG	>100 μM	Kemberling et al./2003/[61]
NBT-II	EGCG	10, 20, or 40 μM/L	Chen et al./2004/[62]
J82	EGCG	70–87 μM	Rieger et al./2007/[63]
UM-UC-3	EGCG	70–87 μM	Rieger et al./2007/[63]
EJ	EGCG	70–87 μM	Rieger et al./2007/[63]
T24	EGCG	70–87 μM 20–100 μg/mL 20–80 μg/mL	Rieger et al./2007/[63]; Qin et al./2007/[64]; Philips et al./2009/[65]
KK47	EGCG	70–87 μM	Rieger et al./2007/[63]
TCCSUP	EGCG	70–87 μM 10–80 μg/mL	Rieger et al./2007/[63]; Philips et al./2009/[65]
TSGH-8301	EGCG	25–100 μM	Chen et al./2011/[66]
MBT-2	EGCG	12.5–50 μM	Hsieh et al./2011/[67]
RT4	EGCG	60–80 μg/mL	Philips et al./2009/[65]
SW780	EGCG	10–80 μg/mL	Philips et al./2009/[65]
Apoptosis induction			
NBT-II	EGCG	10 μM/L	Chen et al./2004/[62]
T24	EGCG	10–80 μg/mL	Qin et al./2007/[64]
TCCSUP	EGCG	40 μg/mL	Philips et al./2009/[65]
TSGH-8301	EGCG	75 μM	Chen et al./2011/[66]
MBT-2	EGCG	50 μM	Hsieh et al./2011/[67]
SW780	EGCG	50–200 μM	Luo et al./2017/[27]
Migration inhibition			
UM-UC-3	EGCG	5 μM	Rieger et al./2007/[63]
EJ	EGCG	5 μM	Rieger et al./2007/[63]
TCCSUP	EGCG	5 μM	Rieger et al./2007/[63]
SW780	EGCG	25–50 μM	Luo et al./2017/[27]
Cell cycle arrest			
NBT-II	EGCG	10, 20, or 40 μM/L	Chen et al./2004/[62]

EGCG: epigallocatechin-3-gallate. GTP: green tea polyphenol.

3.2.1. Cancer Cell Proliferation and Cell Death

In vitro studies have shown that EGCG suppressed cancer cell proliferation and growth in various types of bladder cancer cell lines. Interestingly, one study showed that a high concentration (60 μg/mL) of ECG and ECGC significantly suppressed the proliferation of bladder cancer cell lines (RT4, SW780, TCCSUP, and T24) [65]. However, the same study also showed that a low concentration (10 μg/mL) of ECG could suppress proliferation in SW780, but not in RT4 and T24 [65]. Thus, we speculate that the inhibitory effects of green tea polyphenols on bladder cancer cell proliferation are regulated by complex mechanisms.

In addition to its effects on cancer cell proliferation, EGCG induced apoptosis in various types of bladder cancer cell lines, regardless of the malignant potential and species (Table 3). A study showed that EGCG played an important role in not only the induction of apoptosis, but also the inhibition of growth in a bladder cancer cell line (NBT-II) [62]. However, another study showed that EGCG affected only the apoptosis of bladder cancer cells (SW780), but not cell proliferation or migration [27].

Autophagy is a highly conservative catabolic process used by eukaryotic cells for the degradation of damaged or superfluous proteins and organelles [66]. Although autophagy plays important roles in cell signaling and cellular homeostasis, including physiological cytoprotective or prosurvival mechanisms, completely uncontrolled or excessive autophagy has been associated with cell death [68]. Autophagy is also recognized as an important factor for understanding the pathological characteristics and for planning treatment strategies for many types of cancers [69,70]. This process is stimulated by various stimuli, including nutrients [71,72]. In fact, in bladder cancer cells, autophagy plays an important role in pathological processes and signaling pathways via external stimuli, including natural products [73,74]. With regard to the relationship between autophagy and GTPs, an in vitro study showed that the latter inhibited epirubicin-induced autophagy [75].

Thus, GTPs, especially EGCG, play important roles in cell survival, and affect cell proliferation and cell death in various types of bladder cancer cell lines. On the other hand, as shown in Table 3, the dosage and concentration of EGCG used in in vitro studies varied greatly. Further studies are necessary to judge the optimal dosage and concentration to ascertain the relationship between GTP and bladder cancer cell survival.

3.2.2. Other Cancer-Related Mechanisms

Cancer cell migration and invasion are two key processes for cancer cell dissemination and metastasis in almost all solid tumors, including bladder cancer. As shown in Table 3, in vitro studies have used scratch assays and migration assays to show that EGCG suppressed cell migration and invasion. However, information pertaining to cell migration and invasion is scarce relative to that related to cell survival and death. On the other hand, the concentrations of EGCG that inhibited bladder cancer cell migration were typically lower than those that affected tumor growth and apoptosis (Table 3). More detailed investigations are needed to clarify this issue.

A previous study showed that EGCG caused cell cycle arrest in rat transitional cell cancer [62]. Another study suggested that tea polyphenols can deregulate the cell cycle in bladder cancer cells [46]. Oxidative stress is defined as an imbalance between the cellular production of reactive oxygen species (ROS) and antioxidants; excessive production of ROS causes DNA damage and promotes the activities of oncogenes and/or inhibits tumor suppressor genes [76]. Oxidative stress plays important roles in the aggressiveness of bladder cancer [77]. A previous study has shown that GTPs can protect against oxidative stress in the event of bladder cell death, although this effect was not detected in one of the bladder cancer cell lines (T24) [78].

On the other hand, as shown in Table 3, EGCG has been most widely used for in vitro studies aiming to clarify the relationship between GTPs and various cancer-related functions. Furthermore, other reports have shown that EGCG is the most important component in terms of the health benefits and anticancer effects of green tea [79,80]. Therefore, ECGC has been the focus of discussion in terms of both potential preventative and of therapeutic approaches for bladder cancer.

3.2.3. Cancer-Related Potential Molecular Targets of Green Tea Polyphenols

Next, we evaluate reports on the relationships between GTPs and cancer-related signaling molecules in bladder cancer cell lines (Table 4).

Table 4. Potential molecular targets of green tea polyphenols in bladder cancer cell lines.

Molecules	Cell Line	Author/Year/Reference
Bcl-2 family	T24	Qin et al./2007/61; Gu et al./2017/[68]
	TSGH-8301	Chen et al./2011/[66]
	MBT-2	Hsieh et al./2011/[67]
	SW780	Luo et al./2017/[27]
	BIU87	Gu et al./2017/[68]
Caspase family	TSGH-8301	Chen et al./2011/[66]
	MBT-2	Hsieh et al./2011/[67]
	SW780	Luo et al./2017/[27]
Cyclin D1	NBT-II	Chen et al./2004/[62]
Cyclin-dependent kinase 4/6	NBT-II	Chen et al./2004/[62]
Heat shock protein 27	TSGH-8301	Chen et al./2011/[65]
JNK/Bcl-2/Beclin-1	T24, BIU87	Gu et al./2017/[75]
Matrix metalloproteinase-9	SW780	Luo et al./2017/[27]
N-cadherin	UM-UC-3	Rieger et al./2007/[63]
Nuclear factor-kappa B	TCCSUP	Philips et al./2009/[65]
	SW780	Luo et al./2017/[27]
Phosphatidylinositol 3-kinase /Akt signaling	UM-UC-3	Rieger et al./2007/[63]
	T24	Qin et al./2007/[64]
	TSGH-8301	Chen et al./2011/[66]
Retinoblastoma protein	NBT-II	Chen et al./2004/[62]
Wnt signaling	TCCSUP	Philips et al./2009/[65]

As shown in Table 4, GTPs can regulate the expression and activity of various types of cancer-related molecules. Among them, the bcl-2 and caspase families are well-known important regulators of apoptosis in many types of cancer cells, including bladder cancer cells [81–83]. In addition, phosphatidylinositol 3-kinase (PI3K)/Akt signaling is one of the most important mediators for the regulation of pathological activities such as cell proliferation, apoptosis, and progression in malignancies, including bladder cancer [82,84,85]. Furthermore, a JNK/Bcl-2/Beclin-1-mediated mechanism is associated with autophagy and apoptosis in bladder cancer cells [68]. As a mechanism underlying the pro-apoptotic function, the regulation of nuclear factor-kappa B and matrix metalloproteinase (MMP)-9 has been suggested [27]. Various apoptosis-related molecules have been associated with GTP-induced cell death in bladder cancer cells. Surprisingly, however, there has been no study of the relationship between GTPs and p53 status and function in bladder cancer, even though significant mechanistic associations have been reported in other types of malignancies [86,87]. Therefore, the effects of GTPs on bladder cancer cell proliferation and death require further investigation.

MMP-9 and N-cadherin, which play crucial roles in cancer cell migration and invasion in bladder cancer [88,89], are reportedly modulated by GTPs in bladder cancer cell lines [27,63]. However, there is little information on the effect of GTPs on E-cadherin, which is the best known and classical member of the cadherin family, in bladder cancer. Similarly, the influence of GTPs on MMP-2, which is a strong stimulator of cell invasion and migration, remains unclear. However, there has been a report that a mixture of lysin, proline, arginine, ascorbic acid, and GTEs inhibited cancer cell invasion via the regulation of MMP-2 and MMP-9 production in a bladder cancer cell line (T24) [90].

In a bladder cancer cell line established from Wistar rats (NBT-II), EGCG caused growth inhibition and cell cycle arrest via the downregulation of cyclin D1, cyclin-dependent kinase 4/6, and retinoblastoma protein in terms of regulation of cell cycle progression [62]. As mentioned above, several investigators have reported that GTPs play an important role in cell cycle regulation in bladder cancer cells [46,62]. However, more detailed information on the molecular mechanisms is necessary to understand the antibladder cancer effects of green tea.

Proteomic analysis has shown that EGCG affects the expression levels of heat shock protein 27 in the TSGH-8301 cell line [66]. Interestingly, a recent study showed that heat shock protein 27 expression was significantly associated with clinicopathological features, including the stage and grade, of bladder cancer in 132 patients [91]. The same study also showed no association with clinical outcomes, such as tumor recurrence, progression, and patient survival. Detailed mechanistic links between GTPs and heat shock protein 27 in other diseases, including cancers, have been reported, and knowledge of changes in heat shock protein 27 activities by green tea are important for the evaluation of cancer-related signal pathways and development of new therapeutic strategies [92]. With regard to bladder cancer, more detailed investigations of GTP-induced anticancer effects of heat shock protein 27 are therefore necessary.

In summary, various types of cancer-related molecules are modulated by GTPs. These molecules usually play multiple roles in the malignant behavior of most cancers, including bladder cancer. For example, MMP-9 plays an important role in apoptosis and cell migration, while Wnt signaling plays an important role in cell proliferation, cell cycle regulation, apoptosis, and migration in bladder cancer [93,94]. We propose that identification of detailed molecular mechanisms of anticancer cell effects by GTPs is essential for targeting the key signaling molecules.

3.2.4. Correlation with Genetic Polymorphisms

A previous report has showed that, although the frequency of green tea consumption was not significantly associated with breast cancer risk in all women or in women with the low-activity genotype of the angiotensin-converting enzyme (ACE), a significant decrease in cancer risk with an increase in the frequency of green tea consumption was found in women bearing the high-activity genotype of ACE [95]. Furthermore, the same study group showed that methylenetetrahydrofolate reductase and thymidylate synthase genotypes affected the association between green tea consumption and breast cancer risk [24]. In recent years, several studies on various malignancies have shown the relationship between the anticancer effects of GTPs and genetic polymorphisms [96,97]. With regard to bladder cancer, a study reported that genotype was significantly associated with tea consumption-associated changes in bladder cancer risk [47]. Tea consumption did not decrease the risk of bladder cancer for rs7571337 AA-genotype carriers, whereas it decreased the risk for carriers of the rs7571337 AG+GG genotypes [47]. Unfortunately, the study evaluated the effects of a mix of green tea, black tea, decaffeinated tea, and other herbal teas, rather than those of green tea alone [47]. In another study, lymph node metastasis from urothelial cancer was associated with the methylation status of *DACT1*, which is controlled by polymorphisms in the gene encoding methylenetetrahydrofolate reductase (MTHFR) [98]. Similarly, *MTHFR* 677T polymorphisms were reported to be associated with hypomethylation of insulin-like growth factor-2, the proportion of which was significantly associated with lymph node metastasis [99]. However, such DNA methylation was not significantly associated with green tea consumption [98,99].

In summary, the anticancer effects of GTPs according to genetic polymorphisms in patients with bladder cancer require further studies, with an emphasis on the prevention of carcinogenesis and tumor progression in multiple population groups. Of note, most previous studies were conducted in Asian subjects.

3.3. Anticancer Effects of Green Tea in Animal Models

Various in vivo studies using animal models have shown that GTEs may be useful therapeutic agents for patients with bladder cancer (Table 5).

Table 5. Anticancer effects of green tea in animal models of bladder cancer.

Author/Year/Reference	Agents	Methods	Animal Model	Summary of Results
Sato et al./1999/ [100]	GTE	Drinking	Rat; Chemically induced	Dose-dependently inhibited tumor growth when administered after the carcinogen
Sato et al./2003/ [101]	GTE	Drinking	Rat; Chemically induced	Prevented tumor growth when administered before the carcinogen
Kemberling et al./2003/[61]	EGCG	Intra-vesical	Rat; intravesical implantation	Inhibited the growth of transitional carcinoma cells
Rieger et al./2007/[63]	EGCG	Drinking	Xenograft model	Over 50% decrease in the mean final tumor volume
Sagara et al./2010/[102]	GTE	Drinking	Mouse; Chemically induced	Inhibited tumor growth and invasion via regulation of angiogenesis
Chen et al./2011/[66]	ECGC	Gavage	Mouse; xenograft model	Inhibited tumor growth in a dose-dependent manner
Hsieh et al./2011/[67]	EGCG	Orally, intraperitoneally, intratumor	Mouse; injection of cancer cells	EGCG–gold nanoparticles were more effective than free EGCG in inhibiting tumor growth
Henriques et al./2014/[103]	Whole green tea	Drinking	Mouse; Chemically induced	Influenced inflammation in the urothelium, but not carcinogenesis
Matsuo et al./2017/[104]	GTE	Drinking	Mouse; Chemically induced	Inhibited tumor growth and angiogenesis via human-antigen R-related pathways

ref: reference. GTEs: green tea extracts. ECGC: epigallocatechin-3-gallate.

While one study reported that GTPs inhibited tumor growth and invasion via regulation of angiogenesis in a mouse model of chemically (*N*-butyl-*N*-(4-hydroxybutyl)-nitrosamine; BBN) induced bladder cancer [102], another reported that green tea infusion did not affect the development of bladder cancer after chemical induction in a mouse model [103]. However, the latter study used whole green tea, not GTEs. In another study, GTP intake suppressed the expression of cyclooxygenase-2, hemeoxygenase-1, and human antigen-R (HuR), and this suppression of cancer-related molecules led to the inhibition of cancer cell proliferation and angiogenesis in a mouse model of BBN-induced bladder cancer [104]. Interestingly, the study also found that VEGF-A expression was not directly affected by green tea intake, although it was regulated by green tea intake via HuR regulation [104]. Therefore, green tea intake is speculated to regulate various malignant behaviors through complex mechanisms.

Some rat models of bladder cancer also showed the anticancer effects of green tea. In a study of Fisher 344 rats implanted with urothelial cancer cells (AY-27), 18 of 28 (64%) rats who received intravesical EGCG instillation were free of tumors, whereas all 12 control rats developed tumors [61]. These findings indicated that intravesical EGCG instillation significantly ($p = 0.001$) suppressed the growth of urothelial cell carcinoma in rats [61]. Another study involving a rat model of bladder cancer induced by the intake of drinking water containing BBN showed that the number and volume of tumors were significantly fewer in rats treated with powdered green tea than in control rats that received no such treatment [101]. The same authors also showed dose-dependent anticancer effects of green tea powder intake in a similar rat model of bladder cancer [100]. On the other hand, it has been reported that green tea infusion influences urothelial inflammation, but not carcinogenesis, in a mouse model of BBN-induced bladder cancer [103]. However, in that study, mice treated with BBN only showed no cancer cells.

Taken together, the anticancer effects of GTPs were confirmed in various animal models, and these results support the need for preclinical studies and clinical trials of the use of GTPs in the prevention of recurrence and progression in patients with bladder cancer.

3.4. Bladder Cancer Treatment and Prevention Strategies Based on Green Tea Consumption

Epirubicin is an effective anticancer agent for bladder cancer. Epirubicin reportedly induces this cytoprotective autophagy in bladder cancer cell lines [67]. Interestingly, GTPs inhibited epirubicin-induced autophagy and promoted apoptosis in the same study [67]. Accordingly, it was suggested that GTPs can be used in combination with epirubicin for enhanced epirubicin-based bladder cancer therapy.

Discrepancies in findings regarding the anticancer effects of green tea between epidemiological studies and in vitro studies can be attributed to differences in the concentration of the GTPs used among studies. The concentration of GTPs used in in vivo studies is routinely lower than that used in in vitro studies [105]. In one study, patients with prostate cancer received polyphenon E, which is derived from a hot water extract of green tea leaves (*Camellia sinensis*) and contains 85–95% catechins, including EGCG, for 3–6 weeks before surgery. However, GTP levels in the prostatectomy tissue were low to undetectable [106]. In addition, in a phase II randomized double-blind trial of bladder cancer, polyphenon E or placebo was administered prior to transurethral resection or radical cystectomy, following which tissue EGCG levels were compared between the experimental and placebo groups; there was no significant difference between the two groups [107]. On the basis of these findings, several investigators have shown interest in new technologies and methods that can achieve higher concentrations of GTPs in cancer tissues.

Nanoparticles are recognized as useful drug carriers. The use of EGCG–gold nanoparticles was found to be more effective than the use of free EGCG for treatment in an animal model of bladder cancer [67]. Moreover, EGCG–gold nanoparticles administered orally, intraperitoneally, and intratumorally suppressed tumor growth in C3H/He mice injected with murine bladder cancer cells (MBT-2). The anticancer effects were greater with intraperitoneal and intratumoral administration than with oral administration [67]. Another study showed that Mg(II)-catechin nanocomposite particles had anticancer effects in vitro and in vivo in a rat model of in situ bladder cancer [108]. In that study, Mg(II)-catechin nanocomposite particles that delivered siRNA targeting oncogene eukaryotic translation initiation factor 5A2, showed enhanced antitumor activity [108].

Various new treatment and prevention strategies based on GTPs have been developed in in vitro studies and animal experiments. Some of them have been confirmed to be effective in vivo in bladder cancer animal models. Therefore, there is now a need for translational studies of such in vitro and animal experiments in humans.

3.5. Safety

In general, GTPs are considered to be safe because they are natural compounds. GTPs were found to have no toxic effects on normal cells in the gallbladder [28]. Furthermore, 24-h treatment with 20 μg/mL and 40 μg/mL of EGCG increased the frequency of apoptotic cells in colon cancer cell lines (COLO205), while no significant changes were observed in normal colon epithelial cells (NCM460) [19]. Although green tea and its extracts have a relatively high level of safety for normal cells, it should be noted that "natural" does not always imply safety. In fact, a review on the toxicological effects of green tea showed that various side effects occurred in animal models, healthy volunteers, and patients, with hepatotoxicity, gastrointestinal disorders, and nervous system stimulation being the most important effects, although green tea and its main components are not recognized as major teratogenic, mutagenic, or carcinogenic substances [2]. The study also recommended that green tea should be used with caution in pregnancy, while breast feeding, and in susceptible individuals, as data in these contexts are limited [2].

In normal urothelial cells (UROtsa cell line), GTEs, including ECG and EGCG, were found to inhibit growth in a dose-dependent manner [62]. Another report mentioned that bladder cancer cells (SW780 cell line) were much more sensitive to EGCG than normal bladder epithelial cells (SV-HUC-1 cell line) [27]. In that study, 24-h treatment with EGCG at 100 mM induced cell proliferation inhibition of more than 70% in SW780 cells and of only 7.8% in SV-HUC-1 cells [27]. In addition to anticancer effects, preventive effects against oxidative stress in normal bladder cancer cells have been reported [78].

We previously discussed the anticancer effects of GTPs in a mouse model of BBN-induced bladder cancer [102,104]. When normal urothelial cells in mice treated with GTPs were examined by hematoxylin–eosin staining, abnormal morphological changes were not detected. However, more detailed analyses are necessary to confirm the safety and biological effects of GTPs on normal urothelial cells.

4. Future Direction

The anticancer effects of green tea in bladder cancer have been analyzed using comprehensive methods in epidemiological studies, in vitro studies using bladder cancer cell lines, animal models, and in vivo studies using human tissues. However, some limitations need to be overcome in order to understand the effects of green tea more accurately. Prospective randomized clinical trials with large study populations are yet to be performed to determine the anticancer effects of green tea in Western countries, including the USA, since epidemiological studies have provided some evidence that can serve as a foundation for such trials. On the other hand, such trials are difficult to design because the frequency and amount of green tea consumption in these countries are quite low.

As mentioned above, a combination of conventional chemotherapy and GTPs can be effective in several cancers, including bladder cancer [35,36,67]. In recent years, green tea has come to be known as a radiation sensitizer in prostate cancer [109]. However, there is little information on green tea-induced changes in terms of the anticancer effects of radiotherapy for bladder cancer. At present, immune checkpoint inhibitors are the major therapeutic agents used for patients with advanced/metastatic bladder cancer [110,111], and the usefulness of green tea as a sensitizer of immune checkpoint inhibitors has not yet been investigated. Therefore, more information on the efficacy and safety of combination therapy involving cytotoxic anticancer methods and green tea consumption or GTP intake in bladder cancer is warranted.

Clarification of the extent of the anticancer effects of green tea is difficult, because other bladder cancer-related external factors, such as smoking, exposure to chemical agents, and family history, also play a role [112–115]. In addition, the influence of other beverages, such as coffee, black tea, and oolong tea, and the total fluid intake should be investigated. Furthermore, GTP has complex molecular interactions that could contribute to its potential health benefits [80]. We hope that this review will encourage further investigations of the anticancer effects of green tea that could lead to the development of new treatment and prevention strategies based on green tea consumption and GTP intake, which are relatively safe.

5. Conclusions

In this review, we summarized studies on the potential anticancer effects of green tea consumption and GTP intake in bladder cancer by gathering data from epidemiological, in vivo, and in vitro studies, which have shown conflicting results. In vitro studies using cancer cell lines indicated that GTPs suppress malignant behavior via inhibition of cancer cell proliferation, migration, and invasion and inhibition of apoptosis, and some in vivo studies using animal model also showed similar results. However, some epidemiological studies showed no significant relationship between green tea consumption and the risk of bladder cancer. These discrepancies can be attributed to differences in the race, country, and measurement unit for green tea consumption and/or the influence of other factors, such as smoking, amount of green tea consumption per day, and the intake of other beverages. Therefore, more detailed and wider analyses of larger study populations from various countries, including USA, Europe, and Africa, are necessary to confirm the anticancer effects and usefulness of green tea as an anticancer agent. The anticancer effects of GTPs alone are considered to be limited, whereas a combination of GTPs and other strategies, such as chemotherapy, radiotherapy, immune therapy, and molecular targeted therapy is expected to have some clinical benefit in patients with cancer, including bladder cancer.

Acknowledgments: This study was supported in part by a Grant-in-Aid from the Japan Society for the Promotion of Science (to Yasuyoshi Miyata). No private funding was received for this study.

References

1. Cooper, R.; Morré, D.J.; Morré, D.M. Medicinal benefits of green tea: Part I. Review of noncancer health benefits. *J. Altern. Complement. Med.* **2005**, *11*, 521–528. [CrossRef] [PubMed]
2. Bedrood, Z.; Rameshrad, M.; Hosseinzadeh, H. Toxicological effects of *Camellia sinensis* (green tea): A review. *Phytother. Res.* **2018**, *32*, 1163–1180. [CrossRef] [PubMed]
3. Surh, Y.J. Cancer chemoprevention with dietary phytochemicals. *Nat. Rev. Cancer* **2003**, *3*, 768–780. [CrossRef] [PubMed]
4. Yang, C.S.; Wang, X.; Lu, G.; Picinich, S.C. Cancer prevention by tea: Animal studies, molecular mechanisms and human relevance. *Nat. Rev. Cancer* **2009**, *9*, 429–439. [CrossRef] [PubMed]
5. Bag, A.; Bag, N. Tea polyphenols and prevention of epigenetic aberrations in cancer. *J. Nat. Sci. Biol. Med.* **2018**, *9*, 2–5. [CrossRef] [PubMed]
6. Yang, C.S.; Wang, H.; Li, G.X.; Yang, Z.; Guan, F.; Jin, H. Cancer prevention by tea: Evidence from laboratory studies. *Pharmacol. Res.* **2011**, *64*, 113–122. [CrossRef] [PubMed]
7. Iwasaki, M.; Mizusawa, J.; Kasuga, Y.; Yokoyama, S.; Onuma, H.; Nishimura, H.; Kusama, R.; Tsugane, S. Green tea consumption and breast cancer risk in Japanese women: A case-control study. *Nutr. Cancer* **2014**, *66*, 57–67. [CrossRef] [PubMed]
8. Ogawa, T.; Sawada, N.; Iwasaki, M.; Budhathoki, S.; Hidaka, A.; Yamaji, T.; Shimazu, T.; Sasazuki, S.; Narita, Y.; Tsugane, S. Coffee and green tea consumption in relation to brain tumor risk in a Japanese population. *Int. J. Cancer* **2016**, *139*, 2714–2721. [CrossRef] [PubMed]
9. Zeng, J.L.; Li, Z.H.; Wang, Z.C.; Zhang, H.L. Green tea consumption and risk of pancreatic cancer: A meta-analysis. *Nutrients* **2014**, *6*, 4640–4650. [CrossRef] [PubMed]
10. Sun, C.L.; Yuan, J.M.; Koh, W.P.; Lee, H.P.; Yu, M.C. Green tea and black tea consumption in relation to colorectal cancer risk: The Singapore Chinese Health Study. *Carcinogenesis* **2007**, *28*, 2143–2148. [CrossRef] [PubMed]
11. Oze, I.; Matsuo, K.; Kawakita, D.; Hosono, S.; Ito, H.; Watanabe, M.; Hatooka, S.; Hasegawa, Y.; Shinoda, M.; Tajima, K.; et al. Coffee and green tea consumption is associated with upper aerodigestive tract cancer in Japan. *Int. J. Cancer* **2014**, *135*, 391–400. [CrossRef] [PubMed]
12. Boehm, K.; Borrelli, F.; Ernst, E.; Habacher, G.; Hung, S.K.; Milazzo, S.; Horneber, M. Green tea (*Camellia sinensis*) for the prevention of cancer. *Cochrane Database Syst. Rev.* **2009**, *8*. [CrossRef] [PubMed]
13. Wang, X.; Lin, Y.W.; Wang, S.; Wu, J.; Mao, Q.Q.; Zheng, X.Y.; Xie, L.P. A meta-analysis of tea consumption and the risk of bladder cancer. *Urol. Int.* **2013**, *90*, 10–16. [CrossRef] [PubMed]
14. Tsao, A.S.; Liu, D.; Martin, J.; Tang, X.M.; Lee, J.J.; El-Naggar, A.K.; Wistuba, I.; Culotta, K.S.; Mao, L.; Gillenwater, A.; et al. Phase II randomized, placebo-controlled trial of green tea extract in patients with high-risk oral premalignant lesions. *Cancer Prev. Res.* **2009**, *2*, 931–941. [CrossRef] [PubMed]
15. Singh, B.N.; Shankar, S.; Srivastava, R.K. Green tea catechin, epigallocatechin-3-gallate (EGCG): Mechanisms, perspectives and clinical applications. *Biochem. Pharmacol.* **2011**, *82*, 1807–1821. [CrossRef] [PubMed]
16. Toden, S.; Tran, H.M.; Tovar-Camargo, O.A.; Okugawa, Y.; Goel, A. Epigallocatechin-3-gallate targets cancer stem-like cells and enhances 5-fluorouracil chemosensitivity in colorectal cancer. *Oncotarget* **2016**, *7*, 16158–16171. [CrossRef] [PubMed]
17. Fujiki, H.; Watanabe, T.; Sueoka, E.; Rawangkan, A.; Suganuma, M. Cancer Prevention with Green Tea and Its Principal Constituent, EGCG: From early investigations to current focus on human cancer stem cells. *Mol. Cells* **2018**, *41*, 73–82. [PubMed]
18. Shi, J.; Liu, F.; Zhang, W.; Liu, X.; Lin, B.; Tang, X. Epigallocatechin-3-gallate inhibits nicotine-induced migration and invasion by the suppression of angiogenesis and epithelial-mesenchymal transition in non-small cell lung cancer cells. *Oncol. Rep.* **2015**, *33*, 2972–2980. [CrossRef] [PubMed]
19. Ni, J.; Guo, X.; Wang, H.; Zhou, T.; Wang, X. Differences in the Effects of EGCG on Chromosomal Stability and Cell Growth between Normal and Colon Cancer Cells. *Molecules* **2018**, *23*, 788. [CrossRef] [PubMed]
20. Imai, K.; Suga, K.; Nakachi, K. Cancer-preventive effects of drinking green tea among a Japanese population. *Prev. Med.* **1997**, *26*, 769–775. [CrossRef] [PubMed]
21. Nakachi, K.; Matsuyama, S.; Miyake, S.; Suganuma, M.; Imai, K. Preventive effects of drinking green tea on cancer and cardiovascular disease: epidemiological evidence for multiple targeting prevention. *Biofactors* **2000** *13*, 49–54. [CrossRef] [PubMed]

22. Bettuzzi, S.; Brausi, M.; Rizzi, F.; Castagnetti, G.; Peracchia, G.; Corti, A. Chemoprevention of human prostate cancer by oral administration of green tea catechins in volunteers with high-grade prostate intraepithelial neoplasia: A preliminary report from a one-year proof-of-principle study. *Cancer Res.* **2006**, *66*, 1234–1240. [CrossRef] [PubMed]
23. Nakachi, K.; Suemasu, K.; Suga, K.; Takeo, T.; Imai, K.; Higashi, Y. Influence of drinking green tea on breast cancer malignancy among Japanese patients. *Jpn. J. Cancer Res.* **1998**, *89*, 254–261. [CrossRef] [PubMed]
24. Inoue, M.; Tajima, K.; Mizutani, M.; Iwata, H.; Iwase, T.; Miura, S.; Hirose, K.; Hamajima, N.; Tominaga, S. Regular consumption of green tea and the risk of breast cancer recurrence: Follow-up study from the Hospital-based Epidemiologic Research Program at Aichi Cancer Center (HERPACC), Japan. *Cancer Lett.* **2001**, *167*, 175–182. [CrossRef]
25. Shimizu, M.; Fukutomi, Y.; Ninomiya, M.; Nagura, K.; Kato, T.; Araki, H.; Suganuma, M.; Fujiki, H.; Moriwaki, H. Green tea extracts for the prevention of metachronous colorectal adenomas: A pilot study. *Cancer Epidemiol. Biomarkers Prev.* **2008**, *17*, 3020–3025. [CrossRef] [PubMed]
26. Taniguchi, S.; Fujiki, H.; Kobayashi, H.; Go, H.; Miyado, K.; Sadano, H.; Shimokawa, R. Effect of (−)-epigallocatechin gallate, the main constituent of green tea, on lung metastasis with mouse B16 melanoma cell lines. *Cancer Lett.* **1992**, *65*, 51–54. [CrossRef]
27. Luo, K.W.; Wei, C.; Lung, W.Y.; Wei, X.Y.; Cheng, B.H.; Cai, Z.M.; Huang, W.R. EGCG inhibited bladder cancer SW780 cell proliferation and migration both in vitro and in vivo via down-regulation of NF-κB and MMP-9. *J. Nutr. Biochem.* **2017**, *41*, 56–64. [CrossRef] [PubMed]
28. Wang, J.; Pan, Y.; Hu, J.; Ma, Q.; Xu, Y.; Zhang, Y.; Zhang, F.; Liu, Y. Tea polyphenols induce S phase arrest and apoptosis in gallbladder cancer cells. *Braz. J. Med. Biol. Res.* **2018**, *51*, 6891. [CrossRef] [PubMed]
29. Liu, L.; Hou, L.; Gu, S.; Zuo, X.; Meng, D.; Luo, M.; Zhang, X.; Huang, S.; Zhao, X. Molecular mechanism of epigallocatechin-3-gallate in human esophageal squamous cell carcinoma in vitro and in vivo. *Oncol. Rep.* **2015**, *33*, 297–303. [CrossRef] [PubMed]
30. Zhu, J.; Jiang, Y.; Yang, X.; Wang, S.; Xie, C.; Li, X.; Li, Y.; Chen, Y.; Wang, X.; Meng, Y.; et al. Wnt/β-catenin pathway mediates (−)-Epigallocatechin-3-gallate (EGCG) inhibition of lung cancer stem cells. *Biochem. Biophys. Res. Commun.* **2017**, *482*, 15–21. [CrossRef] [PubMed]
31. Komori, A.; Yatsunami, J.; Okabe, S.; Abe, S.; Hara, K.; Suganuma, M.; Kim, S.J.; Fujiki, H. Anticarcinogenic activity of green tea polyphenols. *Jpn. J. Clin. Oncol.* **1993**, *23*, 186–190. [PubMed]
32. Lecumberri, E.; Dupertuis, Y.M.; Miralbell, R.; Pichard, C. Green tea polyphenol epigallocatechin-3-gallate (EGCG) as adjuvant in cancer therapy. *Clin. Nutr.* **2013**, *32*, 894–903. [CrossRef] [PubMed]
33. Chen, L.; Ye, H.L.; Zhang, G.; Yao, W.M.; Chen, X.Z.; Zhang, F.C.; Liang, G. Autophagy inhibition contributes to the synergistic interaction between EGCG and doxorubicin to kill the hepatoma Hep3B cells. *PLoS ONE* **2014**, *9*, 85771. [CrossRef] [PubMed]
34. Esmaeili, M.A. Combination of siRNA-directed gene silencing with epigallocatechin-3-gallate (EGCG) reverses drug resistance in human breast cancer cells. *J. Chem. Biol.* **2015**, *9*, 41–52. [CrossRef] [PubMed]
35. Suganuma, M.; Saha, A.; Fujiki, H. New cancer treatment strategy using combination of green tea catechins and anticancer drugs. *Cancer Sci.* **2011**, *102*, 317–323. [CrossRef] [PubMed]
36. Fujiki, H.; Sueoka, E.; Watanabe, T.; Suganuma, M. Primary cancer prevention by green tea, and tertiary cancer prevention by the combination of green tea catechins and anticancer compounds. *J. Cancer Prev.* **2015**, *20*, 1–4. [CrossRef] [PubMed]
37. Wang, W.; Chen, D.; Zhu, K. SOX2OT variant 7 contributes to the synergistic interaction between EGCG and Doxorubicin to kill osteosarcoma via autophagy and stemness inhibition. *J. Exp. Lin. Cancer Res.* **2018**, *37*, 37. [CrossRef] [PubMed]
38. Calgarotto, A.K.; Maso, V.; Junior, G.C.F.; Nowill, A.E.; Filho, P.L.; Vassallo, J.; Saad, S.T.O. Antitumor activities of Quercetin and Green Tea in xenografts of human leukemia HL60 cells. *Sci. Rep.* **2018**, *8*, 3459. [CrossRef] [PubMed]
39. Wang, P.; Henning, S.M.; Heber, D.; Vadgama, J.V. Sensitization to docetaxel in prostate cancer cells by green tea and quercetin. *J. Nutr. Biochem.* **2015**, *26*, 408–415. [CrossRef] [PubMed]
40. Chung, J.E.; Tan, S.; Gao, S.J.; Yongvongsoontorn, N.; Kim, S.H.; Lee, J.H.; Choi, H.S.; Yano, H.; Zhuo, L.; Kurisawa, M.; et al. Self-assembled micellar nanocomplexes comprising green tea catechin derivatives and protein drugs for cancer therapy. *Nat. Nanotechnol.* **2014**, *9*, 907–912. [CrossRef] [PubMed]

41. Liang, K.; Chung, J.E.; Gao, S.J.; Yongvongsoontorn, N.; Kurisawa, M. Highly Augmented Drug Loading and Stability of Micellar Nanocomplexes Composed of Doxorubicin and Poly(ethylene glycol)-Green Tea Catechin Conjugate for Cancer Therapy. *Adv. Mater.* **2018**, *30*, 1706963. [CrossRef] [PubMed]
42. Chavan, S.; Bray, F.; Lortet-Tieulent, J.; Goodman, M.; Jemal, A. International variations in bladder cancer incidence and mortality. *Eur. Urol.* **2014**, *66*, 59–73. [CrossRef] [PubMed]
43. Abufaraj, M.; Gust, K.; Moschini, M.; Foerster, B.; Soria, F.; Mathieu, R.; Shariat, S.F. Management of muscle invasive, locally advanced and metastatic urothelial carcinoma of the bladder: A literature review with emphasis on the role of surgery. *Transl. Androl. Urol.* **2016**, *5*, 735–744. [CrossRef] [PubMed]
44. Xu, C.; Zeng, X.T.; Liu, T.Z.; Zhang, C.; Yang, Z.H.; Li, S.; Chen, X.Y. Fruits and vegetables intake and risk of bladder cancer: A PRISMA-compliant systematic review and dose-response meta-analysis of prospective cohort studies. *Medicine (Baltimore)* **2015**, *94*, 759. [CrossRef] [PubMed]
45. Philippou, Y.; Hadjipavlou, M.; Khan, S.; Rane, A. Complementary and alternative medicine (CAM) in prostate and bladder cancer. *BJU Int.* **2013**, *112*, 1073–1079. [CrossRef] [PubMed]
46. Conde, V.R.; Alves, M.G.; Oliveira, P.F.; Silva, B.M. Tea (*Camellia sinensis* (L.)): A putative anticancer agent in bladder carcinoma? *Anticancer Agents Med. Chem.* **2015**, *15*, 26–36. [CrossRef] [PubMed]
47. Wang, J.; Wu, X.; Kamat, A.; Barton, G.H.; Dinney, C.P.; Lin, J. Fluid intake, genetic variants of UDP-glucuronosyltransferases, and bladder cancer risk. *Br. J. Cancer* **2013**, *108*, 2372–2380. [CrossRef] [PubMed]
48. Wakai, K.; Hirose, K.; Takezaki, T.; Hamajima, N.; Ogura, Y.; Nakamura, S.; Hayashi, N.; Tajima, K. Foods and beverages in relation to urothelial cancer: Case-control study in Japan. *Int. J. Urol.* **2004**, *11*, 11–19. [CrossRef] [PubMed]
49. Wilkens, L.R.; Kadir, M.M.; Kolonel, L.N.; Nomura, A.M.; Hankin, J.H. Risk factors for lower urinary tract cancer: the role of total fluid consumption, nitrites and nitrosamines, and selected foods. *Cancer Epidemiol. Biomarkers Prev.* **1996**, *5*, 161–166. [PubMed]
50. Chyou, P.H.; Nomura, A.M.; Stemmermann, G.N. A prospective study of diet, smoking, and lower urinary tract cancer. *Ann. Epidemiol.* **1993**, *3*, 211–216. [CrossRef]
51. Nagano, J.; Kono, S.; Preston, D.L.; Moriwaki, H.; Sharp, G.B.; Koyama, K.; Mabuchi, K. Bladder-cancer incidence in relation to vegetable and fruit consumption: a prospective study of atomic-bomb survivors. *Int. J. Cancer* **2000**, *86*, 132–138. [CrossRef]
52. Kurahashi, N.; Inoue, M.; Iwasaki, M.; Sasazuki, S.; Tsugane, S. Coffee, green tea, and caffeine consumption and subsequent risk of bladder cancer in relation to smoking status: A prospective study in Japan. *Cancer Sci.* **2009**, *100*, 284–291. [CrossRef] [PubMed]
53. Hemelt, M.; Hu, Z.; Zhong, Z.; Xie, L.P.; Wong, Y.C.; Tam, P.C.; Cheng, K.K.; Ye, Z.; Bi, X.; Lu, Q.; et al. Fluid intake and the risk of bladder cancer: Results from the South and East China case-control study on bladder cancer. *Int. J. Cancer* **2010**, *127*, 638–645. [CrossRef] [PubMed]
54. Ros, M.M.; Bas Bueno-de-Mesquita, H.B.; Büchner, F.L.; Aben, K.K.; Kampman, E.; Egevad, L.; Overvad, K.; Tjønneland, A.; Roswall, N.; Clavel-Chapelon, F. Fluid intake and the risk of urothelial cell carcinomas in the European Prospective Investigation into Cancer and Nutrition (EPIC). *Int. J. Cancer* **2011**, *128*, 2695–2708. [CrossRef] [PubMed]
55. Qin, J.; Xie, B.; Mao, Q.; Kong, D.; Lin, Y.; Zheng, X. Tea consumption and risk of bladder cancer: A meta-analysis. *World J. Surg. Oncol.* **2012**, *10*, 172. [CrossRef] [PubMed]
56. Wu, S.; Li, F.; Huang, X.; Hua, Q.; Huang, T.; Liu, Z.; Liu, Z.; Zhang, Z.; Liao, C.; Chen, Y.; et al. The association of tea consumption with bladder cancer risk: A meta-analysis. *Asia Pac. J. Clin. Nutr.* **2013**, *22*, 128–137. [PubMed]
57. Zhang, Y.F.; Xu, Q.; Lu, J.; Wang, P.; Zhang, H.W.; Zhou, L.; Ma, X.Q.; Zhou, Y.H. Tea consumption and the incidence of cancer: A systematic review and meta-analysis of prospective observational studies. *Eur. J. Cancer Prev.* **2015**, *24*, 353–362. [CrossRef] [PubMed]
58. Weng, H.; Zeng, X.T.; Li, S.; Kwong, J.S.; Liu, T.Z.; Wang, X.H. Tea Consumption and Risk of Bladder Cancer: A Dose-Response Meta-Analysis. *Front. Physiol.* **2017**, *7*, 693. [CrossRef] [PubMed]
59. Bai, Y.; Yuan, H.; Li, J.; Tang, Y.; Pu, C.; Han, P. Relationship between bladder cancer and total fluid intake: A meta-analysis of epidemiological evidence. *World J. Surg. Oncol.* **2014**, *12*, 223. [CrossRef] [PubMed]
60. Khan, N.; Afaq, F.; Saleem, M.; Ahmad, N.; Mukhtar, H. Targeting multiple signaling pathways by green tea polyphenol (−)-epigallocatechin-3-gallate. *Cancer Res.* **2006**, *66*, 2500–2505. [CrossRef] [PubMed]

61. Kemberling, J.K.; Hampton, J.A.; Keck, R.W.; Gomez, M.A.; Selman, S.H. Inhibition of bladder tumor growth by the green tea derivative epigallocatechin-3-gallate. *J. Urol.* **2003**, *170*, 773–776. [CrossRef] [PubMed]
62. Chen, J.J.; Ye, Z.Q.; Koo, M.W. Growth inhibition and cell cycle arrest effects of epigallocatechin gallate in the NBT-II bladder tumour cell line. *BJU Int.* **2004**, *93*, 1082–1086. [CrossRef] [PubMed]
63. Rieger-Christ, K.M.; Hanley, R.; Lodowsky, C.; Bernier, T.; Vemulapalli, P.; Roth, M.; Kim, J.; Yee, A.S.; Le, S.M.; Marie, P.J.; et al. The green tea compound, (−)-epigallocatechin-3-gallate downregulates N-cadherin and suppresses migration of bladder carcinoma cells. *J. Cell Biochem.* **2007**, *102*, 377–388. [CrossRef] [PubMed]
64. Qin, J.; Xie, L.P.; Zheng, X.Y.; Wang, Y.B.; Bai, Y.; Shen, H.F.; Li, L.C.; Dahiya, R. A component of green tea, (-)-epigallocatechin-3-gallate, promotes apoptosis in T24 human bladder cancer cells via modulation of the PI3K/Akt pathway and Bcl-2 family proteins. *Biochem. Biophys. Res. Commun.* **2007**, *354*, 852–857. [CrossRef] [PubMed]
65. Philips, B.J.; Coyle, C.H.; Morrisroe, S.N.; Chancellor, M.B.; Yoshimura, N. Induction of apoptosis in human bladder cancer cells by green tea catechins. *Biomed. Res.* **2009**, *4*, 207–215. [CrossRef]
66. Chen, N.G.; Lu, C.C.; Lin, Y.H.; Shen, W.C.; Lai, C.H.; Ho, Y.J.; Chung, J.G.; Lin, T.H.; Lin, Y.C.; Yang, J.S. Proteomic approaches to study epigallocatechin gallate-provoked apoptosis of TSGH-8301 human urinary bladder carcinoma cells: Roles of AKT and heat shock protein 27-modulated intrinsic apoptotic pathways. *Oncol. Rep.* **2011**, *26*, 939–947. [PubMed]
67. Hsieh, D.S.; Wang, H.; Tan, S.W.; Huang, Y.H.; Tsai, C.Y.; Yeh, M.K.; Wu, C.J. The treatment of bladder cancer in a mouse model by epigallocatechin-3-gallate-gold nanoparticles. *Biomaterials* **2011**, *32*, 7633–7640. [CrossRef] [PubMed]
68. Galluzzi, L.; Morselli, E.; Vicencio, J.M.; Kepp, O.; Joza, N.; Tajeddine, N.; Kroemer, G. Life, death and burial: Multifaceted impact of autophagy. *Biochem. Soc. Trans.* **2008**, *36*, 786–790. [CrossRef] [PubMed]
69. Dower, C.M.; Wills, C.A.; Frisch, S.M.; Wang, H.G. Mechanisms and context underlying the role of autophagy in cancer metastasis. *Autophagy* **2018**, in press. [CrossRef] [PubMed]
70. Wilde, L.; Tanson, K.; Curry, J.; Martinez-Outschoorn, U. Autophagy in cancer: A complex relationship. *Biochem. J.* **2018**, *475*, 1939–1954. [CrossRef] [PubMed]
71. Kroemer, G.; Mariño, G.; Levine, B. Autophagy and the integrated stress response. *Mol. Cell* **2010**, *40*, 280–293. [CrossRef] [PubMed]
72. Liuzzi, J.P.; Guo, L.; Yoo, C.; Stewart, T.S. Zinc and autophagy. *BioMetals* **2014**, *27*, 1087–1096. [CrossRef] [PubMed]
73. Fan, B.; Zhang, X.; Ma, Y.; Zhang, A. Fangchinoline Induces Apoptosis, Autophagy and Energetic Impairment in Bladder Cancer. *Cell Physiol. Biochem.* **2017**, *43*, 1003–1011. [CrossRef] [PubMed]
74. Kou, B.; Liu, W.; Xu, X.; Yang, Y.; Yi, Q.; Guo, F.; Li, J.; Zhou, J.; Kou, Q. Autophagy induction enhances tetrandrine-induced apoptosis via the AMPK/mTOR pathway in human bladder cancer cells. *Oncol. Rep.* **2017**, *38*, 3137–3143. [CrossRef] [PubMed]
75. Gu, W.; Lin, Y.; Gou, X.; He, W. Tea Polyphenol inhibits autophagy to sensitize Epirubicin-induced apoptosis in human bladder cancer cells. *Neoplasma* **2017**, *64*, 674–680. [CrossRef] [PubMed]
76. Sies, H. Oxidative stress: Oxidants and antioxidants. *Exp. Physiol.* **1997**, *82*, 291–295. [CrossRef] [PubMed]
77. Miyata, Y.; Matsuo, T.; Sagara, Y.; Ohba, K.; Ohyama, K.; Sakai, H. A Mini-Review of Reactive Oxygen Species in Urological Cancer: Correlation with NADPH Oxidases, Angiogenesis, and Apoptosis. *Int. J. Mol. Sci.* **2017**, *18*, 2214. [CrossRef] [PubMed]
78. Coyle, C.H.; Philips, B.J.; Morrisroe, S.N.; Chancellor, M.B.; Yoshimura, N. Antioxidant effects of green tea and its polyphenols on bladder cells. *Life Sci.* **2008**, *83*, 12–18. [CrossRef] [PubMed]
79. Haque, I.; Subramanian, A.; Huang, C.H.; Godwin, A.K.; Van Veldhuizen, P.J.; Banerjee, S.; Banerjee, S.K. The Role of Compounds Derived from Natural Supplement as Anticancer Agents in Renal Cell Carcinoma: A Review. *Int. J. Mol. Sci.* **2017**, *19*, 107. [CrossRef] [PubMed]
80. Saeki, K.; Hayakawa, S.; Nakano, S.; Ito, S.; Oishi, Y.; Suzuki, Y.; Isemura, M. In Vitro and In Silico Studies of the Molecular Interactions of Epigallocatechin-3-*O*-gallate (EGCG) with Proteins That Explain the Health Benefits of Green Tea. *Molecules* **2018**, *23*, 1295. [CrossRef] [PubMed]
81. Duggan, B.J.; Gray, S.; Johnston, S.R.; Williamson, K.; Miyaki, H.; Gleave, M. The role of antisense oligonucleotides in the treatment of bladder cancer. *Urol. Res.* **2002**, *30*, 137–147. [CrossRef] [PubMed]
82. Shin, D.Y.; Kim, G.Y.; Hwang, H.J.; Kim, W.J.; Choi, Y.H. Diallyl trisulfide-induced apoptosis of bladder

cancer cells is caspase-dependent and regulated by PI3K/Akt and JNK pathways. *Environ. Toxicol. Pharmacol.* **2014**, *37*, 74–83. [CrossRef] [PubMed]

83. Campbell, K.J.; Tait, S.W.G. Targeting BCL-2 regulated apoptosis in cancer. *Open Biol.* **2018**, *8*, 180002. [CrossRef] [PubMed]
84. Wu, X.; Obata, T.; Khan, Q.; Highshaw, R.A.; De Vere White, R.; Sweeney, C. The phosphatidylinositol-3 kinase pathway regulates bladder cancer cell invasion. *BJU Int.* **2004**, *93*, 143–150. [CrossRef] [PubMed]
85. Ahn, K.I.; Choi, E.O.; Kwon, D.H.; HwangBo, H.; Kim, M.Y.; Kim, H.J.; Ji, S.Y.; Hong, S.H.; Jeong, J.W.; Park, C.; et al. Induction of apoptosis by ethanol extract of Citrus unshiu Markovich peel in human bladder cancer T24 cells through ROS-mediated inactivation of the PI3K/Akt pathway. *Biosci. Trends* **2017**, *11*, 565–573. [CrossRef] [PubMed]
86. Fang, C.Y.; Wu, C.C.; Hsu, H.Y.; Chuang, H.Y.; Huang, S.Y.; Tsai, C.H.; Chang, Y.; Tsao, G.S.; Chen, C.L.; Chen, J.Y. EGCG inhibits proliferation, invasiveness and tumor growth by up-regulation of adhesion molecules, suppression of gelatinases activity, and induction of apoptosis in nasopharyngeal carcinoma cells. *Int. J. Mol. Sci.* **2015**, *16*, 2530–2558. [CrossRef] [PubMed]
87. Prasad, R.; Katiyar, S.K. Polyphenols from green tea inhibit the growth of melanoma cells through inhibition of class I histone deacetylases and induction of DNA damage. *Gene. Cancer.* **2015**, *6*, 49–61.
88. Bryan, R.T. Cell adhesion and urothelial bladder cancer: the role of cadherin switching and related phenomena. *Philos. Trans R. Soc. Lond B Biol. Sci.* **2015**, *370*. [CrossRef] [PubMed]
89. Wu, G.J.; Bao, J.S.; Yue, Z.J.; Zeng, F.C.; Cen, S.; Tang, Z.Y.; Kang, X.L. Elevated expression of matrix metalloproteinase-9 is associated with bladder cancer pathogenesis. *J Cancer Res. Ther.* **2018**, *14*, 54–59.
90. Roomi, M.W.; Ivanov, V.; Kalinovsky, T.; Niedzwiecki, A.; Rath, M. Antitumor effect of ascorbic acid, lysine, proline, arginine, and green tea extract on bladder cancer cell line T-24. *Int. J. Urol.* **2006**, *4*, 415–419. [CrossRef] [PubMed]
91. Lee, M.S.; Lee, J.; Lee, S.; Yoo, S M.; Kim, J.H.; Kim, W.T.; Kim, W.J.; Park, J. Clinical, prognostic, and therapeutic significance of heat shock protein 27 in bladder cancer. *Oncotarget* **2018**, *9*, 7961–7974. [CrossRef] [PubMed]
92. Zhang, L.; Pang, E.; Loo, R.R.; Rao, J.; Go, V.L.; Loo, J.A.; Lu, Q.Y. Concomitant inhibition of HSP90, its mitochondrial localized homologue TRAP1 and HSP27 by green tea in pancreatic cancer HPAF-II cells. *Proteomics* **2011**, *11*, 4638–4647. [CrossRef] [PubMed]
93. Casadevall, D.; Kilian, A.Y.; Bellmunt, J. The prognostic role of epigenetic dysregulation in bladder cancer: A systematic review. *Cancer Treat. Rev.* **2017**, *61*, 82–93. [CrossRef] [PubMed]
94. Yoshida, T.; Sopko, N.A.; Kates, M.; Liu, X.; Joice, G.; McConkey, D.J.; Bivalacqua, T.J. Three-dimensional organoid culture reveals involvement of Wnt/β-catenin pathway in proliferation of bladder cancer cells. *Oncotarget* **2018**, *9*, 11060–11070. [CrossRef] [PubMed]
95. Yuan, J.M.; Koh, W.P.; Sun, C.L.; Lee, H.P.; Yu, M.C. Green tea intake, ACE gene polymorphism and breast cancer risk among Chinese women in Singapore. *Carcinogenesis* **2005**, *26*, 1389–1394. [CrossRef] [PubMed]
96. Liu, P.; Zhang, M.; Xie, X.; Jin, J.; Holman, C.D. Green tea consumption and glutathione S-transferases genetic polymorphisms on the risk of adult leukemia. *Eur. J. Nutr.* **2017**, *56*, 603–612. [CrossRef] [PubMed]
97. Scholl, C.; Lepper, A.; Lehr, T.; Hanke, N.; Schneider, K.L.; Brockmöller, J.; Seufferlein, T.; Stingl, J.C. Population nutrikinetics of green tea extract. *PLoS ONE* **2018**, *13*, 0193074. [CrossRef] [PubMed]
98. Cheng, H.; Lu, M.; Mao, L.J.; Wang, J.Q.; Li, W.; Wen, R.M.; Chen, J.C. Relationships among MTHFR a1298c gene polymorphisms and methylation status of Dact1 gene in transitional cell carcinomas. *Asian Pac. J. Cancer Prev.* **2012**, *13*, 5069–5074. [CrossRef] [PubMed]
99. Cheng, H.; Deng, Z.; Wang, Z.; Zhang, W.; Su, J. MTHFR C677T polymorphisms are associated with aberrant methylation of the IGF-2 gene in transitional cell carcinoma of the bladder. *J. Biomed. Res.* **2012**, *26*, 77–83. [CrossRef]
100. Sato, D. Inhibition of urinary bladder tumors induced by *N*-butyl-*N*-(4-hydroxybutyl)-nitrosamine in rats by green tea. *Int. J. Urol.* **1999**, *6*, 93–99. [CrossRef] [PubMed]
101. Sato, D.; Matsushima, M. Preventive effects of urinary bladder tumors induced by *N*-butyl-*N*-(4-hydroxybutyl)-nitrosamine in rat by green tea leaves. *Int. J. Urol.* **2003**, *10*, 160–166. [CrossRef] [PubMed]
102. Sagara, Y.; Miyata, Y.; Nomata, K.; Hayashi, T.; Kanetake, H. Green tea polyphenol suppresses tumor invasion and angiogenesis in *N*-butyl-(-4-hydroxybutyl) nitrosamine-induced bladder cancer. *Cancer Epidemiol.* **2010**, *34*, 350–354. [CrossRef] [PubMed]

103. Henriques, A.; Arantes-Rodrigues, R.; Faustino-Rocha, A.I.; Teixeira-Guedes, C.I.; Pinho-Oliveira, J.; Talhada, D.; Teixeira, J.H.; Andrade, A.; Colaço, B.; Paiva-Cardoso, M.N.; et al. The effects of whole green tea infusion on mouse urinary bladder chemical carcinogenesis. *Iran. J. Basic Med. Sci.* **2014**, *17*, 145–148. [PubMed]
104. Matsuo, T.; Miyata, Y.; Asai, A.; Sagara, Y.; Furusato, B.; Fukuoka, J.; Sakai, H. Green Tea Polyphenol Induces Changes in Cancer-Related Factors in an Animal Model of Bladder Cancer. *PLoS ONE* **2017**, *12*, 0171091. [CrossRef] [PubMed]
105. Bailey, H.H.; Mukhtar, H. Green tea polyphenols and cancer chemoprevention of genitourinary cancer. *Am. Soc. Clin. Oncol. Educ. Book* **2013**, 92–96. [CrossRef] [PubMed]
106. Nguyen, M.M.; Ahmann, F.R.; Nagle, R.B.; Hsu, C.H.; Tangrea, J.A.; Parnes, H.L.; Sokoloff, M.H.; Gretzer, M.B.; Chow, H.H. Randomized, double-blind, placebo-controlled trial of polyphenon E in prostate cancer patients before prostatectomy: evaluation of potential chemopreventive activities. *Cancer Prev. Res.* **2012**, *5*, 290–298. [CrossRef] [PubMed]
107. Gee, J.R.; Saltzstein, D.R.; Kim, K.; Kolesar, J.; Huang, W.; Havighurst, T.C.; Wollmer, B.W.; Stublaski, J.; Downs, T.; Mukhtar, H.; et al. A Phase II Randomized, Double-blind, Presurgical Trial of Polyphenon E in Bladder Cancer Patients to Evaluate Pharmacodynamics and Bladder Tissue Biomarkers. *Cancer Prev. Res.* **2017**, *10*, 298–307. [CrossRef] [PubMed]
108. Chen, Z.; Yu, T.; Zhou, B.; Wei, J.; Fang, Y.; Lu, J.; Guo, L.; Chen, W.; Liu, Z.P.; Luo, J. Mg(II)-Catechin nanoparticles delivering siRNA targeting EIF5A2 inhibit bladder cancer cell growth in vitro and in vivo. *Biomaterials* **2016**, *81*, 125–134. [CrossRef] [PubMed]
109. Schroeder, A.C.; Xiao, H.; Zhu, Z.; Li, Q.; Bai, Q.; Wakefield, M.R.; Mann, J.D.; Fang, Y. A Potential Role for Green Tea as a Radiation Sensitizer for Prostate Cancer. *Pathol. Oncol. Res.* **2017**, in press. [CrossRef] [PubMed]
110. Bellmunt, J.; de Wit, R.; Vaughn, D.J.; Fradet, Y.; Lee, J.L.; Fong, L.; Vogelzang, N.J.; Climent, M.A.; Petrylak, D.P.; Choueiri, T.K.; et al. Pembrolizumab as second-line therapy for advanced urothelial carcinoma. *N. Engl. J. Med.* **2017**, *376*, 1015–1026. [CrossRef] [PubMed]
111. Rouanne, M.; Roumiguié, M.; Houédé, N.; Masson-Lecomte, A.; Colin, P.; Pignot, G.; Larré, S.; Xylinas, E.; Rouprêt, M.; Neuzillet, Y. Development of immunotherapy in bladder cancer: present and future on targeting PD(L)1 and CTLA-4 pathways. *World J. Urol.* **2018**, in press. [CrossRef] [PubMed]
112. Meyer, J.; Rohrmann, S.; Bopp, M.; Faeh, D. Swiss National Cohort Study Group. Impact of smoking and excess body weight on overall and site-specific cancer mortality risk. *Cancer Epidemiol. Biomarkers Prev.* **2015**, *24*, 1516–1522. [CrossRef] [PubMed]
113. Aben, K.K.; Witjes, J.A.; Schoenberg, M.P.; Hulsbergen-van de, K.C.; Verbeek, A.L.; Kiemeney, L.A. Familial aggregation of urothelial cell carcinoma. *Int. J. Cancer* **2002**, *98*, 274–278. [CrossRef] [PubMed]
114. Espina, C.; Straif, K.; Friis, S.; Kogevinas, M.; Saracci, R.; Vainio, H.; Schüz, J. European Code against Cancer 4th Edition: Environment, occupation and cancer. *Cancer Epidemiol.* **2015**, *39*, 84–92. [CrossRef] [PubMed]
115. Wu, W.; Tong, Y.; Zhao, Q.; Yu, G.; Wei, X.; Lu, Q. Coffee consumption and bladder cancer: a meta-analysis of observational studies. *Sci. Rep.* **2015**, *5*, 9051. [CrossRef] [PubMed]

Permissions

All chapters in this book were first published by MDPI; hereby published with permission under the Creative Commons Attribution License or equivalent. Every chapter published in this book has been scrutinized by our experts. Their significance has been extensively debated. The topics covered herein carry significant findings which will fuel the growth of the discipline. They may even be implemented as practical applications or may be referred to as a beginning point for another development.

The contributors of this book come from diverse backgrounds, making this book a truly international effort. This book will bring forth new frontiers with its revolutionizing research information and detailed analysis of the nascent developments around the world.

We would like to thank all the contributing authors for lending their expertise to make the book truly unique. They have played a crucial role in the development of this book. Without their invaluable contributions this book wouldn't have been possible. They have made vital efforts to compile up to date information on the varied aspects of this subject to make this book a valuable addition to the collection of many professionals and students.

This book was conceptualized with the vision of imparting up-to-date information and advanced data in this field. To ensure the same, a matchless editorial board was set up. Every individual on the board went through rigorous rounds of assessment to prove their worth. After which they invested a large part of their time researching and compiling the most relevant data for our readers.

The editorial board has been involved in producing this book since its inception. They have spent rigorous hours researching and exploring the diverse topics which have resulted in the successful publishing of this book. They have passed on their knowledge of decades through this book. To expedite this challenging task, the publisher supported the team at every step. A small team of assistant editors was also appointed to further simplify the editing procedure and attain best results for the readers.

Apart from the editorial board, the designing team has also invested a significant amount of their time in understanding the subject and creating the most relevant covers. They scrutinized every image to scout for the most suitable representation of the subject and create an appropriate cover for the book.

The publishing team has been an ardent support to the editorial, designing and production team. Their endless efforts to recruit the best for this project, has resulted in the accomplishment of this book. They are a veteran in the field of academics and their pool of knowledge is as vast as their experience in printing. Their expertise and guidance has proved useful at every step. Their uncompromising quality standards have made this book an exceptional effort. Their encouragement from time to time has been an inspiration for everyone.

The publisher and the editorial board hope that this book will prove to be a valuable piece of knowledge for researchers, students, practitioners and scholars across the globe.

List of Contributors

Przemysław Sitarek
Department of Biology and Pharmaceutical Botany, Medical University of Lodz, 90-151 Lodz, Poland

Anna Merecz-Sadowska and Radosław Zajdel
Department of Economic Informatics, University of Lodz, 90-214 Lodz, Poland

Tomasz Śliwiński
Laboratory of Medical Genetics, Faculty of Biology and Environmental Protection, University of Lodz, 90-236 Lodz, Poland

Tomasz Kowalczyk
Department of Molecular Biotechnology and Genetics, University of Lodz, 90-237 Lodz, Poland

Paul D. Roach
School of Environmental and Life Sciences, University of Newcastle, Ourimbah, NSW 2258, Australia

Anh V. Le
School of Environmental and Life Sciences, University of Newcastle, Ourimbah, NSW 2258, Australia
Faculty of Bio-Food Technology and Environment, University of Technology (HUTECH), Ho Chi Minh City 700000, Vietnam

Tien T. Huynh
School of Science, RMIT University, Bundoora, VIC 3083, Australia

Sophie E. Parks
School of Environmental and Life Sciences, University of Newcastle, Ourimbah, NSW 2258, Australia
Central Coast Primary Industries Centre, NSW Department of Primary Industries, Ourimbah, NSW 2258, Australia

Minh H. Nguyen
School of Environmental and Life Sciences, University of Newcastle, Ourimbah, NSW 2258, Australia
School of Science and Health, Western Sydney University, Penrith, NSW 2751, Australia

Kaushiki Chatterjee and Jimmie E. Fata
Doctoral Program in Biology, CUNY Graduate Center, New York, NY 10016, USA
Department of Biology, College of Staten Island, New York, NY 10314, USA

Dina AlSharif, Christina Mazza, Palwasha Syar and Mohamed Al Sharif
Department of Biology, College of Staten Island, New York, NY 10314, USA

Daniel Pereira Bezerra
Instituto Gonçalo Moniz, Fundação Oswaldo Cruz (IGM-FIOCRUZ/BA), Salvador 40296-710, Bahia, Brazil

Gardenia Carmen Gadelha Militão
Departamento de Fisiologia, Universidade Federal de Pernambuco, Recife 50670-901, Pernambuco, Brazil

Mayara Castro de Morais and Damião Pergentino de Sousa
Departamento de Ciências Farmacêuticas, Universidade Federal da Paraíba, João Pessoa 58051-970, Paraíba, Brazil

Tung-chin Chiang
Department of Environmental and Occupational Health, University of Arkansas for Medical Sciences, Little Rock, AR 72205, USA

Brian Koss and Aaron Storey
Department of Biochemistry & Molecular Biology, University of Arkansas for Medical Sciences, Little Rock, AR 72205, USA

L. Joseph Su
Winthrop P. Rockefeller Cancer Institute, Cancer Prevention and Population Sciences Program & Department of Epidemiology, University of Arkansas for Medical Sciences, Little Rock, AR 72205, USA

Charity L. Washam, Stephanie D. Byrum and Alan J. Tackett
Department of Biochemistry & Molecular Biology, University of Arkansas for Medical Sciences, Little Rock, AR 72205, USA
Arkansas Children's Research Institute, Little Rock, AR 72202, USA

Amit Kumar Singh and Abhay K. Pandey
Department of Biochemistry, University of Allahabad, Allahabad 211 002, Uttar Pradesh, India

María Herranz-López, María Losada-Echeberría and Enrique Barrajón-Catalán
Instituto de Biología Molecular y Celular (IBMC) and Instituto de Investigación, Desarrollo e Innovación en Biotecnología Sanitaria de Elche (IDiBE), Universitas Miguel Hernández 03202 Elche, Spain

Gautam Sethi
Department for Management of Science and Technology Development, Ton Duc Thang University, Ho Chi Minh City 700000, Vietnam
Faculty of Pharmacy, Ton Duc Thang University, Ho Chi Minh City 700000, Vietnam
Department of Pharmacology, Yong Loo Lin School of Medicine, National University of Singapore, Singapore 117600, Singapore

Muthu K. Shanmugam, Myriam Merarchi and Alan Prem Kumar
Department of Pharmacology, Yong Loo Lin School of Medicine, National University of Singapore, Singapore 117600, Singapore

Sudha Warrier
Division of Cancer Stem Cells and Cardiovascular Regeneration, Manipal Institute of Regenerative Medicine, Manipal University, Bangalore 560065, India

Frank Arfuso
Stem Cell and Cancer Biology Laboratory, School of Biomedical Sciences, Curtin Health Innovation Research Institute, Curtin University, Perth, WA 6102, Australia

Anupam Bishayee
Department of Pharmaceutical Sciences, College of Pharmacy, Larkin University, 18301 N. Miami Avenue, Miami, FL 33169, USA

Fataneh Jafari, Leila Hosseinzadeh and Mohammad Hosein Farzaei
Pharmaceutical Sciences Research Center, School of Pharmacy, Kermanshah University of Medical Sciences, Kermanshah 67146, Iran

Yalda Shokoohinia
Pharmaceutical Sciences Research Center, School of Pharmacy, Kermanshah University of Medical Sciences, Kermanshah 67146, Iran
Department of Pharmacognosy and Biotechnology, School of Pharmacy, Kermanshah University of Medical Sciences, Kermanshah 67146, Iran

Zeynab Mohammadi and Leili Bazvandi
Students Research Committee, School of Pharmacy, Kermanshah University of Medical Sciences, Kermanshah 67146, Iran

Nicholas Chow
Department of Clinical and Administrative Sciences, College of Pharmacy, Larkin University, Miami, FL 33169, USA

Piyali Bhattacharyya
School of Health Sciences, University of Turabo, Gurabo, PR 00778, USA

Ammad Ahmad Farooqi
Laboratory for Translational Oncology and Personalized Medicine, Rashid Latif Medical College, Lahore 54000, Pakistan

Seyed Mohammad Nabavi
Applied Biotechnology Research Center, Baqiyatallah University of Medical Sciences, Tehran 1435916471, Iran

Mükerrem Betül Yerer
Department of Pharmacology, Faculty of Pharmacy, University of Erciyes, 38039 Kayseri, Turkey

Yasuyoshi Miyata, Tomohiro Matsuo, Kyohei Araki, Yuichiro Nakamura, Yuji Sagara, Kojiro Ohba and Hideki Sakai
Department of Urology, Nagasaki University Graduate School of Biomedical Sciences, Nagasaki 852-8501, Japan

Index

www.ingramcontent.com/pod-product-compliance
Lightning Source LLC
LaVergne TN
LVHW082214200926
848484LV00008B/2254